NEUROLOGICAL EXAMINATION
FOR PHYSIOTHERAPISTS

NEUROLOGICAL EXAMINATION FOR PHYSIOTHERAPISTS

Chaitali Shah
Incharge Principal
Parul Institute of Physiotherapy
Parul University
Vadodara, Gujarat, India

Foreword
Nilima Patel

JAYPEE BROTHERS MEDICAL PUBLISHERS
The Health Sciences Publisher
New Delhi | London

JAYPEE **Jaypee Brothers Medical Publishers (P) Ltd**

Headquarters
EMCA House
23/23-B, Ansari Road, Daryaganj
New Delhi 110 002, India
Landline: +91-11-23272143, +91-11-23272703
+91-11-23282021, +91-11-23245672
E-mail: jaypee@jaypeebrothers.com

Corporate Office
4838/24, Ansari Road, Daryaganj
New Delhi 110 002, India
Phone: +91-11-43574357
Fax: +91-11-43574314
E-mail: jaypee@jaypeebrothers.com

Overseas Office
J.P. Medical Ltd
83, Victoria Street, London
SW1H 0HW (UK)
Phone: +44 20 3170 8910
E-mail: info@jpmedpub.com

EU GPSR Authorised Representative
Logos Europe, 9 rue Nicolas Poussin
17000, La Rochelle, France
Phone: +33 (0) 6 67 93 73 78
E-mail: contact@logoseurope.eu

Website: www.jaypeebrothers.com
Website: www.jaypeedigital.com

Inquiries for bulk sales may be solicited at: jaypee@jaypeebrothers.com

Neurological Examination for Physiotherapists

First Edition: 2018, *Reprint:* **2025**

ISBN: 978-93-5270-322-7

Printed in India

Dedicated to

All my Teachers and Students

Foreword

In recent years, there has been a great interest among clinicians regarding the tremendous expansion of research in the field of neuromotor control and the implications of this research to clinical practice. In my humble opinion, Dr Chaitali Shah is like one of those, a Bachelor of Physiotherapy (BPT) from Maharaja Sayajirao University, Vadodara, Gujarat and Master of Physiotherapy (MPT) (Neurology) from Chaudhary Charan Singh University, Meerut, Uttar Pradesh, India, is a dynamic professional with around 9 years of experience as an academician and clinician. She has been working as the Senior Lecturer in the Parul Institute of Physiotherapy, Parul University, Vadodara, Gujarat, India.

She is an effective communicator with excellent relationship in management skills and strong analytical, leadership, decision-making, problem-solving and organizational abilities. She is looking after the management of academic schedule, coordination with external professors, and management of internal and external examinations, and she is also the Organizer and Planner for extra-curriculum for physiotherapy students related to their academics.

She has to her credit, the publications of her study on neurological conditions in national and international journals. Her participation in conferences, workshops, and seminars reflects her zeal to learn, update herself and teach constructively.

Her exemplary dedication, well-defined, disciplined and controlled life, full faith in neuro-assessment and rehabilitation and a very deep-rooted strong desire to learn it as well as possible, enabled her to understand the intricacies of neuro-assessment extremely well. She has learnt a great deal about both theoretical and practical aspects of neurological disorders. This has resulted in the application of her knowledge of neuro-assessment for the betterment of hundreds of her patients and students. She will be able to use it further and will also guide others to use it most advantageously in physiotherapy.

Her objective is to succeed in an environment of growth and excellence and earn a job, which provides her satisfaction and self-development to help her to achieve organizational goal.

My heartiest congratulations to Dr Chaitali Shah for so successfully completing this book at a very early age of her career, for the welfare of students and patients. This should be, I feel, considered as her innovation in physiotherapy.

May Goddess *Maa Paraamba* bless her with the choicest blessings and grant her the desired success in all her efforts to serve humanity. May She bless her with all happiness, peace and prosperity and lead her on the path to reach the apogee of this field with the hands that cures and the touch that heals.

Nilima Patel
PhD (AM and Rehabilitation)
Fellow of Physiotherapy (IAP)
Incharge Head and Principal
College of Physiotherapy
Sir Sayajirao General Hospital
Vadodara, Gujarat, India

Preface

Assessment forms important part in management of neurological patients. Students have general ideas about general points covered in neurological examination but are uncertain of best methods of carrying out various tests, of the purpose lies behind them, of true meaning of abnormal findings and of how to overcome technical difficulties and to avoid arriving at false conclusion.

This book is aimed to provide a simple framework for physiotherapy students to perform a straightforward neurological examination.

Neurological examination is used as an investigative tool in patients when a neurological abnormality is found on screening or when an abnormality can be expected from history.

There is no ideal neurological examination technique. There are conventional ways to perform an examination. Most neurologists have developed their own system for examination—a variation on conventional techniques. This book teaches the necessary mental and manual skills for neurological examination.

Assessment of all neurological conditions dealt by the physiotherapists has been included in the book which will be of great use for the users.

This book is written keeping in mind the graduate as well as the postgraduate students of physiotherapy who want to carry out basic neurological assessments. It mainly focuses on basic assessment only not the differential diagnosis.

Scales used for general neurological examination as well as disease-specific scales used by physiotherapists are also included in the book, which will be very helpful for postgraduate students.

I hope that this book will provide fundamental knowledge about neurological assessments and will be of great use for the physiotherapy students.

Chaitali Shah

Acknowledgments

First and foremost, I would like to thank God. In the process of putting the book together, I realized how true this gift of writing is for me. God has given me the power to believe in my passion and pursue my dreams. I could never have done this without the faith I have in God, the almighty.

I would like to express my gratitude to the many people who saw me through this book; to all those who provided support, talked things over, read, wrote, offered comments, allowed me to quote their remarks and assisted in the editing, proofreading and designing.

Hearty thanks to my teachers, mentors, colleagues, and friends who had directly or indirectly supported me.

My great thanks to my both parents and family members who supported and encouraged me in their own way to write the book.

To my husband, Jaimin Shah: what can I say? I am so thankful that I have you in my corner pushing me for this book. All the good that comes from this book, I look forward to sharing with you! Thanks for not just believing, but knowing that I could do this!

To my lovely son, Manush Shah: I am so grateful for you. You are the one person in this world, I would like give my life for. The hard work that went into making this book a reality is like our boy.

Most grateful thanks to my publishers, M/s Jaypee Brothers Medical Publishers, New Delhi, India, who has given me opportunity to publish my efforts in front of all readers and physiotherapists. Due to them, I am going to complete my first success and dream of my life.

Last but not least, I beg forgiveness of all those who have been with me over the course of the years and whose names I have failed to mention.

Contents

1 History

STRUCTURE AND PURPOSE OF HEALTH HISTORY

- Purpose of interview is to gather information from the patient.
- To establish trusting and supporting relationship with the patient.
- To offer information and counseling.
- *Identifying data*:
  - Such as age, birthplace, occupation
  - It will give you basic information about the person and what the likely problem might be.
- *Source of referral*:
  - It helps in understanding the patient's possible motivation.
  - Introductory information also includes the date and in rapidly changing circumstances the time.
  - The source of history whether it be the patient, family, friends.
  - A letter of referral or the past medical record also deserves comment. It helps the therapist to assess the value and possible biases of information.
- *Chief complaints*:
  - These are one or more symptoms or other concerns for which the patient is seeking care or advice.
  - Use simple words in patient's own language.
  - Main aim of asking is to make the patient independent in his day-to-day life and hence chief complaints are given as inability to eat, difficulty in dressing, difficulty in walking.
  - Complaints will consist of the ultimate outcome of all abnormality.
  - Nothing can give more pleasure to the patient than getting rid of the chief complaints.
  - Complete relief from chief complaint is main aim of any intervention towards which whole assessment gets directed.
- *Present illness*:
  - It includes how the patient thinks and feels about the illness.
  - How the illness has affected the patient's daily life and function.

- *Past history*:
  - Patient's childhood illness and any history of adult medical illness.
  - It includes previously done surgeries, obstetric or gynecologic events, psychiatric condition, accidents and injuries, transfusions, etc.
- *Health maintenance*:
  - Includes immunizations and screening, examinations, lifestyle issues and safety practices.
- *Family history*:
  - Helps to assess the patient's risk of developing certain diseases and may also suggest family experiences relevant to the patient's concern.
  - Many neurological problems have genetic basis so a detailed family history is very important in making the diagnosis.
- *Personal and social history*:
  - It suggests contributory factors in patient's illness and helps the therapist to evaluate the patient's source of support, likely reaction to illness, coping mechanism, strength and fears.
  - For these, the environment in which the patient normally lives, his/her financial circumstances, family and carers in the community, are all important to the current and future care.
- *Review of the systems*:
  - Therapist should ask for common symptoms in each major body system and, thus, try to identify problems that the patient has not mentioned.
  - A fairly general question that introduces each system or subsystem is helpful, e.g.
    - How are your ears and hearing?
    - How about your lungs and breathing?
    - Any trouble with your heart?
    - How is your digestion?

IMPORTANT CONSIDERATIONS DURING INTERVIEW

Things to be considered before beginning the interview:

- *Reviewing the chart*:
  - Medical chart may give you valuable information about past diagnosis and treatment.
  - Therapist should look at identifying data, the problems list, medication list and other specific detail such as documentation of allergies.

- *Therapist's task*:
  - Therapist must clarify goals for the interview.
- *Therapist's behavior*:
  - Just as therapist observe the patient throughout the interview, the patient could be watching the therapist. Therapist send message through her words and behavior.
  - Posture, gesture, eye contact and words can all express interest, acceptance, attention and understanding.
  - Negative reaction such as this is normal and undustable, should not be expressed. Guard against them not only when talking with the patient but also when discussing the patient with the colleagues in the hall or at other public place.
- *Therapist's appearance*: Cleanliness, neatness, conservative dress and a name tag are necessary to the patient.
- *Note taking*: Note taking should not divert therapist's attention from the patient. When patient is talking about sensitive or disturbing material put your pen down and, especially be aware of maintaining eye contact.
- *The environment*: As private and, comfortable as possible.

THE STAGES OF INTERVIEW

- Greeting the patient and establishing rapport.
- Inviting patient story.
- Establishing agenda for interview.
- Generating and testing hypothesis about nature of problem by expanding and clarifying the patient's story.
- Creating shared understanding of problem.
- Negotiating a plan of further diagnostic evaluation, treatment and patient education.
- Planning for follow-up and closing interview.

KEY POINTS WHILE TAKING HISTORY

- Ask open-ended question like what concerns bring you here today?
- How can I help you?
- At the initial part of the interview using responses called continue works best. They include nonverbal cues such as head nodding and verbal phrases such as go on or I see.
- Question should proceed from general to specific.

- Use the language that is uneatable and appropriate to the patient.
- In general, an interview moves back and forth from open-ended question to direct question and then onto another question.

ATTRIBUTES OF SYMPTOM

- Location
  Where is it? Does it radiate?
- Its quality
  What is it like?
- Its quantity or severity
  How bad is it?
- Its timing
  When did it start? How long does it last?
- The setting in which it occurs, including environmental factors, personal activities, emotional reactions or other circumstances that may have contributed to the illness.
- Factors that make it better or worse.
- Associated manifestation.

ELICITING THE PATIENT'S PERSPECTIVE

- Patient's thoughts about the nature and cause of problem.
- Patient's feeling about the problem especially fear.
- Patient's expectation.
- Effect of problem on patient's life.
- Similar experiences in patient's personal or family history.
- Any step that the patient has taken to address the problem.

SOAP PROTOCOL FOR ASSESSMENT

The SOAP note (an acronym for Subjective, Objective, Assessment, and Plan) is a method of documentation employed by healthcare providers to write out notes in a patient's chart, along with other common formats, such as the admission note.

- *Subjective component*:
  - Initially, it is the patient's chief complaint. This is a very brief statement of the patient (quoted) as to the purpose of the office visit or hospitalization.

- If this is the first time a therapist is seeing a patient, the therapist will take a history of present illness. This describes the patient's current condition in the narrative form.
- The history or states of experienced symptoms is/are recorded in the patient's own words. All information pertaining to subjective information is communicated to the healthcare provider by the patient or his/her representative.
- It will include all pertinent and negative symptoms under review of body systems. Pertinent medical history, surgical history, family history, and social history, along with the current medications, smoking status, drug/alcohol/caffeine use, level of physical activity and allergies, are also recorded.

A SAMPLE history is one method of obtaining this information from a patient.

Subsequent visits for the same problem briefly summarize the history of present illness (HPI), including pertinent testing, results, referrals, treatments, outcomes and follow-ups.

The mnemonic below refers to the information a physician should elicit before referring to the patient's 'old charts' or 'old carts'.
- **O**nset, **L**ocation, **D**uration, **C**haracter (sharp, dull)
- Alleviating/aggravating factors
- Radiation
- Location onset (when and mechanism of injury—if applicable) Chronology (better or worse since onset, episodic, variable, constant, etc.), Quality (sharp, dull)
- *Severity*:
  - Modifying factors (what aggravates/reduces the symptoms—activities, postures, drugs, etc.). Additional symptoms (unrelated or significant symptoms to the chief complaint). Treatment (has the patient seen another provider for this symptom?)

- *Objective components*:
  - The objective section of the SOAP includes information that the healthcare provider observes or measures from the patient's current presentation. The objective component includes: vital signs and measurements, such as weight.
  - Findings from physical examinations, including basic cardiac and respiratory systems, the affected systems, possible involvement of other systems, pertinent normal findings and abnormalities.

  - Results from laboratory and other diagnostic tests already completed.
  - Medication list obtained from pharmacy or medical record.
- *Assessment*:
  - A medical diagnosis for the purpose of the medical visit on the given date of the note written is a quick summary of the patient with main symptoms/diagnosis, including a differential diagnosis, a list of other possible diagnoses usually in order of most likely to least likely.
  - The assessment will also include possible and likely etiologies of the patient's problem. It is the patient's progress since the last visit, and overall progress towards the patient's goal from the physician's perspective.
  - In a pharmacist's SOAP note, the assessment will identify what the drug-related/induced problem is likely to be and the reasoning/evidence behind it.
  - This will include etiology and risk factors, assessments of the need for therapy, current therapy, and therapy options. When used in a problem-oriented medical record, relevant problem numbers or headings are included as subheadings in the assessment.
- *Plan*:
  - The plan is what the healthcare provider will do to treat the patient's concerns, such as ordering further lab, radiological work up, referrals given, procedures performed, medications given and education provided.
  - The plan will also include goals of therapy and patient-specific drug and disease-state monitoring parameters. This should address each item of the differential diagnosis.
  - For patients who have multiple health problems that are addressed in the SOAP note, a plan is developed for each problem and is numbered accordingly, based on severity and urgency for a therapy.
  - A note of what was discussed or advised with the patient as well as timings for further review or follow-up are generally included.
  - Often the assessment and plan sections are grouped together.

2 Speech

BACKGROUND

Language: All modes of expression (spoken speech, gestures).

Abnormality of speech needs to be considered first as this may interfere with history taking and subsequent ability to assess the higher function and perform rest of the examination.

Preliminary Information

Physiotherapist should first know the patient's nationality, native language and educational level, his previous ability to read, write, spell and calculate his handedness.

Therapist must find if there is any mental deterioration, hemianopia or hemiparesis, which might confuse the tests.

Abnormality of speech can reflect abnormalities anywhere along the following chain.

Process	*Abnormality*
Hearing	Deafness
Understanding thoughts and word findings	Aphasia
Voice production	Dysphonia
Articulation	Dysarthria

APHASIA

- All disorders of understanding thoughts and word findings.
- Aphasia means absence of speech.

Types of Aphasia

- *Broca's/expressive/motor aphasia*:
  - Speech is nonfluent
  - Preserved comprehension

- Poor repetition
- Poor naming ability
- Distinct breakdown of correct syntax (grammar)
- Repeated and incorrect use of words.

Usual cause: An infarct in territory of anterior part of left middle cerebral artery.

- *Wernicke's/receptive/sensory aphasia*:
  - Comprehension affected
  - Repetition impaired
  - Poor naming
  - Patient fails to produce correct words or syntax

Usual cause: Posterior left middle cerebral artery infarction with damage to posterior third of superior temporal gyrus.

- *Conductive aphasia*:
  - Loss of repetition
  - Preserved comprehension and output
  - Grammatical confrontation defective
- *Transcortical sensory aphasia*:
  - As in Wernicke's aphasia but preserved repetition
  - Poor comprehension
  - Fluent but meaningless speech
  - Preserved repetition
- *Transcortical motor aphasia*:
  - As in Broca's aphasia but preserved repetition
  - Preserved comprehension
  - Nonfluent speech
  - Preserved repetition
- *Global aphasia*:
  - Lesion affecting both Broca's and Wernicke's area
  - Nonfluent, mute
  - Impaired repetition
  - Automatic emotional speech intact
- *Nominal aphasia*:
  - Lesion in angular gyrus
  - Fluent spontaneous speech
  - Normal verbal output
  - Normal auditory comprehension
  - Impaired naming
  - Normal reading
  - Normal writing

Assessment of Aphasia

Spontaneous Speech

Most information is gained from just listening to the patient.

Let the patient try to tell his story without his relative interrupting.

Is the speech fluent or nonfluent? Listen carefully to construction of each word and sentence. Are they correct? Is he making sense?

Is he using wrong words or words which are nearly normal but not exactly right (paraphasia)? Is he repatriating same words after having once used them (preservation)?

Same time, the examiner has to find if he understands the question, ask to him and the instruction given during course of the examination.

- *Observe grammar*:
  - *Telegraphic*: Unable to produce grammatically correct sentences but able to convey thoughts and ideas well.
  - *Jargon*: Able to construct sentences but unable to convey thoughts and ideas meaningfully.
  - *Paraphasia*: Use of wrong words.
  - *Neologism*: Use of nonexistent words.
- *Observe prosody (emotional component of speech)*:
  - *Normal prosody*: Quality of speech, rate of speech, length of phrases, pauses in between.
  - *Dysprosodic speech*: Prosodic excess or prosodic insufficiency.

Comprehension

[*Note*: Patients reaction and answer to ordinary conversation are normal and appropriate. Exception of some patients with conductive aphasia most severely affected patients should be able to answer questions designed to require an answer yes or no. for example, it is true that it is raining outside?]

Give series of verbal command and observe for comprehension.

Naming Object

Patient is asked about names of common objects such as watch, comb, key, pen, pencil. Then go to component part of object such as strap, buckle and second hand of watch. If he fails to give a name, can he choose right one from a list?

Repetition

Ability to repeat word or phrases is important. Ask patient to repeat complex phrase and if fails simpler phrases or even single words.

Reading

Assess patient's normal capacity in relation to age, education and visual acuity. Give individual word to read out first then sentences, then longer passages and finally instruction to perform certain action. This will link motor and sensory side.

Writing

Dysphasia is disorder of language, not just speech. Patient may be able to write his name and address but not construct linguistic correct sentences.

Calculation

Ask patient to perform simple sums. Start simply by easy addition, subtractions.

DYSARTHRIA

- Voice production requires coordination of breathing, vocal cords, larynx, palate, tongue and lips. Dysarthria can reflect difficulty at different levels.
- Lesion of upper motor neuron type, of extra-pyramidal system and cerebellar lesion disturb the integration process of speech production and tend to disturb rhythm of speech.
- Lesion of one or several of cranial nerves tend to produce characteristic distortion of certain parts of speech but the rhythm is normal.

Types of Dysarthria

- *Spastic dysarthria*:
  - Caused by bilateral upper motor neuron disease
  - The tongue is small and spastic
  - The speech is slurred
  - Excursion of mouth limited

- The letter p, b, d and t suffer particularly
- The impression is that patient is trying to talk from back of mouth
- Jaw jerk exaggerated
- *Phonation*: Strained voice tremor
- *Prosody*: Excess or insufficient
- *Nasality*: Hypo or hyper
- *Loudness*: Harsh or monotonus
- *Rate*: Slow.
    - *Common causes*
        - Pseudo-bulbar palsy
        - Motor neuron disease
        - Upper brainstem tumor
- *Rigid dysarthria*:
    - Caused by lesion of extra-pyramidal system producing rigidity of face or tongue muscle without wasting and exaggeration of reflexes
    - Speech is monotonous
    - Excursion of tongue and lips are greatly reduced
    - In severe case the phenomenon of palilalia, i.e. repetition of a particular syllable, may be heard.
        - *Common cause:* Parkinsonism
- *Ataxic dysarthria*:
    - Incoordination of muscle of speech including respiratory muscle
    - Speech is irregular, slurred and drunken
    - Sometimes too loud or too soft
    - Words run into each other
        - *Common causes*
            - Multiple sclerosis
            - Cerebellar disease or tumors
            - Hereditary ataxia
            - Chorea
            - Anticonvulsant and other drug toxicity

Dysarthria due to Lesion of Lower Motor Neuron or Muscle

Speech well preserved, but individual words and sounds cause difficulty, the distribution and extent of muscle weakness governing the particular variety of defect produced.

- Facial paralysis causes difficulty with labials such as p, b, m, and w.
- Tongue paralysis affects a large number of sounds, particularly those involving the letters l, d, n, s, t, x, z and speech is distorted.
- Palatal paralysis produces nasal speech. B and d become m, n and g become rh and k sounds like ng. The patient's speech being worse when the head is bent forward.

Myasthenic Dysarthria

- Voice may be normal at beginning of each sentence but abnormality develops as sentence progresses.
- Hoarseness of voice due to palatal weakness.
- After few minutes of rest voice will become normal.
- The abnormality temporarily cures by injection of neostigmine or edrophonium chloride.

Dysarthria in Dysphasic States

A combination of dysphasia and dysarthria may accompany internal carotid artery thrombosis or other vessels of the neck are diseased as well.

Dysphasia occurs due to lesion of dominant hemisphere, whereas dysarthria occur due to any site.

Examination

- Listen to clarity of patient's enunciation during history taking.
- Ask patient to repeat certain phrases. Many tongue twisters are used. Start with easy words.
- Ask person to read a paragraph from a simple book.
- Ask patient to count successively to 30 or above to test for muscle fatigue.

Listen to the words, heather they slur into one another whether the rhythm is jerky, explosive, monotonous whether speech is too loud or too soft whether particular letters present particular difficulty, and which they are, whether there is a nasal tone to speech, whether the disturbance is constant throughout, variable or increasing towards end of each sentence or on prolong continuing.

DYSPHONIA

This is disturbance of voice production and may reflect either local vocal cord pathology, an abnormality of nerve supply via the vagus, or occasionally a psychological disturbance.

Examination

If the patient is able to give his name and address but unable to produce normal volume of sound or speaks in whisper, this is dysphonia.
- Ask patient to cough and listen quality of cough.
- Ask patient to say a sustained e..e..e does it fatigue?

Findings

- *Normal cough*: Motor supply to vocal cord is intact.
- *Dysphonia with normal cough*: Local laryngeal problem or hysteria.
- *Cough lacks explosive start-bovine cough*: Vocal cord palsy.
- *The note cannot be sustained and fatigues*: Consider myasthenia.

METHOD OF DIFFERENTIATION

- Patient is conscious but making no attempt to speak or make sound, this is mutism.
- If the patient though speaking fails to produce any volume of sound or merely whispers, this is aphonia due to disorder of larynx or vocal cord.
- If volume of sound and content of speech is normal but articulation and enunciation of individual word and phrase is distorted this is dysarthria.
- If patient is failing to put into properly constructed words or phrases the thoughts he wishes to express even if articulation is adequate this is dysarthria.

Disorder of Speech

- *Lesion in central mechanism*:
  - *Slurred speech*: Diffuse cerebral speech.
  - *Scanning speech*: Cerebellar disease.

  - *Staccato speech*: Cerebellar disease.
  - *Monotonus speech*: Parkinsonism.
  - *Hiccup speech*: Chorea, myoclonus.
  - In multiple sclerosis speech is ataxic there are explosive and staccato elements with slowness, stumbling, slurring and cerebellar type of speech ataxia.
  - In Friedrich's ataxia the ataxic, staccato and explosive elements predominates. Speech is clumsy often scanning and pitch may suddenly change in the middle of sentence.
- *Lesion in peripheral mechanism*:
  - *Palatal*: Nasal speech as with a bad cold.
  - *Tongue*: Distorted speech specially letters t, s, and d.
  - *Facial*: Difficulty with b, p, m, w.
  - *Dysphonia*: Disorder of function of larynx in which phonation is low even though articulation is preserved.
  - Ask patient to cough listen quality of cough.
  - Ask patient to say sustain e..e..e. Does it fatigue?
  - *Dysarthria*: Symbolic formulation of word is normal, phonation is preserved. Lesion in cranial nerve related to articulation or in its central regulation of nerve leads to interference with clear enunciation.

3 Mental State and Higher Functions

HIGHER MENTAL FUNCTIONS

Purpose of Assessment

- It interferes with patient's ability to carry out functional activity.
- Functional loss unexplained by motor deficit, sensory deficit or deficient comprehension.
- It is done to determine with cognitive and perceptual abilities are intact and which are limited.

Factors Influencing Assessment

- Education, economic status
- Patient is confused
- Rapid and frequent mood changes
- Low frustration tolerance
- Poor judgment
- Fatigue
- Prior expectation
- *Anxiety*: Reduced receptive and expressive communication skills, depression, fatigue.
- Premorbid intellectual ability should be ascertained from interview of family or friends.
- *Vision*: Homonymous hemianopia, poor visual acuity, diplopia/double vision, due to defective function of ocular muscle in both eyes, visual field deficits.
- *Mental state*: The mental state relates to mood and thoughts of a patient.

Abnormalities May Reflect

- Neurological disease, such as frontal lobe disease or dementia
- Psychiatric illness which may be causing neurological symptoms (e.g. anxiety leading to panic attack).

Mental state examination attempt to distinguish:

- Focal neurological deficit
- Diffuse neurological deficit
- Primary psychiatric illness
- Illness secondary to, or associated with, neurological disease.

MENTAL STATE

Appearance and Behavior

- Watch the patient while taking history.
  - Depression is characterized by furrowed brow, immobile, downcast faces, and slow monotonus speech.
  - Anxious patient will be restless in appearance. Symptoms of anxiety include palpitation, sweating and hyperventilation.
  - If mood of patients changes rapidly it suggests emotional lability.

Mood

- Ask patients are you ever able to cheer up?
- Do you see any hope in future?
  - Patient with depression says they find it difficult to cheer up and see little hope in future.
  - Patient with schizophrenia have lack of mood, smiling when you expect them to be sad.
  - Manic patients are Euphoric.

Vegetative Symptoms

- Weight loss or gain
- Sleep disturbance
- Appetite
- Libido
- Constipation

Delusions

- A delusion is firmly held belief, not altered by rational argument, and not a conventional belief within the culture and society of the patient.
- It cannot be elicited in history by direct questioning.
- Delusions are seen in acute confessional state and psychotic illness.

Hallucinations

- It is a perception experienced without external stimuli that is indistinguishable from perception of a real external stimulus.
- Temporal lobe lesion produce well-organized hallucination, occipital lobe visual hallucinations are ill formed.
- Patient with nondominant hemisphere lesion are able to describe hallucination more clearly and in detail.

Illusions

- It is misinterpretation of external stimuli and it is common in patient with altered consciousness.
- For example, confuse patient says that he can see a giant fist shaking outside of window, which is in fact tree blowing in the wind outside.

HIGHER FUNCTIONS

It is use to encompass thoughts, memory, understanding, perception and intellect.

Attention

It is awareness of environment or responsiveness to stimulus or task without being distracted by other stimuli.

It is inability to attend to a specific stimulus while simultaneously suppressing extraneous stimuli.

- Sustained attention is capacity to attend relevant information during activity.
- Person can maintain consistent response during conscious activity.
- Selective attention is capacity to attend to a task despite environmental visual or auditory stimuli.
- Alternating attention is the capacity to move flexibly between tasks and respond appropriately to demand of each task.
- Divided attention is capacity to respond simultaneously to two or more task or stimuli when all stimuli are relevant.
- Patient has to stop dressing activity to talk to may show difficulty in focus attention.
- Patient distracted by music or other background noise may show difficulty in focus attention.
- Problem with focus attention may refer as distractibility.

- Affection of reticular formation and limbic and frontal region.
- Stroop test and trail making test is use to check attention.

Orientation

Determine whether patient knows his name, address, where he is, who the doctor and nurse are?

It refers to patient's awareness of time, person and place. Oriented × 3 refers to 3 parameters of time, person and place. If patient is not fully oriented to one or more domains, then oriented × 2 (time) or oriented × 1 (time, place).

Sample questions to assess orientation

- *Time*
  - What time is it?
  - What year is it?
- *Person*
  - What is your name?
  - How old are you?
- *Place*
  - Do you know name of your city?
  - Do you know where you are right now?

Memory

- Mental process that allows the individual to store experiences and perceptions for recall at a later time. Memory comprises acquisition or learning, storage or retention and retrieval or recall.
- *Immediate recall*: Retention of information that has been stored for few seconds.
- Short-term memory mediate retention of events or learning that has taken place within few minutes, hours or days.
  - Patient with problem in immediate recall may *have problem in following instruction given by.*
- *Long-term memory:*
  - Early experience and information acquired over period of years.
  - Patient who do not have long-term memory are often described as having amnesia.
  - Patient is having problem in recall.
  - Common in brain injury and Alzheimer's disease but are not commonly seen in stroke patients.

Executive Function

- *Volition*: It is capacity to determine what one needs and wants to do.
  - It includes goal planning, task initiation, self-awareness, and awareness of environment.
- *Planning*: Identification and organization of steps and elements need to carry out an intention or achieved goal.
- *Purposive action*: It includes productivity and self regulation, which encompasses ability to initiate, maintain, switch and stop complex action in orderly manner to realize goal.
- *Effective performance*: Capacity for quality control including ability to self-monitor and self correct one's behavior because inability to self-monitor and self-control patient cannot perceive their mistakes whereas other may identify them but take no action to correct.

It is associated with frontal, prefrontal cortex and reciprocal connection with other cortical and sub-cortical region.

- Impulsiveness
  - Poor judgment
  - Poor planning ability
  - Lack of foresight

Cognition: It is defined as process of knowing and includes both awareness and judgment.

Three areas for testing cognition dependent function:
1. Fund of knowledge.
2. Calculation ability.
3. Proverb interpretation.

Fund of Knowledge

- It is defined as the sum total of an individual's learning and experience in life.
- To check fund of knowledge therapist can ask questions like who is current Vice President of India.

Calculation Ability

- It assesses foundational mathematical abilities.
- Two associated terms are dyscalculia or acalculia.

Proverb Interpretation

- It tests the patients ability to interpret use of words outside of their usual context or meaning. This is sophisticated cognitive function.
- *Samples for proverbs are*:
  - A stitch in time saves nine.
  - A rolling stone has no mass.

Approaches used for treatment:
- *Remedial approach*: Providing structure feedback performance can be enhanced unless patient has awareness about problem remedial approach will not be effective.
- *Adaptive approach*: Can use other intact cognitive function and modify environment beeper or alarm use to overcome initiation problem.

Perception

Definition: Integration of sensory impression into information which is psychologically meaningful.

It is ability to select those stimuli that require attention and action to integrate those stimuli with each other and with prior information and finally to interpret them.

Sensation: It is defined as appreciation of stimuli through organ of special sense.

Clinical Indicators

- Inability to do simple task independently
- Difficulty in initiating or completing task
- Difficulty in switching from one task to next
- They have inability to follow instruction
- They make same mistake over and over
- Frequently inattentive to one side of body

Body Scheme/Body Image

- *Body image*: It is visual or mental image of one's body that includes feeling about one's body in relation to health and disease.
- *Body scheme*: Postural model of body includes relationship of body part to each other or to environment.

Unilateral Neglect

Inability to register and integrate stimuli and perception from one side of body and environment or hemispace which is not due to sensory loss.

It is not due to homonymous hemianopsia or hemisensory loss.

In severe cases patient appears totally indifferent to left side of body and environment and may deny left extremity belong to him/her.

Clinically

- Patient has difficulty in dressing and forgot to put on sleeve or pent.
- Woman may neglect to put make-up.
- Patient may not eat from left half of plate, read newspaper from midline.
  - *Lesion*: Inferior-posterior regions of right parietal lobe.
  - *Assessment technique*:
    - Behavior inattention test (BIT)
  - Patient asked to copy simple drawing **(Figs 3.1A and B)**.

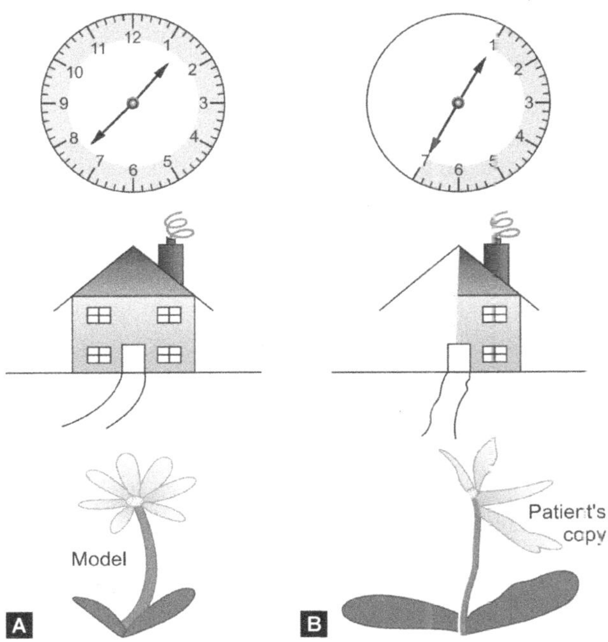

Figs 3.1A and B (A) Normal drawing; (B) Drawing by patient with unilateral neglect

- Patient asked to perform ADL like dressing.
  - *Treatment*: Remedial approach
- Stimuli that are specialize for right side of brain such as shapes and blocks should be used to enhance activation.
- Stimuli which activate left side brain such as letters and numbers should be minimized simply clenching and declutching fist can improve attention.
- *Compensation*: Turning towards left look in mirror and touch both faces.
- *Functional approach*: Repeated practice of transfer from wheelchair or eating.
  - Activity broken in parts and component performed.
  - Verbal self-cueing.
- *Adaptive environment*: Call button telephone on unaffected side.
- *Sensory motor approach*: Stimulate left side with rough cloth, ice or other material.
- *Transfer of training*: Patient participates in task and make necessary to look towards affected side.

Anosognosia

- Severe condition includes denial and lack of awareness of presence of severity and one's paralysis.
- Limits patient's ability to recognize need for and thus to use compensatory technique.
- Disown paralysis of limb and refuse to accept responsibility for their limb has mind of its own and it is at home or in closet.

Assessment: Ask patient what happens to the arm or leg whether it is paralyzed.

Patient denies paralysis.

Treatment: Difficult to treat. Safety is very important. Patient does not know about disability.

Somatoagnosia

Lack of awareness of body structure and relationship of body parts to oneself or others.

Autopognosia/simple body agnosia: Patient has difficulty in performing transfer activities.

Assessment Technique

- Patient requested to point different body parts. For example, show me your knees, show me your feet.
- Patient is asked to imitate movement of therapist touches his or her cheeks, mirror image response is accepted.
- Patient requested to answer questions. For example, are your knees below head? Which is on top of your head, feet or hairs?

Treatment

1. *Sensory motor approach*: Sensory stimulation to affected body part. Rub body part with rough cloth.
2. *Transfer of training approach*: Verbally identifies body part or points picture of them.
   - *Right or left discrimination*: It is inability to identify right or left part of one's body or that of.
     - Clinically patient cannot tell which is right and which is left and patient is unable to use instruction which include right and left word.

Lesion: Usually lesion to left hemisphere. If in right hemisphere than with aphasia.

- Patient is asked to point body parts. For example, right ear, left foot, right arm.
- Six responses should be elicited on patient's own body, on or on human model.

Treatment

- Giving instruction with right and left word should be avoided.
- Instead of that give instruction like arm with watch.

Adaptive Environment

Shoes or clothing should be marked with red tape.

Finger Agnosia

It is inability to identify finger of one's own hand or that of examiner. Difficulty in naming finger on command. Middle three fingers are more commonly affected.

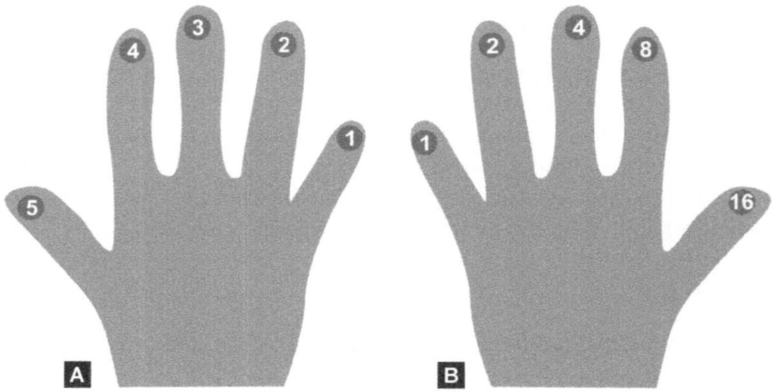

Figs 3.2A and B Finger agnosia: (A) Spare; (B) Disturbed

Lesion

Bilateral finger agnosia, agraphia, acalculia, right and left discrimination problem. This all are called Gerstmann's syndrome.

Assessment

- Patient is asked to name finger touched by the therapist.
- Patient is asked to point finger named by the therapist.
- Patient is asked to point finger to equivalent finger on life size picture **(Figs 3.2A and B)**.
- Patient is asked to imitate finger movement.

Treatment

- Apply sensory stimulation
- Rub dorsal surface
- Transfer of training
- Patient is quizzed on finger identification.

SPATIAL RELATIONS DISORDER

Figure Ground Discrimination

- Inability to visually distinguish figure from the ground in which it is embedded.

- Patient cannot locate item in a pocket book or drawer, locate buttons on shirt or distinguish armhole.

Lesion: Parieto-occipital lesion right hemisphere.

Assessment: Ayres figure ground test.

Functional test: White towel on white sheet.

Treatment

Comprehension: Use of other intact sense learning lock wheelchairs.

Adaptation and simplification of environment: Red tape.

Functional approach: Repeated practice.

Transfer of training: Visually locating object.

Form Discrimination

- Inability to perceive or attend subtle differences in form and shape.
- Patient confuse with pen and tooth brush, vase and water pitcher.

Assessment

Number of items similar in shape and size like paper clip, coin, key, ring.

Treatment

- *Transfer of training*: Differentiating cues.
- Encourage use of vision, touch and self-verbalization.

Spatial Relations

Inability to perceive relation of one object in space to other.

Difficulty in spoon, cutlery, plate:
- *Lesion*: Inferior parietal lobe.
- *Assessment*:
  - Picture of clock and ask the patient to fill number.
  - Two or three object on piece of paper in a particular pattern.
  - Improve validity
  - Unilateral neglect and hemianopsia ruled out.

- *Treatment:*
  Give simple command like:
  - Go behind table
  - Sit next to me
  - Step over line
  - *Sensory motor approach*: If patient avoid using midline give midline activity.

Position in Space

Inability to perceive special concept such as in, out, up, down.

Difficulty in range of motion:
- *Lesion*: Non-dominant parietal lobe
- *Assessment*: Shoe and shoe box
- *Treatment*: Transfer of training and sensory motor approach.

Topographic Disorientation

Difficulty in understanding and remembering relationship of one location to another.

Patient is unable to get from one location to another.

Clinically patient cannot find way from his or her room to physical therapy clinic despite of shown repeatedly.
- *Lesion*: Inferior parietal lobe, occipital associated cortex.
- *Assessment*:
  - Patient is asked to draw or describe familiar route.
- *Treatment*:
  - *Transfer of training approach*: Use of verbal cues.
  - *Functional approach*: Repeated practice.
  - *Adaptation to environment*: Frequently traveled routes are marked with color dots.
  - Gradual increase in distance between two dots and then eliminate them.
  - *Cognitive awareness*: Not to leave clinic, room or home unattended.

Depth and Distance Perception

Inaccurate judgment of direction, depth and distance.

Patient has difficulty in navigating stairs, may miss chair on attempting to sit, and may continue pouring glass.

- *Lesion*: Posterior right hemisphere, visual association cortex.
- *Assessment*:
  - Patient is asked to take or grasp object from table. Patient may overshoot or undershoot it.
  - *Assess depth perception*: Patient can be ask to fill glass of water. Patient with depth perception deficit may over pouring it.
- *Treatment*:
  - Become aware of deficit and take precaution while walking.
  - *Transfer of training approach*: Patient is asked to place feet on designated spots during gait training.
  - *Functional approach*: Compensate through intrinsic mechanism.

Vertical Disorientation

- Disorder of perception of what is vertical.
- It contributes to disturb motor performance, posture and gait **(Figs 3.3A and B)**.
- It is not influenced by presence of homonymus hemianopsia.
- *Lesion*: Non-dominant parietal lobe.
- *Assessment*: Holds cane vertically and then turns sideway to horizontal plane.
  - Patient handed cane and asked to turn it back to original position.
  - If patient's concept is wrong patient will hold it to particular angle.
- *Treatment*:
  - Patient is made aware of disability and should be instructed to compensate by using touch for self-orientation especially when going doorways.

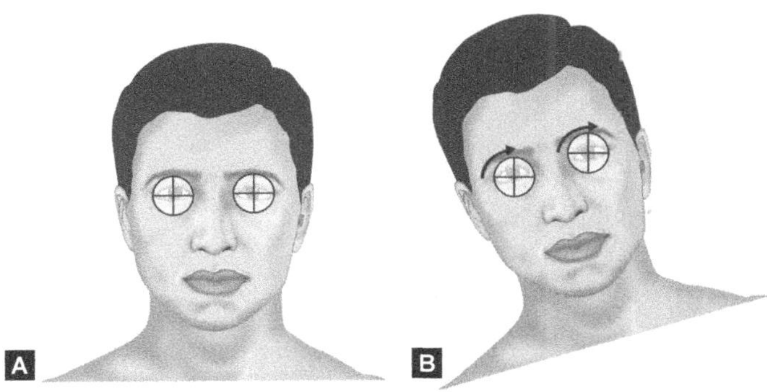

Figs 3.3A and B (A) Normal visual field; (B) Visual field with vertical disorientation

AGNOSIAS

It is inability to recognize or make sense of incoming information despite intact sensory capacity.

Visual Object Agnosia

It is inability to recognize familiar object despite of normal function of eyes and optic tracts.

The patient may not recognize people, possessions and common objects.

- *Simultanagnosia—Balint's syndrome*: Inability to perceive visual stimuli as whole.
- *Lesion*: Dominant occipital lobe.
- *Prosopagnosia*: Inability to identify familiar faces.
  - It is accompanied by visual field defect.
  - *Lesion*: Bilateral symmetric occipital lesion.
- *Color agnosia*: Inability to recognize colors, it is not color blindness.
  - Occipito-temporo-parito association cortex.
- *Assessment:* Several common objects place infront of patient. Patient is ask to name object. It is important to rule out aphasia and apraxia.
- *Treatment*
  - *Transfer of training approach*: Discriminate between faces that are important to patient using photographs.
  - Silent visual cues for relating names to faces.
  - *Use of intact sensory modalities*: Such as touch or audition.

Auditory Agnosia

Inability to recognize non-specific sound or to discriminate between the patient cannot discriminate between ring of doorbell and that of telephone.

- *Lesion*: Dominant temporal lobe.
- *Assessment*: Taken by speech and language pathologist.
- *Treatment*: Drilling patient on sounds.

Tactile Agnosia/Astereognosis

It is inability to recognize forms by handling them inspite of intact tactile, proprioceptive and thermal sensation.

Patient is handed an object with vision occluded, patient will fail to recognize it.

- *Lesion*: Parito-temporo-occipital lobe.
- *Assessment*: Patient is ask to identify object place in hand by examining them.
- *Treatment:*
  - Transfer of training
  - Feeling shapes and texture with vision occluded. Cognitive awareness.

APRAXIA

- Disorder of volitional skilled learns movement.
- Inability to perform purposeful movement which cannot be accounted for inadequate strength, loss of co-ordination, impaired sensation, additional difficulties, abnormal tone, movement disorder or uncooperativeness.
- *Lesion*: Dominant hemisphere.

Ideomotor Apraxia

- Break down between concept and performance, disconnection between idea and movements and its motor execution.
- Patient is able to carry out habitual task automatically and describe how they are done but unable to imitate gesture or perform it on command.
- Patient will fail to walk when requested on traditional manner.
- Male patient is asked to comb hair, he may able to identify comb, tell its uses but not use comb appropriately but he comb hair automatically.

Lesion: Left dominant hemisphere.

Assessment

- Patient is asked to brush teeth.
- Then sits in front of the patient. Patient is asked to imitate different posture of limb.
- Patient with apraxia will unable to imitate posture.

Treatment

- Speaks slowly and use shortest possible sentence.
- One command is given at a time and second command is not given until one task is completed.

- Task should be broken down into its component part.
- When all individual units are mastered an attempt to combine them should be made.
- Repetition is necessary.
- Family member should use approach which is successful.

Sensory motor approach: Sensory input use on affected body parts to produce appropriate motor response.

Ideational Apraxia

- Failure in conceptualization of task.
- It is inability to perform motor act either automatically or on command because patient no longer understand purpose of task or cannot formulate motor pattern require for that.
- Patient cannot verbally describe process to perform task.
- Patient is given toothbrush and toothpaste and told to brush teeth.
- Patient puts tube of toothpaste in mouth or tries to put toothpaste on toothbrush without removing cap.
- Patient is unable to describe verbally
  - *Lesion*: Dominant parietal lobe.
  - Seen in cerebral arteriosclerosis.
  - *Treatment*: Same as ideomotor aprexia.

Constructional Apraxia

- Characterize by faulty spatial analysis and conceptualization of task.
- Encompass capacity to understand relationship of parts to a whole.
- It is critical in activities such as drawing, dressing, building from model, copying block designs and the like.
- Patient has problem in two or three dimensional drawing, construction or arranging block.
- Patient cannot place individual component in corrective manner.
- Patient who understands all about sandwiches and what they are for but unable to assemble one.
- *Lesion*: Posterior parietal lobe.
- *Assessment technique*
- Drawing of house, flower or clock.
- Patient is requested to copy geometric design.
- Right and left sided lesion demonstrable qualitative difference.

Table 3.1: Perceptual problem due to dominant and nondominant hemisphere involvement

	Dominant	*Nondominant*	*Either*
Body scheme/ body image	Somatoagnosia	• Unilateral neglect • Anosognosia	• Right or left discrimination • Finger agnosia
Spatial relation		• Figure ground discrimination • Position in space • Depth and distance • Vertical disorientation	

- *Right sided damage* **(Table 3.1)**:
  - Patient will draw diagonal and will neglect left side of page.
  - Patient will draw pieces of picture without any coherence relationship.
  - Drawing complex and unrecognizable.
  - Patient will have immense difficulty in copying or constructing anything in three dimensions.
- *Left hemisphere damage* **(Table 3.1)**
  - Figure more recognizable.
  - Characterized by great simplicity.
- *Treatment:*
  - Transfer of training approach.
  - Copy drawings.
  - Simple patterns are used and then gradually progress to more complex.

APPROACHES USED FOR MANAGEMENT

Transfer of Training Approach (Retraining)

- Practice in one task will enhance performance of other task with similar perceptual demand
- Disruption in brain region has impact on brain function
- Peg board activity will result in improving functional task
- Visual cancellation task result in improvement in reading and writing although no training in writing was offered
- Patient's capacity to learn must be evaluated and learning capacity is key to patient's ability to generalize material learned in one situation to others

- It is used for maintenance of sitting or standing balance, weight baring exercises or functional use of affected extremities.

Sensory Integrative Approach

- It defines pattern of sensory integrative dysfunction and suggest treatment techniques
- It is defined as organization of sensation for use.
- *Proprioceptive sensation*: Bouncing, pushing
- *Vestibular system*: Rocking chairs, rolling.
- *Learning new skills involving movement*: Swimming, building blocks, skipping.
  - It proceeds in developmental sequence normal child within context of goal directed, meaningful activity.
  - It helps in high level adaptive behavior.
  - Offering opportunity for control sensory input can affect CNS processing of sensory information, decrease result in desire motor response.
  - Performance of adaptive response decrease in turn influence the way in which the brain organizes and process sensation. Enhancing ability to learn
  - Rubbing or icing provides sensory input
  - Resistance and weight-bearing provide proprioceptive input
  - Use of spinning to provide vestibular input
  - In young children use of compensatory or splinter skills is avoided in favor of remediating underlying deficits
  - In addition specific assessment and treatment requirement have been developed for and standardized on children who sufficiently have plastic nervous system to be influence by form of therapy
  - A mature adult with diffuse cerebral damage may have other complicating medical concerns and deficits in mobility that actually contraindicate use of equipment that is essential to treatment process.

Neurodevelopment Approach (NDT)

- This approach is aimed at maximize function and minimizes impairment
- It is problem-solving approach
- Perception is facilitated during normal infant neuromotor development by kinesthetic, proprioceptive, tactile and vestibular feedback received through normal movement experience

- Utilize this sensation as a progression from early physiological flexion movement against gravity for sitting, crawling, kneeling, standing and initial walking
- It provides sense of midline orientation awareness of two side of body and total body awareness
- Weight-bearing enhance proprioception
- Bilateral activity enhances total body awareness and diminished unilateral neglect.

Functional Approach (Rehabilitative/Compensatory)

Difficulty in generalizing and learning from dissimilar task. Direct repetitive practice of functional skill is impaired. For example, depth perception difficulty and difficulty in climbing stairs with visual cues

- *Compensation*: Change that need to be made in patient's approach to task.
- *Adaption*: Alteration made in human and physical environment in order to facilitate relearning skill. Patient need to teach to attend the cues from environment helps in identifying cues and call up on new cues.
- *General suggestion for adaptation*
  - Use simple direction
  - Establish and carry out routine.
  - Do each activity in consistent manner
  - Employ repetition as much as necessary. For example, difficulty in right and left discrimination. Give red tape on left shoes.

ADVANTAGE

- Therapist concentrate on outcome directed real life functional activity
- Intervention directed towards specific functional outcome
- Activities are age appropriate, concrete and relevant to patient's concern
- Task can incorporate in daily routine.

LIMITATION

Method learned in one task is not typically generalized to performance of another task.

4 Cranial Nerve Examination

Causes for cranial nerve abnormality.
- From specific lesion to the nerve
- From lesion in the nucleus
- In communicating pathways to and from the cortex, cerebellum or other parts of brainstem
- As generalized problem of nerve and muscle.

Causes for more than one cranial nerve abnormality:
- If there is lesion where several cranial nerves run together either in brainstem or within the skull
- When affected by generalized disorder (e.g. Myasthenia gravis)
- Following multiple lesions (e.g. Multiple sclerosis, basal meningitis).

CRANIAL NERVE-I OLFACTORY NERVE

This is rarely tested in clinical practice.

Procedure

- Take a bedside object—a piece of fruit, a juice bottle and ask patient if it smells normal.
- Agent often use include peppermint, camphor and rosewater. The subject is asked to identify these smells.
- Each nostril is tested separately.

Findings

- If patient is able to identify smell properly—normal
- The patient is unable to recognize scents offered but recognizes ammonia—anosmia.
- This finding is limited to one nostril—unilateral anosmia.
- The patient recognize no smells, including ammonia—consider that the loss may not be entirely organic.

Causes

- *Anosmia in both nostrils*: Loss of sense of smell
- Blocked nasal passages
- Trauma
- Aging
- Parkinsonism.

Unilateral Anosmia

- Blocked nostrils
- Unilateral frontal lesion.

CRANIAL NERVE-II OPTIC NERVE

- General
- Pupils
- Acuity
- Field
- Fundi.

General

- Look at patient's eyes and note any difference between two sides.
- Look if any asymmetry.
- If an eyelid is lower than other this is referred as ptosis.
- It can be partial or complete.
  If eyelid is higher than normal usually above the top of eyrish this is described as lid retraction.

Causes of Ptosis

- Horner's syndrome
- Third nerve palsy
- Age related
- Myasthenia gravis.

Causes of Exophthalmos/Lid Retraction

Dysthyroid eye.

Pupils

- *Pupillary light reaction*:
  - *Afferent*: Optic
  - *Efferent*: Parasympathetic component of third nerve on both side
- *Accommodation reaction*:
  - *Afferent*: Arises in frontal lobe
  - *Efferent*: As for light reaction

Pupil Examination

- Size
- Outline
- Holes in Irish/foreign bodies.
- Shine a bright light in one eye
  - *Direct reflex*: Look at reaction of eye.
  - *Consensual reflex*: Look at reaction in other eye.
- Place your finger 10 cm in front of the patient's nose.
  - Ask patient to look into distance and then at your finger.
- *Swinging light test*:
  - Shine a bright light into one eye and then the other at about 1 sec interval. Swing the light repeatedly between the two.

Findings

- Pupil constrict as the light is shown into it repeatedly is known as normal response.
- Pupil on one side constrict when light is shown in it and pupil on other side dilate when light is shown into it.
- This is known as Marcus-Gunn pupil.

Acuity

- *Ocular problem*: Such as dense cataract not correctable with glasses identifiable on ophthalmoscopy.
- Optical problems:
- Abnormalities of focusing system in the eye commonly called long or shorty sightness. It can be corrected by glasses.

Retinal or Neuroorbital Abnormality

- Cannot correct by using lenses. Visible on ophthalmoscopy.
- Ask patient to put glasses if used. Cover one eye of the patient.

Using Snellen's Chart

- Stand the patient 6 meter from a well-lit chart. Ask him to read down from largest letter to the smallest.
- Record the result. Distance in meters/feets from the chart.

Using Near Vision Chart

- Hold the chart 30 cm from the patient and ask him to read section of print.
- Record smallest print size to read.
- Ensure reading glasses are used if needed.

Using Bedside Material

- Newspaper headlines
- Count fingers
- See hand movements
- Perceive light
- Findings
- Visual acuity
- Correctable by glasses-ocular defect.

Fields

- The visual fields are divided vertically through the point of fixation into temporal and nasal fields.
- Something on your right as you look ahead is in the temporal field of your right eye and nasal field of your left eye.
- Field defect are said to be homonymous if the same part of the visual field is affected in both eyes.
  - Acuity
  - Fields
    - Ask patient to look with both eyes at your eyes.
    - Put your hands out on both sides approximately 50 cm apart and 30 cm above your level.
    - Ask patient to indicate which index finger you move right, left or both.
    - Repeat with hands approximately 30 cm below eye level.

Test each eye individually:

- Large objects more easily seen than small objects. White object more easily seen than red. Central vision is colored (cones) peripheral vision is monochrome (rods)
  - White hat pin is use for peripheral visual field defect. Red pin use to assess defect of central vision.
- Sit just one arm length away from the patient at the same level. Cover patient's right eye and ask him to look at your right eye with his left eye. Tilt patient's head to get eyebrows and nose out of the way.
- When using white pin imagine sphere of radius 30 cm centered on patient's eye. Bring a white pin in towards the line of fixation along an arc of sphere. Ensure pin cannot be seen when you start. Ask patient to tell you when he first sees the pin. Initially bring the pin slowly from four directions. Northeast, Northwest, Southeast, Southwest.
  - When using red pin imagine there is a plane like a vertical sheet of glass, halfway between you and the patient. You are going to compare your visual field on that plane. The field of red is about 30–40° from the point of fixation.
- Hold the red pin within that plane beyond where you can see it as red. Move it within the place towards the point of fixation. Ask patient to tell you when he can see it as red. Bring the pin slowly from all four directions.

Causes for central field defect:

- Scotoma
- Blind spot.

Findings:

- Defect limited to one eye
  - Tubular vision
  - Scotoma
- Defect affecting both eye
  - Bitemporal hemianopia.

CRANIAL NERVE-III, IV, VI OCULOMOTOR, TROCHLEAR, ABDUCENS

Eye movements can be divided into four types:

1. *Saccadic eye movements (frontal lobe):* The rapid movement from one point of fixation to another. For example, movement to look from page to someone in room if you were told to look up **(Fig. 4.1)**.

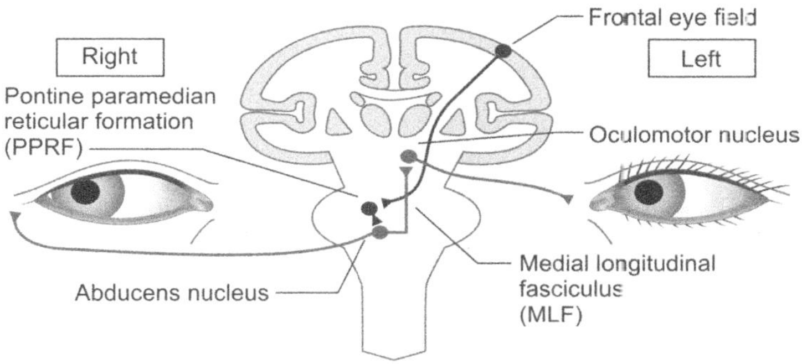

Fig. 4.1 Saccadic eye movements

2. *Pursuit eye movement (occipital lobe)*: Slow eye movement use to maintain fixation on a moving object e.g. to maintain eye contact as a person moved across a room.
3. *Vestibulo-ocular reflex (cerebellar vestibular nucleus)*: The eye movement that compensate for movement of head to maintain fixation.
4. *Convergence*: Midbrain **(Fig. 4.2)**
   - The movement that maintain fixation as object is brought close to the face.

- *Cover test*: For lateral squint
  - Ask patient to look with both eyes at your right eye then cover his left eye. Then uncover the left eye rapidly and cover right eye. Look to see if the left eye has corrected to look back at your eye.
  - *Findings*: One eye has to correct as it is uncovered.
- *Test the eye movement to pursuit*:
  - Hold a pen vertically about 50 cm away from the patient in center of his gaze. Ask him to follow it with his eyes without moving his head and tell you if he sees double. Hold his chin lightly to prevent head movement.
  - Move the pen slowly and ask the patient to tell you if he sees double.
- *Test saccadic eye movement*:
  - Ask the patient to look to the right to the left then up and down.
  - Look at speed of adduction
- *Test convergence*: Ask the patient to look into distance and then look at your finger placed 50 cm in front of him.

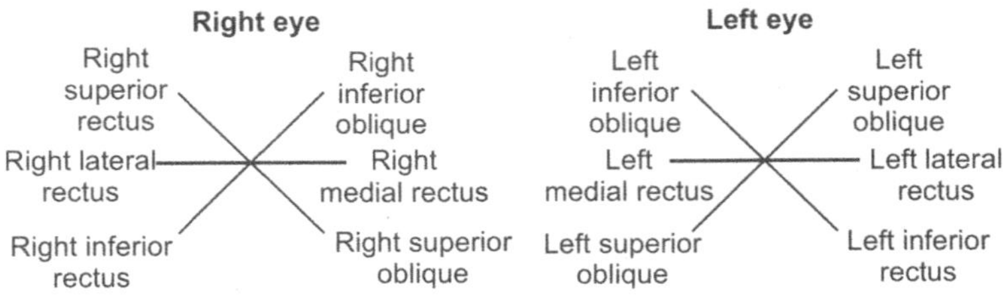

Fig. 4.2 Muscles producing movement of eyeball

- *Vestibulo-ocular reflex*: Use for unconscious patient. Ask patient to look into the distance at a fix point then his head to the left and then the right and flex the neck and extend the neck.

Findings

- One eye deviated down and out with ptosis (Third nerve palsy)
- Eyes aligned in different vertical planes (skew deviation).

CRANIAL NERVE-V TRIGEMINAL

While palpating the temporal and masseter muscle in turn ask the patient to clench his or her teeth. Note the strength of muscle contraction **(Fig. 4.3)**.

Sensory

- Ophthalmic (V_1) supplies cornea
- Maxillary (V_2) cheek
- Mandibular (V_3) lower lip.

After explaining what you plan to do test the forehead cheecks and jaw on each side for pain sensation. Patient's eye should be closed. Test light touch, pain, temperature (hot and ice water).

- For vibratory sensation tuning fork is used.
- Ask patient to respond whenever you touch the skin **(Fig. 4.4)**.

Test Corneal Reflex

Ask the patient to look up and away from you. Approach from other side out of patient's line of vision. Touch the cornea lightly with a fine wisp of cotton **(Fig. 4.5)**.

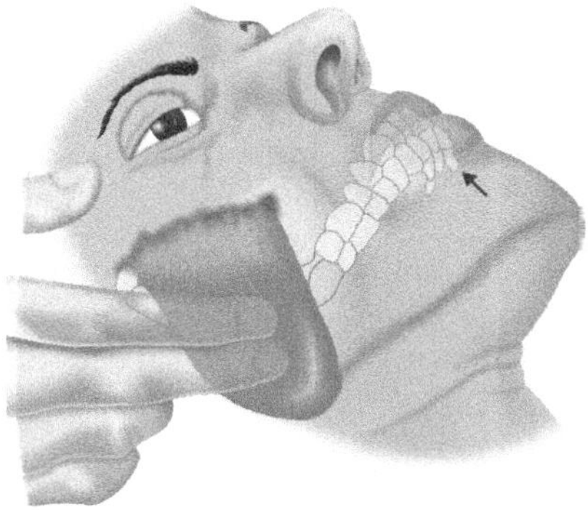

Fig. 4.3 Palpation of masseter

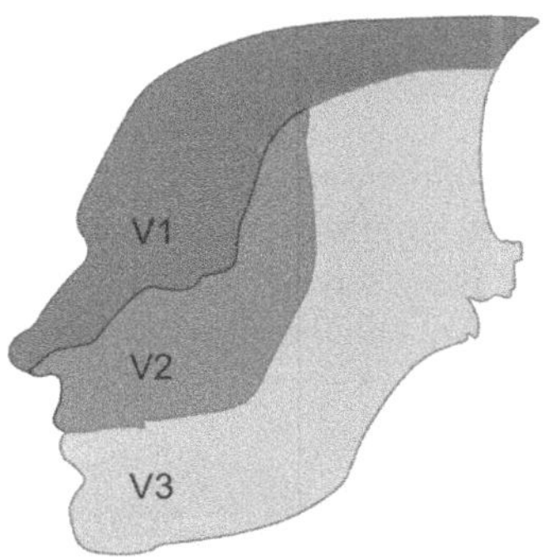

Fig. 4.4 Sensory distribution of trigeminal nerve over face

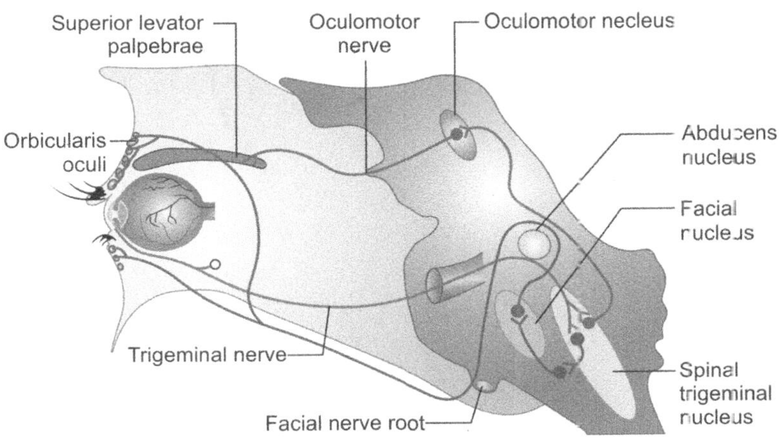

Fig. 4.5 Pathway for corneal reflex

Findings

Blinking response of eye.

Jaw Jerk

Ask the patient to let his mouth hang loosely open. Place your finger on his chin. Percuss your finger with the hammer feel and observe jaw movement **(Fig. 4.6)**.

- Wasting of muscle in MND.
- Facioscapulohumeral dystrophy.

CRANIAL NERVE-VII FACIAL NERVE

- *Face*: Muscle of facial expression.
- *Ear*: Stapedius
- *Taste*: Anterior 2/3rd of the tongue.
- *Tear*: Parasympathetic supply to parotid gland.
  - In UMN forehead is preserved.
  - In LMN all muscles of facial expression are affected.

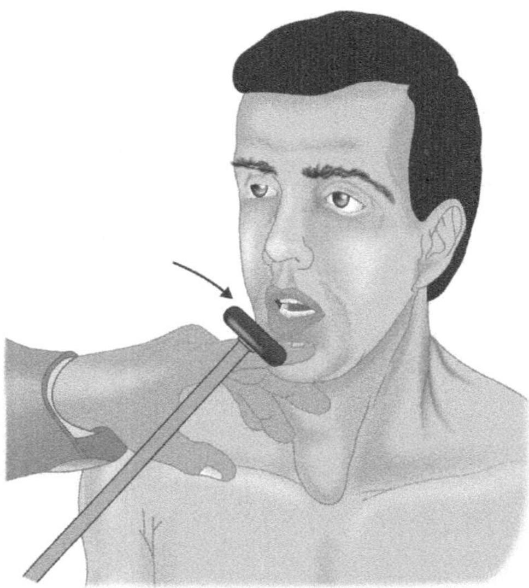

Fig. 4.6 Jaw jerk

Observation

Look at symmetry of face:
- Nasolabial folds
- Forehead wrinkles.

Bell's Phenomena

Eye turned upward on attempted closure **(Figs 4.7A and B)**.

Ask the patient to:
- Raise eyebrows
- Frown
- Close both eyes tightly and then try to open it
- Show both upper and lower teeth
- Smile
- Puff out both cheeks
  - Note any weakness or asymmetry
  - Taste sensation over anterior 2/3rd of tongue.

Causes for unilateral LMN weakness:
- Bell's palsy
- Herpetic infection (Ramsay Hunt syndrome)

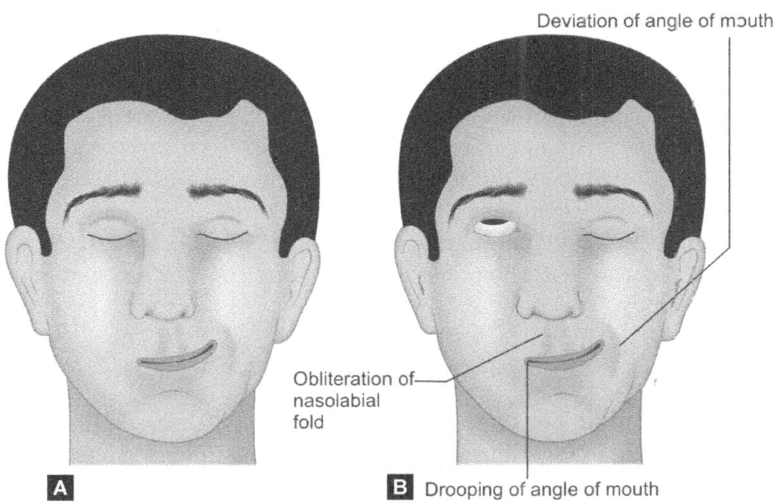

Figs 4.7A and B (A) Normal closure of eye; (B) Bell's phenomenon

- Basal meningitis
- Parotid tumors

Bilateral LMN weakness:
- GBS
- Sarcoidosis
- Myasthenia gravis
- Myopathies.

Unilateral upper motor neuron (UMN)
Cerebrovascular accident

Bilateral UMN:
- Motor neuron disease (MND)
- Pseudobulbar palsy.

Emotional paralysis: Parkinsonism.

CRANIAL NERVE-VIII VESTIBULOCOCHLEAR NERVE

- Test the hearing.
- Test one ear at a time block the opposite ear.
- Hold your watch by patient's ear. Discuss how far away from the ear it is still heard.

Rinne's Test

- The Rinne's test is a hearing test, primarily for evaluating loss of hearing in one ear (unilateral hearing loss). It compares perception of sounds transmitted by air conduction to those transmitted by bone conduction through the mastoid. Thus, one can quickly screen for the presence of conductive hearing loss.
- A Rinne test should always be accompanied by a Weber test to also detect sensorineural hearing loss and thus confirm the nature of hearing loss.

Procedure

The Rinne test is performed by placing a high frequency (512 Hz) vibrating tuning fork against the patient's mastoid bone and asking the patient to tell you when the sound is no longer heard. Once they signal they cannot hear it, quickly position the still vibrating tuning fork 1–2 cm

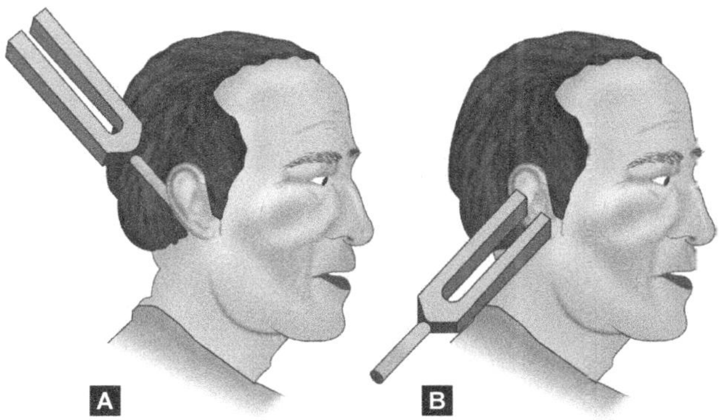

Figs 4.8A and B Rinne's test: (A) Bone conduction; (B) Air conduction

from the auditory canal, and again ask the patient to tell you if they are able to hear the tuning fork **(Figs 4.8A and B)**.

Result

- *Normal hearing*: Air conduction should be greater than bone conduction and so the patient should be able to hear the tuning fork next to the pinna (outer ear) after they can no longer hear it when held against the mastoid.
- *Abnormal hearing*:
  - If they are not able to hear the tuning fork after the mastoid test, it means that their bone conduction is greater than their air conduction. This indicates there is something inhibiting the passage of sound waves from the ear canal, through the middle ear apparatus and into the cochlea (i.e. there is a conductive hearing loss).
  - In sensorineural hearing loss the ability to sense the tuning fork by both bone and air conduction is equally diminished, implying they will hear the tuning fork by air conduction after they can no longer hear it through bone conduction. This pattern is similar to what is found in people with normal hearing, but patients with sensorineural hearing loss will indicate that the sound has stopped much earlier. This can be revealed by the investigator (with normal hearing) placing the fork close to her own ear after the patient indicates that the sound has subsided, noting that the sound from the fork is still loud and clear to a normal ear **(Table 4.1)**.

Table 4.1: Rinne's test and Weber's test for conductive deafness

Rinne		*Weber*				
Left	*Right*	*Lateralizes to left*		*No lateralization*	*Lateralizes to right*	
		Left ear	*Right ear*	*Both ears*	*Left ear*	*Right ear*
(+)	(+)	Normal	Sensorineural loss	Normal Sensorineural loss	Sensorineural loss	Normal
(–)	(+)	Conductive loss	Normal		Combined loss	Normal
(+)	(–)	Normal	Combined loss		Normal	Conductive loss
(–)	(–)	Conductive loss	Combined loss	Conductive loss	Combined loss	Conductive loss
Combined loss = conductive and sensorineural loss						

Weber's Test

The Weber test is a quick screening test for hearing. It can detect unilateral (one-sided) conductive hearing loss (middle ear hearing loss) and unilateral sensorineural hearing loss (inner ear hearing loss) **(Fig. 4.9)**.

Conductive hearing ability is mediated by the middle ear composed of the ossicles: incus, malleus, stapes. Sensorineural hearing ability is mediated by the inner ear composed of the cochlea with its internal basilar membrane and attached cochlear nerve (cranial nerve VIII).

The outer ear consisting of the pinna, ear canal, and ear drum or tympanic membrane transmits sounds to the middle ear but does not contribute to the conduction or sensorineural hearing ability save for hearing transmissions limited by cerumen impaction (wax collection in the ear canal).

The Weber and the Rinne test are typically performed together with the results of each combined to determine the location and nature of any hearing losses detected.

Procedure

In the Weber test a vibrating tuning fork is placed in the middle of the forehead, above the upper lip under the nose over the teeth, or on top

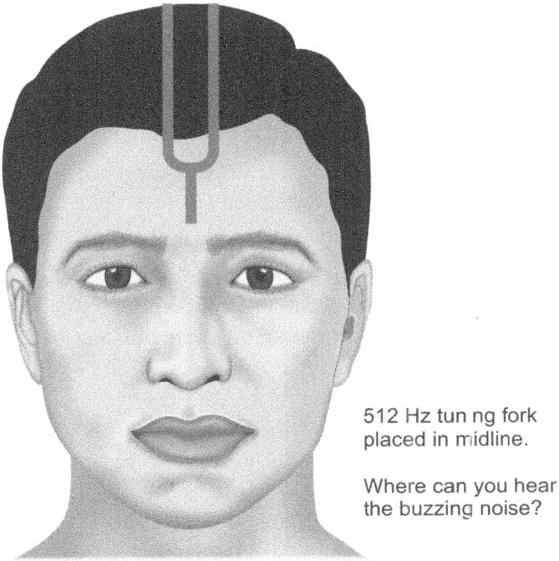

Fig. 4.9 Weber's test

of the head equidistant from the patient's ears on top of thin skin in contact with the bone. The patient is asked to report in which ear the sound is heard louder.

Result

A normal Weber test has a patient reporting the sound heard equally in both sides.

In an affected patient, if the defective ear hears the Weber tuning fork louder, the finding indicates a conductive hearing loss in the defective ear.

In an affected patient, if the normal ear hears the tuning fork sound better, there is sensorineural hearing loss on the other (defective) ear.

In a normal patient, the Weber tuning fork sound is heard equally loudly in both ears, with no one ear hearing the sound louder than the other (lateralization). Similarly, a patient with symmetrical hearing loss will hear the Weber tuning fork sound equally well, with diagnostic utility only in asymmetric (one-sided) hearing losses. In a patient with hearing loss, the Weber tuning fork sound is heard louder in one ear (lateralization) than the other. This clinical finding should be confirmed by repeating the procedure and having the patient occlude one ear with a finger; the sound should be heard best in the occluded ear.

The results of both tests are noted and compared accordingly below to localize and characterize the nature of any detected hearing losses.

Note: The Weber and Rinne are screening tests that are not replacements for formal audiometry hearing tests **(*See* Table 4.1)**.

Vestibular Assessment

The vestibular system is not easy to examine at the bedside because it is difficult to test part of system or even one side in isolation.

- *Gait*: Always heel-toe walking.
- Gait is unsteady.
- *Nystagmus*: Slow drift in one direction with fast correction in the opposite direction.

Hallpike's Test

The Dix–Hallpike test is performed with the patient sitting upright on the examination table with the legs extended. The patient's head is then rotated to one side by approximately 45°. The clinician helps the patient to lie down backwards quickly with the head held in approximately 20° of extension. This extension may either be achieved by having the clinician supporting the head as it hangs off the table or by placing a pillow under their upper back. The patient's eyes are then observed for about 45 seconds as there is a characteristic 5–10 second period of latency prior to the onset of *nystagmus*. If rotational nystagmus occurs then the test is considered positive for benign positional vertigo. During a positive test, the fast phase of the rotatory nystagmus is toward the affected ear, which is the ear closer to the ground. The direction of the fast phase is defined by the rotation of the top of the eye, either clockwise or counter-clockwise. Home devices are available to assist in the performance of the Dix–Hallpike maneuver for patients with a diagnosis of benign paroxysmal positional vertigo (BPPV) **(Fig. 4.10)**.

There are several key characteristics of a positive test:

- Latency of onset (usually 5–10 seconds)
- Tensional (rotational) nystagmus. If no tensional nystagmus occurs but there is upbeating or downbeating nystagmus, a central nervous system (CNS) dysfunction is indicated.

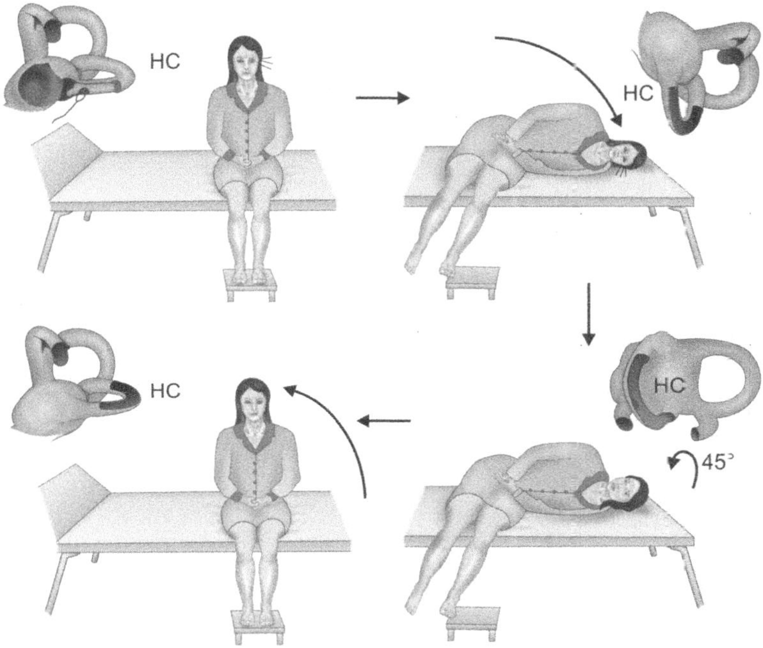

Fig. 4.10 Dix-Hallpike test

- *Upbeating or downbeating nystagmus*: Upbeating nystagmus indicates that the vertigo is present in the posterior semicircular canal of the tested (lower ear) side. Downbeating nystagmus indicates that the vertigo is in the anterior semicircular canal of the contralateral (upper ear) side.
- *Fatigable nystagmus*: Multiple repetition of the test will result in less and less nystagmus.
- *Reversal*: Upon sitting after a positive maneuver the direction of nystagmus should reverse for a brief period of time.

To complete the test, the patient is brought back to the seated position, and the eyes are examined again to see if reversal occurs. The *nystagmus* may come in paroxysms and may be delayed by several seconds after the maneuver is performed.

If the test is negative, it makes benign positional vertigo a less likely diagnosis and *central nervous system* involvement should be considered.

Turning Test

- Ask the patient to stand facing you.
- Ask patient to point both arms straight out in front of him towards the therapist.
- Ask patient to walk on the spot when he is doing this. He should then close his eyes.
- Watch his position.
- *Findings*: Patient gradually turns to one side and may turn to 180°. This indicates a lesion on the side he turns towards.

CRANIAL NERVE-IX GLOSSOPHARYNGEAL NERVE

- *Sensory*: Posterior 1/3rd of tongue, pharynx, middle ear
- *Motor*: Stylopharyngeus
- *Autonomic*: Salivary gland.

Gag Reflex

- *Afferent*: Glossopharyngeal
- *Efferent*: Vagus
- *Procedure*: Touch pharyngeal wall. Watch uvula, it should lift following stimulus.

Findings

- Uvula moves to one side. UMN or LMN of vagus on other side.
- Uvula does not move on saying Ahh or Gag suggest bilateral palatal muscle paralysis.
- Uvula moves on saying ahh but not on Gag with reduced sensation of Pharynx. IX cranial nerve palsy.

Examination of Larynx

- *Procedure*: Ask patient to cough. Listen onset is explosive or gradual.
- Listen to speech.
- *Normal response*: The palate should elevate symmetrically both when sustaining AH and in response to stimulation on either side. Patient should also be asked if they feel stimulus.
- *Finding*: With unilateral palatal weakness, the palate fails to elevate on the weak side and gag reflex will be absent on weak side.

Examination of Pharynx

- *Procedure*: Note position of uvula
- If not seen use tongue depressor
- Ask patient to say Ahh
- Observe that does it moves centrally or to one side?
- Ask patient to swallow
- Watch smooth coordination of action.

Finding

- Gradual onset cough-vocal cord palsy.
- Bubbly voice and cough combine cord palsy and pharyngeal pooling.

Testing Reflexes

- *Oculocardiac reflex*: Is bradycardia caused by pressure on eyeball. It may also be induced by painful stimulation of skin on the side of neck. The reflex is inconstant, unstandardized and influence by emotion. Usually the pulse is not slowed than more than 5–8 beat per minute.
- *Vomiting reflex*: It produces reverse peristalsis in esophagus and stomach, with forceful ejection of material from the stomach. Vomiting occurs for many reasons. Stimulation of pharynx, palate, esophagus, stomach, duodenum or lower GI tract may activate the reflex.
- *Hiccup*: It is sudden reflex contraction of the diaphragm causing forceful inspiration. Associated laryngeal spasm cause the glottis to snap shut, causing sudden arrest of inspiration and the characteristic sound. The phrenic nerves are major pathway but cranial nerve X contributes.
- *Yawning*: It is complex respiratory reflex with deep prolong inspiration, usually involuntary, through the open mouth. It typically occurs during sleepiness and fatigue but also be brought on by suggestion or boredom. Yawning can occur in neurological disease as well.
- *Carotid sinus reflex*: It is produced by stimulation of carotid sinus or carotid body by pressure at carotid bifurcation. It causes slowing of heart rate, a fall in blood pressure, a decrease in cardiac output, and peripheral vasodilatation. When the response is exaggerated there may be syncope. The afferent limb is carried over cranial nerve IX and the efferent over cranial nerve X.

CRANIAL NERVE-X VAGUS NERVE

- *Sensory*: Tympanic membrane
  - External auditory canal, external ear
- *Motor*: Muscles of palate, pharynx, larynx
- *Autonomic*: Afferent from carotid baroreceptor
  - Parasympathetic supply to and from thorax and abdomen.

CRANIAL NERVE-XI SPINAL ACCESSORY NERVE

- Look at neck
  - Wasting/fasciculation of sternocleidomastoid
  - Hypertrophy of sternocleidomastoid
  - Position of head.

Manual Muscle Testing

Sternocleidomastoid

- Ask the patient to lift his head forward against resistance and look at both sternocleidomastoid.
- Ask patient to turn his head to one side against resistance and watch opposite sternocleidomastoid (SCM).

Trapezius

Ask patient to shrug his shoulders. Watch for symmetry.

Findings

- Weakness of SCM and trapezius on same side.
  - Peripheral accessory palsy
- Weakness of ipsilateral SCM and contralateral trapezius.
  - Upper motor neuron (UMN) weakness on ipsilateral side.
- Bilateral wasting and weakness of SCM
  - Myopathy
  - Motor neuron disease (MND).
- Abnormal head position.
  - Cervical dystonia.

CRANIAL NERVE-XII HYPOGLOSSAL NERVE

- *Sensory*: None
- *Motor*: Intrinsic muscles of tongue
- Observe tongue for size, color, texture, any fasciculation.
- *Procedure*: To assess weakness
- Ask the patient to push his tongue into his cheek and test the power by pushing against it. Repeat on both sides.
- Test repeated movements:
  - Ask patient to put his tongue in and out as fast as he can move it from side-to-side
  - Ask patient to say ticker, ticker, and ticker as fast as he can.
  - Test speech.

Table 4.2: Cranial nerves, its type, area innervated and its function

Cranial nerve	*Fibers*	*Structures innervated*	*Functions*	*Brainstem nucleus*
I olfactory	Sensory	Olfactory epithelium (via olfactory bulb)	Olfaction	----------------
II optic	Sensory	Retina	Vision	----------------
III oculomotor	Motor	Superior/middle/inferior rectus, inferior oblique, levator palpebrae	Movement of eye ball	Oculomotor nucleus
	Parasympathetic	Pupillary constrictor, ciliary muscle of eyeball. Both via the ciliary ganglion	Pupillary constriction and accommodation	Oculomotor nucleus
IV trochlear	Motor	Superior oblique	Movement of eyeball	Trochlear nucleus
V trigeminal	Sensory	Face, scalp, cornea, nasal and oral cavities, cranial dura mater	General sensation	Trigeminal sensory nucleus
	Motor	Muscles of mastication	Opening/closing mouth	Trigeminal motor nucleus
		Tensor tympani muscle	Tension of tympanic membrane	Trigeminal motor nucleus
VI abducens	Motor	Lateral rectus	Movement of eyeball	Abducens nucleus
VII facial	Sensory	Anterior 2/3 of tongue	Taste	Nucleus solitarius
	Motor	Muscles of facial expression	Facial movement	Facial motor nucleus
		Stapedius muscle	Tension of ossicles	Facial motor nucleus
	Parasympathetic	Salivary and lacrimal glands via submandibular and pterygopalatine ganglia	Salivation and lacrimation	Superior salivatory nucleus

Contd...

Contd...

Cranial nerve	*Fibers*	*Structures innervated*	*Functions*	*Brainstem nucleus*
VIII vestibulocochlear	Sensory	Cochlea	Hearing	Cochlear nucleus
		Vestibular apparatus	Proprioception of head, balance	Vestibular nucleus
IX glossopharyngeal	Sensory	Eustachian tube, middle ear	General sensation	Trigeminal sensory nucleus
		Carotid body, and sinus	Chemo/baroreception	
		Pharynx, posterior 1/3 of tongue	Taste	Nucleus solitarius
	Motor	Stylopharyngeus	Swallowing	
	Parasympathetic	Salivary glands via the otic ganglion	Salivation	Inferior salivatory nucleus
X vagus	Sensory	Pharynx, larynx, esophagus, extemalear	General sensation	Trigeminal sensory nucleus˙
		Aortic bodies and arch	Chemo/baroreception	
		Thoracic and abdominal viscera	Visceral sensation	Nucleus solitarius
	Motor	Soft plate, larynx, pharynx, upper esophagus	Speech, swallowing	Nucleus ambiguus
	Parasympathetic	Cardiovascular, respiratory and gastrointestinal systems	Control of these systems	Dorsal motor nucleus of vagus
XI accessory	Motor	Sternomastoid, trapezius	Movement of head and shoulders	Nucleus ambiguus, cranial nerves
XII hypoglossal	Motor	Intrinsic and extrinsic muscles of tongue	Movement of tongue	Hypoglossal nucleus

5 Motor System Examination

OVERVIEW OF MOTOR FUNCTION

Motor control evolves from a complex set of neural, physical, and behavioral processes that govern posture and movement.

Some movements like reflex pattern have a genetic basis and predominate and immerge through process of normal growth and development.

Motor skills are learned through interaction and exploration of the environment.

Important Definitions

- *Motor program*: An abstract representation when initiated result in production of a coordinated movement sequence.
- *Motor plan*: It is an idea or plan for purposeful movement that is made up of several component motor programs.
- *Feedback*: It is a response produced information received during or after the movement and is used to monitor output for corrective action.
- *Feed forward*: Sending of signals in advance of movement to ready the sensory motor systems, allows for anticipatory adjustment in postural activity.
- *Coordination*: Ability to execute smooth, accurate, and controlled motor responses.

Examination of motor function:
- Patient history
- Review of relevant system
- Specific tests and measures
  - *Joint integrity and mobility*: Long standing immobilization results in contracture, fix resistance.
  - *Arthrokinematics*: It assess movement of joint surfaces.

- Osteokinematics by goniometry (Both active range of motion (AROM) and passive range of motion (PROM) are measured)
- Causes of limitation
- End feel
- Ligaments, muscle contractures, muscle shortening, muscle tension

Therapist should determine:
- Presence of pain with motion
- Pattern and quality of movement
- Movement of associated joints
- Postural stabilization
- Cause of limitation

TONE

Tone is defined as resistance of muscle to passive elongation or stretch when an individual attempts to maintain muscle relaxation.

Tone may be due to:
- Physical inertia
- Intrinsic mechanical elastic stiffness of muscles and connective tissues
- Reflex muscle contraction

Postural tone: It describes a pattern of muscular tension that exists throughout the body and affects group of muscles.

Dynamic evaluation of tone: Muscle imbalance across a joint while performing a functional task.

Dynamic tone is assess by:
- *Observation of movement pattern*
  - Equinus gait
  - Scissor gait
  - Upper extremity flexion/adduction
  - Mass movement postures.
- *Observation tips*:
  - Try observing with and without orthoses or ambulation aids
  - Videotaping can be helpful

Static evaluation of tone: Passive testing of muscle tone at a single joint level.

Static tone can be assessed by:

- Ashworth scale and modified Ashworth scale
- Tardieu scale
- Spasm frequency scale
- EMG/ H reflex

Testing tone: Patient should be in supported comfortable position.

Testing Tone in the Upper Limbs

Pronator test: Ask the patient to hold his arms out in front with his palms facing upward and close his eyes tightly.

Findings

- One arm pronates and drifts downwards indicate weakness on that side.
- Both arm drifts indicates bilateral weakness.
- Arm rises suggest cerebellar disease.
- Finger continuously move up and down.
- Pseudoathetosis indicates deficits of joint position sense.

Testing Tone in Lower Limbs

Tone at hip: Patient is lying with straight legs. Roll the knee from side to side.

Tone at knee: Put your hand behind the knee and lift it rapidly. Watch the heel. Hold knee and ankle. Flex and extend knee.

Tone at ankle: Hold ankle and plantarflex and dorsiflex the foot.

Findings

- *Normal*: Slight resistance through whole range of movements.
- *Decrease tone (Hypotonia)*:
  - Loss of resistance through the movement. Heel does not lift off the bed when knee is lifted quickly. Marked loss of tone flaccidity.
  - The muscles are lax; they assume a pendulous shape when allowed to hang freely, offer diminish resistance to passive movement and so widen the range of movement at a joint.
- *Increased tone*:
  - *Resistance increase suddenly, the heel leaves the bed when knee is lifted quickly*: Spasticity.

Table 5.1: Clinical rating scale for tone		
Grade	*Response*	*Cause*
0	No response (flaccidity)	Complete loss of neuromuscular integrity (LMN lesion)
1	Decrease response (Hypotonia)	Decrease neuromuscular integrity
2	Normal response	Normal neuromuscular function
3	Exaggerated response (Mild to moderate hypertonia)	UMN or extra-pyramidal lesion
4	Sustained response (severe hypertonia)	UMN or extra-pyramidal lesion

- *Increase through whole range, as if bending lead pipe*: Lead pipe rigidity.
- *Regular intermittent break in tone through whole range*: Cogwheel rigidity.

Note: Patient should be relaxed while checking tone. It can be done by asking the patient to count down from 100.

Tonal abnormalities are categorized as **(Table 5.1)**:
- Hypertonia (increased above normal resting levels)
- Hypotonia (decreased below normal resting levels)
- Dystonia (impaired or disordered tonicity).

TONAL ABNORMALITIES

Hypertonia

- *Spasticity*
  - Spasticity is a hypertonic motor disorder characterized by velocity-dependent resistance to passive stretch.
  - It arises from injury to corticospinal pathways and occurs as a part of upper motor neuron (UMN) syndrome.
  - Loss of inhibitory control on lower motor neuron (LMN) results in disordered spinal segmental reflexes, including increased alpha motoneuron excitability, increased flexor reflex, altered synaptic activity, decreased presynaptic inhibition.
  - *The signs and symptoms of UMN syndrome include:*
    - Hyperactive stretch reflexes
    - Involuntary flexor and extensor spasms

- Clonus
- Babinski's sign
- Exaggerated cutaneous reflexes
- Loss of precise autonomic control

Dyssynergic movement patterns also occur, including co-activation of agonist and antagonist muscle groups, abnormal timing, paresis, loss of dexterity, and fatigability.

Effects of chronic spasticity:

- Contracture
- Abnormal posturing
- Deformity
- Functional limitation and disability

Resistance increases with increasing velocity of larger and quicker stretch; stronger resistance of spastic muscles.

Clasp knife response is seen.

Clonus

- Sudden stretching of hypertonic muscle produces reflex contraction. If the stretch is maintained during subsequent relaxation, further reflex contraction will occur and this continues indefinitely, unless the stretch stimulus is released.
- Clonus is characterized by cyclic, spasmodic alteration of muscle contraction and relaxation. It is common in plantar flexors, jaw or wrist.

Demonstration of clonus:

- *At the ankle*: It is most easily demonstrated by dorsiflexing the ankle; maintain foot in position and a rhythmic contraction may be found. More than 3 beats is abnormal **(Fig. 5.1)**.
- *At the knee*: With the knee straight take the patella and bring it briskly downwards, rhythmic contraction noted it is always abnormal **(Fig. 5.2)**.
- *At the wrist*: Relax arm, hand and wrist. Wrist prone. Snap wrist back into extension. Look for—Shaking of upper extremity.
  - It may present at any joint. It represents an increase in reflex excitability and may be present in very tense patient.
  - The Babinski's sign is dorsiflexion of the great toe with fanning of the other toes on stimulation of lateral side of foot.

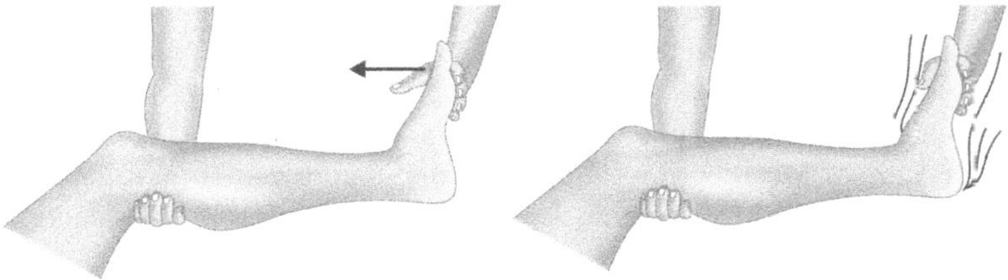

Fig. 5.1 Checking of ankle clonus

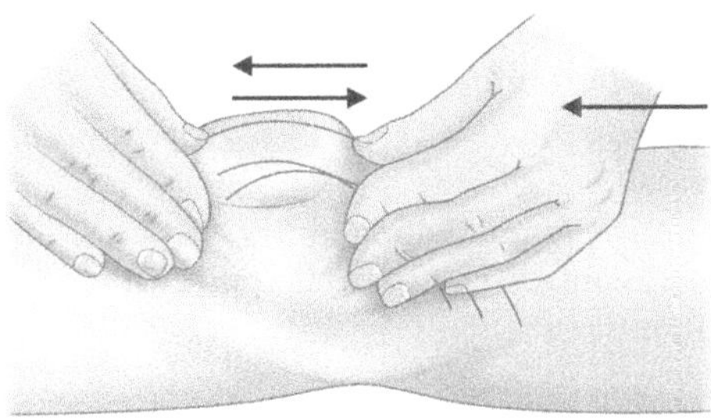

Fig. 5.2 Checking of patellar clonus

Table 5.2: Modified Ashworth scale for spasticity

Grade	*Description*
0	No increase in muscle tone
1	Slight increase in muscle tone, manifested by a catch and release or by minimal resistance at the end of the ROM when the affected part(s) is moved in flexion or extension.
1+	Slight increase in muscle tone, manifested by a catch, followed by minimal resistance throughout the remainder (less than half) of the ROM.
2	More marked increase in muscle tone through most of the ROM, but affected part(s) easily moved.
3	Considerable increase in muscle tone, passive movement difficult.
4	Affected part(s) rigid in flexion or extension.

- Spasticity grading is done by modified Ashworth scale (MAS) **(Table 5.2)**.

Tardieu scale for spasticity:

- This test is performed with patient in supine position, with head in midline.
- Measurement takes place at three velocities (V1, V2, and V3)
- Responses are recorded at each velocity as X/Y with X indicating 0 to 5 rating and Y indicating degree of angle at which muscle reaction occurs
- By moving limb at different velocities response to stretch can be more easily judged since stretch reflex responds differently to velocity.

Velocities

- V1: As slow as possible, slower than natural drop of limb segment under gravity.
- V2: Speed of limb segment falling under gravity.
- V3: As fast as possible, faster than the rate of the natural drop of the limb segment under gravity.

Scoring

- No resistance throughout the course of the passive movement.
- Slight resistance throughout the course of the passive movement, no clear catch at precise angle.
- Clear catch at precise angle interrupting the passive movement followed by release.
- Fatigable clonus with <10 seconds when maintaining the pressure and appearing at the precise angle.
- Unfatigable clonus with >10 seconds when maintaining the pressure and appearing at the precise angle.
- Joint is immovable.

Hypotonia

Hypotonia and flaccidity are the term used to define decreased or absent muscular tone. Resistance to passive movement is diminished, stretch reflexes are dampened or absent, and limbs are easily moved (floppy). Hyper extensibility of joints is common.

Common Causes

- Lesion of the motor side of the reflex arc. Anterior horn cell disease, neuropathies, peripheral nerve injuries.
- Lesion of the sensory side of the reflex arc. Neuropathies, tabes dorsalis, herpes zoster.
- Combined motor and sensory lesions.
- Syringomyelia, cord or root compression, gross cord destruction.
- Lesion of muscle itself.
- Myopathies, spinal muscle atrophy, myasthenia gravis.
- States of neurological shock.

Earliest stages of a severe cord lesion or a profound hemiplegic. This is temporary unless destruction is extreme.

Lower motor neuron (LMN) results from lesions that affect the anterior horn cell and peripheral nerve. It produces symptoms of decreased or absent tone, decreased or absent reflexes, paresis, muscle fasciculation and fibrillations with denervation, and neurogenic atrophy.

Mild decrease in tone along with asthenia can also be seen in cerebella lesions. Temporary states of flaccidity or hypotonia, termed spinal shock or cerebral shock depending on the location of the lesion, can be seen with UMN lesions.

Chorea in Sydenham's chorea, the involuntary movements are associated with marked hyper extensibility of joints, especially wrist and fingers, but reflexes are often retained.

Dystonia

It is a hyperkinetic movement disorder characterized by disordered tone and involuntary movements involving large portions of the body. The movements are similar to athetoid.

Movements with typical twisting or writhing motions.

Dystonic posturing refers to sustained abnormal postures caused by co-contraction of muscles that may last for several minutes, hours, or permanently.

Dystonia results from a CNS lesion (commonly in the basal ganglia) and can be inherited (primary idiopathic dystonia), associated with neurodegenerative disorders (Wilson's disease, Parkinson's disease on excessive L-dopa therapy), or metabolic disorders.

Dystonia can affect only one part of the body (focal dystonia) or two or more adjacent areas (segmental dystonia).

Rigidity

- Rigidity is a hypertonic state characterized by increased uniform resistance that persists throughout the whole ROM and is independent of the velocity of movement (lead pipe rigidity).
- It is associated with lesions of the basal ganglia system (extra pyramidal syndromes) and is seen in Parkinson's disease.
- It involves both agonist and antagonist. Rigidity is the result of excessive supraspinal drive (UMN facilitation) acting on alpha motor neurons; spinal reflex mechanisms are normal. Patients demonstrate stiffness, inflexibility, and significant functional limitation.
- Cogwheel rigidity refers to a hypertonic state with superimposed rachetlike jerkiness and is commonly seen in upper extremity movements and in patients with Parkinson's disease.
- Tremor, bradykinesia, and loss of postural stability are also associated motor deficits in patients with Parkinson's disease.

Decorticate Rigidity

- Abnormal flexor response **(Fig. 5.3A)**
- Refers to sustained contraction and posturing of trunk and lower limb in extension and upper limbs in flexion
- Indicates corticospinal tract lesion at the level of diencephalon.

Decerebrate Rigidity

- Abnormal extensor response **(Fig. 5.3B)**

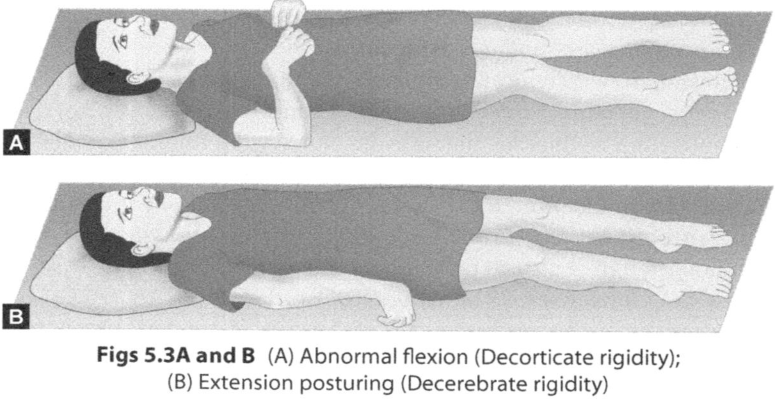

Figs 5.3A and B (A) Abnormal flexion (Decorticate rigidity); (B) Extension posturing (Decerebrate rigidity)

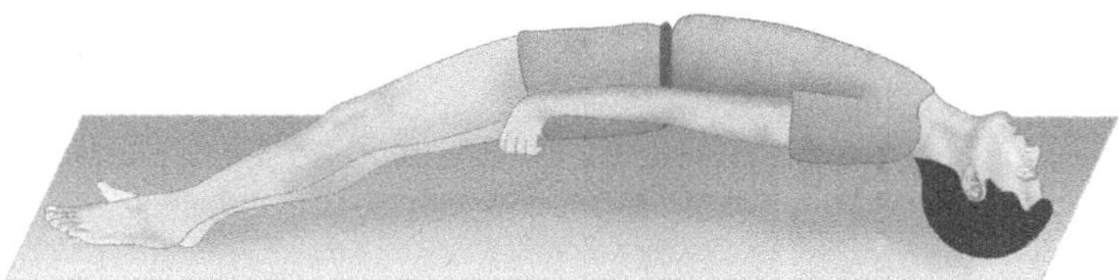

Fig. 5.4 Opisthotonus posture

- Refers to sustained contraction and positioning of trunk and lower limb in position of full extension
- Indicates a corticospinal brainstem lesion between the superior colliculus and vestibular nucleus.

Opisthotonus

It is strong and sustained contraction of the extensor muscles of neck and trunk. The patient assumes a rigid hyper extended posture **(Fig. 5.4)**.

Synergy

Synergy patterns are abnormal, stereotyped, primitive, mass movement pattern associated with spasticity and which can be triggered either reflexively and voluntarily. Synergy can be either flexor or extensor. They involve the action of certain muscles in combination that gives rise to abnormal pattern not useful for functional activities.

ABNORMAL SYNERGY IN UPPER AND LOWER LIMBS (TABLE 5.3)

- *Flexion synergy for upper limbs*: Shoulder girdle retraction and elevation, shoulder abduction external rotation, supination, flexion of elbow, wrist and finger flexion **(Fig. 5.5A)**.
- *Flexion synergy for lower limbs*: Hip flexion abduction and lateral rotation, knee flexion, dorsiflexion and inversion **(Fig. 5.6A)**.
- *Extension synergy*: For upper limbs—shoulder girdle protraction and depression, shoulder adduction, internal rotation, elbow extension, pronation, wrist and finger flexion **(Fig. 5.5B)**.
- *Extension synergy*: For lower limbs—hip extension, adduction, internal rotation, knee extension, ankle plantar flexion, inversion, and plantar flexion **(Fig. 5.6B)**.

Table 5.3: Abnormal synergy patterns

	Flexion synergy	*Extenson synergy*
Upper extremity	• Scapular retraction and elevation • Shoulder abduction, external rotation • Elbow flexion • Forearm supination • Wrist/finger flexion	• Scapular protraction • Shoulder adduction • Internal rotation • Elbow extension • Forearm pronation • Wrist/finger flexion
Lower extremity	• Hip flexion, abduction • External rotation • Knee flexion • Ankle dorsiflexion, inversion • Toe dorsiflexion	• Hip extension adduction • Internal rotation • Knee extension • Ankle PF, inversion • Toe plantar flexion

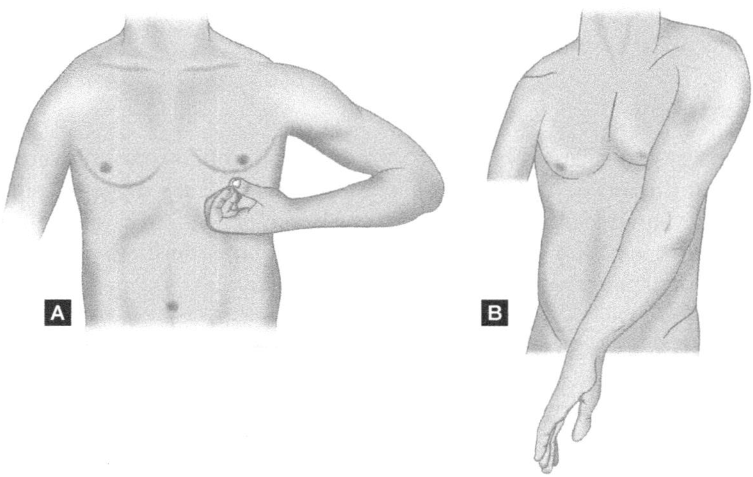

Figs 5.5A and B Upper limb synergy pattern: (A) Flexor synergy; (B) Extensor synergy

Thus is can observed that the following muscle does not take part in either of the synergies:

- Latissimus dorsi
- Teres major
- Serratus anterior

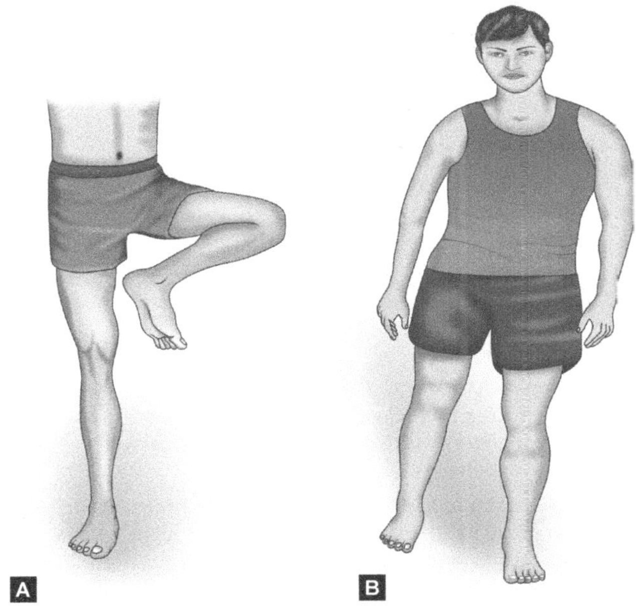

Figs 5.6A and B Lower limb synergy pattern: (A) Flexor synergy; (B) Extensor synergy

- Wrist and finger extensors
- Ankle evertors

Voluntary Control Grading for Assessing Synergy Patterns

- *Grade 0*: No contraction.
- *Grade 1*: Flicker of contraction present or initiation of movement.
- *Grade 2*: Half range of motion in synergy or abnormal pattern.
- *Grade 3*: Full range of motion in synergy or abnormal pattern.
- *Grade 4*: Initial half range is performed in isolation and the latter half in pattern.
- *Grade 5*: Full range of motion in isolation but goes into pattern when resistance is offered.
- *Grade 6*: Full range of motion isolation against resistance.

Motor examination of arm: Pyramidal weakness predominantly affects finger extension, elbow extension and shoulder abduction **(Table 5.4)**.

Table 5.4: Strength testing for upper limb

Movement	*Command*	*Muscle*	*Nerve*	*Root*
Shoulder abduction	Ask patient to lift both his elbows out to the side. Ask him to push up	Deltoid	Axillary	C5
Elbow flexion	Hold patients elbow and wrist. Ask him to pull his hand towards his face	Biceps brachii **(Fig. 5.7)**	Musculo-cutaneous	C5,6
Elbow extension	Hold patients elbow and wrist. Ask him to extend elbow	Triceps **(Fig. 5.7)**	Radial nerve	C6,7,8
Finger extension	Fix patient's hand. Ask him to keep his fingers straight. Press against extended fingers	Extensor digitorum **(Fig. 5.8D)**	Posterior interosseous nerve	C7
Finger flexion	Ask patient to grip your finger and attempt to open patients grip	FDS, FDP **(Fig. 5.8C)**	Median and ulnar nerves	C8
Finger abduction	Ask patient to spread his fingers out. Ensure palm is in line with the fingers	Dorsal interosseous **(Fig. 5.8A)**	Ulnar nerve	T1
Finger adduction	Ask patient to bring his fingers together make sure fingers are straight	Palmar interosseous **(Fig. 5.8B)**	Ulnar nerve	T1
Thumb abduction	Ask patient to place his palm flat with supinated arm. Ask him then to bring his thumb towards his nose	Abductor pollicis brevis	Median nerve	T1
Pushing of arm	Stand behind patient in front of wall. Ask him to push against wall with his arms straight and hands at shoulder level. Look at position of scapula. If the muscle is weak the scapula lifts off the chest wall	Serratus anterior	Long thoracic nerve	C5,6,7

Contd...

Contd...

Movement	*Command*	*Muscle*	*Nerve*	*Root*
Retraction of scapula	Ask patient to put his hands on hips. Hold his elbows and ask him to bring his elbows backwards	Rhomboids	Nerve to rhomboids	C4,5
Raise the arm	Stand behind patient. Ask him to lift his arm from the side against resistance	Supraspinatus	Suprascapular nerve	C5
	Stand behind the patient, hold his elbow against his side with elbows flexed, asking him to keep his elbow in and move his hand out to side	Infraspinatus	Suprascapular nerve	C5,6
	Hold the patient's forearm and wrist with semi-pronated. Ask patient to pull his hand towards his face	Brachioradialis	Radial nerve	C6

Muscles are innervated by more than one nerve root. The exact distribution varied between individuals.

Manual muscle testing: In UMN lesion MMT is performed bilaterally for comparison for muscle strength assessment. If voluntary control testing is more than or equal to Grade-4 (Brunstrom) then only MMT is performed **(Tables 5.5 to 5.9)**.

- *Check for weakness*:
  - Weakness of trunk
  - Weakness of extremities
- *Check for loss of control*:
  - Control of extremities
  - Trunk control
- *Check for muscle activation deficits*:
  - Improper initiation of movement
  - Improper muscle selection for task
  - Inappropriate sequencing.
- *Excessive force production*

Strength testing of shoulder abduction

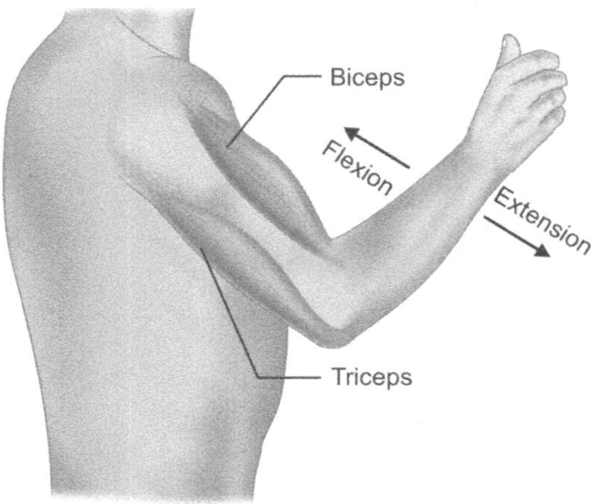

Fig. 5.7 Strength testing of biceps and triceps

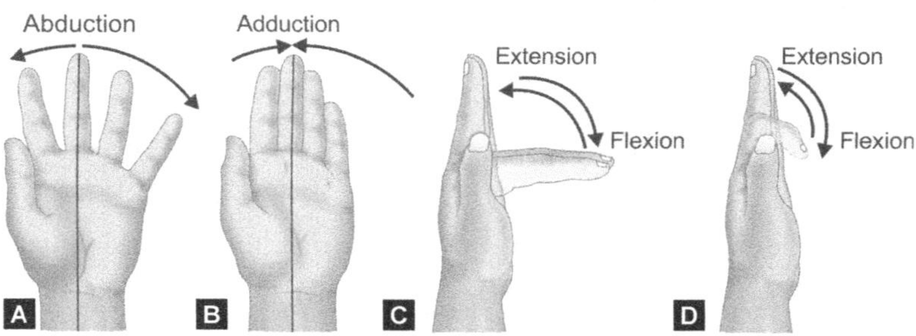

Figs 5.8A to D Strength testing of finger abduction, adduction, flexion, extension

Table 5.5: Stages of motor recovery (Brunstrom)	
I	Flaccid limb
II	Some spasticity with weak flexion and extension synergy
III	Prominent spasticity; voluntary motion occur within synergy pattern
VI	Some selective activation of muscle outside of synergy pattern, spasticity reduced
V	Most limb movement independent from synergy; spasticity further reduced but still present with rapid movement
VI	Near normal coordination with isolated movement
VII	Restoration to normal

Table 5.6: Root innervations (Myotomes)

Root	*Movements*	*Reflex*
C5	Shoulder abduction, elbow flexion	Biceps
C6	Elbow flexion (semipronated)	Supinator
C7	Finger extension, elbow extension	Triceps
C8	Finger flexion	Finger
T1	Small muscles of hand	No reflex

Resisted motion	*Myotome*
Shoulder shrug	C2, C3, C4
Arm abduction (Deltoids)	C5
Elbow flexion	C6
Elbow extension	C7
Wrist extension	C6, C7
Wrist flexion	C7
Thumb extension	C8
Finger abduction and adduction	T1

Table 5.7: Strength testing for lower limb

Movement	*Command*	*Muscle*	*Nerve*	*Root*
Hip flexion	Ask patient to lift his knee towards his chest. When the knee is at 90° ask him to pull it as hard as he can, put your hand against his knee and try to overcome this	Iliopsoas	Lumbar sacral plexus	L1, 2
Hip extension	Patient is lying flat with his legs straight. Put your hand under his heel and ask him to push down to press your hand	Gluteus maximus **(Fig. 5.9A)**	Inferior gluteal nerve	L5, S1
Knee extension	Ask patient to bend his knee. When it is flexed at 90° support the knee with one hand and place other hand at his ankle and ask him to straighten his leg	Quadriceps femoris **(Fig. 5.9C)**	Femoral nerve	L3, 4

Contd...

Contd...

Movement	*Command*	*Muscle*	*Nerve*	*Root*
Knee flexion	Ask patient to bend his knee and bring his heel towards his bottom. When the knee is at 90° try to straighten the leg while holding the knee. Watch the hamstring muscle	Hamstrings	Sciatic nerve	L4, 5
Foot dorsiflexion	Ask patient to cock his ankle back and bring his toes towards his head	Tibialis anterior	Deep peroneal nerve	L4,5
Plantar flexion	Ask patient to point his toes with his leg straight. Try to overcome this	Gastrocnemius **(Fig. 5.9D)**	Posterior tibial nerve	S1
Big toe extension	Ask the patient to pull his big toe up towards his face. Try to push the distal phalanx of his big toe down	Extensor hallucis longus	Deep peroneal nerve	L5
Extension of toes	Ask the patient to bring all his toes towards his head. Press against proximal part of his toes	Extensor digitorum brevis	Deep peroneal nerve	L5, S1
Hip abductors	Fix one ankle, ask patient to push other leg out at the side and resist this movement by holding the other ankle	Gluteus medius and minimus **(Fig. 5.9B)**	Superior gluteal nerve	L4,5
Hip adductors	Ask the patient to keep his ankles together. Fix one ankle and try to pull the other ankle out	Adductors	Obturator nerve	L2,3
Foot inversion	With the ankle 90° ask patient to turn his foot inwards	Tibialis posterior	Tibial nerve	L4,5
Foot eversion	Ask patient to turn his foot out to the side	Peroneus longus and brevis	Superficial peroneal nerve	L5, S1

Table 5.8: Root innervations (Myotomes)	
Resisted motion	*Myotome*
Hip flexion	L1, L2
Knee extension	L3, L4
Ankle dorsiflexion	L4, L5
Extension of big toe	L5
Ankle plantar flexion	S1

Table 5.9: Medical Research Council Scale is used for grading of power	
Grade	*Description*
5	Normal power
4+	Sub-maximal movement against resistance
4	Moderate movement against resistance
4–	Slight movement against resistance
3	Moves against gravity but not resistance
2	Moves with gravity eliminated
1	Flicker
0	No movement

Preferred Testing Order of Muscle Groups

- *Sitting*:
  - Trapezius (shoulder elevators)
  - Deltoid (shoulder abductors)
  - Biceps brachii (elbow flexors)
  - Wrist extensors (Extensor carpi ulnaris/radialis)
  - Wrist flexors (flexor carpi ulnaris/radialis)
  - Iliopsoas (Hip flexors)
  - Quadriceps femoris (knee extensors)
  - Ankle dorsiflexors (tibialis anterior)
- *Supine*:
  - Neck flexors (scalene, sternocleidomastoid)
  - Trapezius
  - Deltoid
  - Gluteus medius

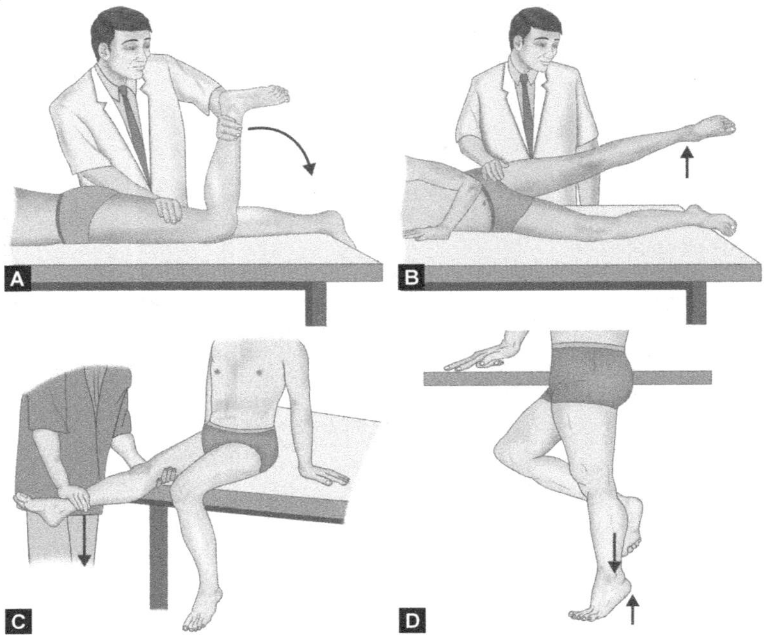

Figs 5.9A to D (A) Strength testing of hip extensors; (B) Strength testing of hip abductors; (C) Strength testing of knee extensors; (D) Strength testing of ankle plantar flexors

- *Side lying*: (Lying on left side right muscles tested)
  - Gluteus medius
  - Iliopsoas
  - Gluteus maximus
  - Hamstrings
  - Biceps brachii
  - Neck flexors
  - Neck extensors
- *Prone lying*:
  - Neck extensors (semispinalis, iliocostalis, splenius cervicis)
  - Gluteus maximus (hip extensor)
  - Hamstrings (knee flexor)
  - Ankle plantar flexors (gastronomies)
- *Side lying*: (Lying on right side left muscles tested)
  - Gluteus medius
  - Iliopsoas

- Gluteus maximus
- Hamstrings
- Biceps brachii
- *Standing*:
  - Ankle plantar flexors
- *Grading power*:

GRADING METHODS FOR MANUAL MUSCLE TESTING (TABLES 5.11 AND 5.12)

- *Oxford method*:
  - 0 = No contraction of muscle
  - 1 = Flicker (Slight) contraction with no movement
  - 2 = Movement in full range in gravity minimal (eliminated) position
  - 3 = Movement in full range against gravity
  - 4 = Movement in full range against gravity with moderate resistance
  - 5 = Movement in full range against gravity with maximal resistance (Normal movement)
- *Lovett method*:
  - Normal = Normal
  - Good = Muscle is able to overcome gravity with slight resistance
  - Fair = Muscle is able to overcome gravity
  - Poor = Muscle is able to overcome friction in gravity minimal (eliminated) position
  - Trace = Muscle only contracts but do not produce movement
  - Zero = Muscle is unable to show any contraction.
- *Brunnstrom*: Dennen method
  - *Normal*: Normal movement taking age, sex and general muscular development of individual into consideration.
  - *Normal*: Normal ROM with almost normal strength.
  - *Good*: Movement against gravity with slight resistance. At least 10 movements completed without fatigue.
  - *Good*$^{+}$: Same as good but the resistance is more.
  - *Good*$^{-}$: Movement against gravity with slight resistance. At least 5 movements performed without fatigue.
  - *Fair*: 50% of normal ROM performed against gravity and after few repetitions, patient becomes fatigue.

- *Fair*$^{+}$: More than 50% ROM against gravity and patient performs it at least 10 times without the sign of fatigue.
- *Poor*: At least 50% of ROM with gravity eliminated. Patient does it at least 5 times.
- *Poor*$^{+}$: 50% of ROM or more done with gravity eliminated with slight resistance and at least 5 times.
- *Poor*: Few degree of ROM done with gravity eliminated.
- *Trace*: Flickering of muscle fibers can be palpated when movement is attempted.
- *Zero*: No contraction in any of the muscle which performs movement.

- *Grading of small muscles*:
  - The conventional grading cannot be employed for measuring strength of small muscles such as muscles of face. In this case following grades are used.
  - *Functional*: Normal or only slight impairment
  - *Weak functional*: Moderate impairment that affects the degree of active motion
  - *Non-functional*: Severe impairment
  - *Zero*: Absent.

Inference from Manual Muscle Testing

Weakness/Paresis (Table 5.10)

- Usually seen in contralateral side of lesion
- MCA stroke are more common so weakness is largely seen in UL in clinical practice
- Distal muscles are more affected than proximal muscles
- Mild weakness of ipsilateral side.

Muscle Activation Deficits

- *Improper initiation of movement*: It occurs when the client attempt to move arm or leg in space and substitute the stronger proximal muscle than weaker distal muscles.

  Example 1: If we ask a client to lift hemiplegic arm and reach forward for an object, he or she often initiates the movement proximally instead of distally with the hand and forearm using the stronger elevator or abductor instead of weaker hand and forearm muscle.

  This is also seen during walking.

Example 2: The client initiates the swing phase of gait proximally instead of distally using stronger pelvic elevators or rotators instead of weaker ankle and foot muscles.

- *Inappropriate muscle selection*: When the client substitute strong muscle group for a paralyzed muscle although it is inappropriate for the function.
  Example 1: When the hamstrings are weak the client may use the quadriceps to lift the leg up a step. This result in strong over shifting in the trunk and makes balance precarious.
- *Inappropriate sequencing*: Includes improper initiation and excessive co-contraction. Excessive co-contraction occurs when the client activates too many muscles either at the same time or out of the sequence for the task.
- *Excessive force production*: Occurs when patient activates muscle with inappropriate effort during voluntary movement.
  When force is excessive movement pattern is slow and the extremity feels stiff. Frequently these muscles fatigue and extremity slowly fall back to the starting position.

Table 5.10: Distribution of weakness according to location of lesions

Location of lesion	*Distribution of weakness*
Middle cerebral artery	Contralateral arm and face > leg
Anterior cerebral artery	Contralateral leg > arm and face
Internal capsule	Contralateral face = arm = leg
Brainstem	Ipsilateral cranial nerve and contralateral body
Cervical cord (transverse)	Both arms and both legs
Thoracic cord (transverse)	Both legs
Cauda equine	Both legs, asymmetric, multiple root pattern
Anterior horn cell	Focal early, generalize late
Single nerve root	Muscle of affected myotome
Plexus	Plexus pattern, complete or partial
Mononeuropathy	Muscles of affected nerve
Polyneuropathy	Distal > proximal
Neuromuscular junction	Bulbar, proximal extremities
Muscle	Proximal > distal

Table 5.11: Manual muscle testing chart

Muscle group	*Muscle power grade*	
Shoulder	*Right*	*Left*
Flexors		
Extensors		
Abductors		
Adductors		
External rotators		
Internal rotators		
Elbow		
Flexors		
Extensors		
Radio ulnar		
Supinators		
Pronators		
Wrist		
Flexors		
Extensors		
Radial deviators		
Ulnar deviators		
CMC		
1st CMC flexors		
Abductors		
MP-flexors		
1st		
2nd		
3rd		
4th		
5th		
MP-abduction		
2nd		
3rd right		
3rd left		
4th		
5th		
PIP extension to flexion		
1st		
2nd		

Contd...

Contd...

Muscle group	*Muscle power grade*	
3rd		
4th		
5th		
DIP extension to flexion		
2nd		
3rd		
4th		
5th		
Cervical spine		
Neck flexors		
Neck extensors		
Thoracolumbar spine		
Trunk extensors		
Trunk flexors		
Side flexors		
Rotators		
Hip joint		
Flexors		
Extensors		
Abductors		
Adductors		
External rotators		
Internal rotators		
Knee joint		
Flexors		
Extensors		
Ankle joint		
Plantar flexors		
Dorsi flexors		
Invertors		
Evertors		
Great toe		
Extensor hallucis longus		
Flexor hallucis longus		
2nd to 5th toes		
Extensor digitorum longus and brevis		
Flexor digitorum longus and brevis		
Lumbricals		

These movements are label spastic pattern and intervene with inhibition techniques.

Range of Motion (Tables 5.12 to 5.14)

- *Active movement in upper limbs*:
  - General quality of movement is observed
  - Is movement smooth, ataxic, weak, patterned?
  - Movement analysis includes a combined functional assessment
  - Other bimanual task and specific assessment of active movement components
  - Assessment of functional movement is based on subjective finding regarding arm and hand use
  - Assess active or attempted movement in supine or sitting as appropriate
  - Describe movements and problems
  - How much assistance required
  - Were these movement performed in isolation
  - Was there any influence of abnormal pattern?
  - Record presence of movements and limiting factors on chart.

Supine	*Sitting*
Shoulder protraction	Hand to mouth raise arm forward to
Shoulder horizontal abduction	90° hand to sacrum, hand to top of head, raise arm overhead
Shoulder horizontal adduction	Radial deviation with wrist extension
Shoulder flexion	Wrist extension while holding an object
Shoulder extension	Grasp thumb abduction with wrist in radial deviation and extension
Elbow flexion	Opposition thumb to finger
Elbow extension	

- *Active movements in lower limbs*:
  - Movements are tested in appropriate position
  - Describe about assistance required
  - Where the movement perform in isolation
  - Was the influence of an abnormal pattern?
  - Did loss of muscle length or joint range affect active movement?
  - Did sensory loss affect movement?
  - Record other factor influencing movement
  - After active ROM check for passive ROM

Table 5.12: Range of movements—upper limb

Joint movements	*Active ROM*		*Passive ROM*	
Shoulder	*Right*	*Left*	*Right*	*Left*
Flexion (180)				
Extension (60)				
Abduction (180)				
Adduction (70)				
External rotation (90)				
Internal rotation (80)				
Elbow				
Flexion (150)				
Extension (0)				
Radio ulnar				
Supination (80)				
Pronation (80)				
Wrist				
Flexion (80)				
Extension (70)				
Radial reviation (20)				
Ulnar deviation (30)				
1st digit				
CMC				
CMC flexion (15)				
CMC extension (20)				
Abduction (70)				
MCP				
Flexion (50)				
Extension (0)				
IP joint				
Flexion (80)				
Extension (20)				
2nd-5th Digit				
MCP				
Flexion (90)				
Extension (45)				
Abduction				
PIP				
Flexion (100)				
Extension (0)				
DIP				
Flexion (90)				
Extension (0)				

Table 5.13: Range of motion TM joint and spine		
Joint movements	*Active ROM*	*Passive ROM*
TM joint		
Depression (43)		
Anterior protrusion (7)		
Lateral deviation (9)		
Cervical spine		
Flexion (45)		
Extension (45)		
Lateral flexion (45)		
Rotation (60)		
Thoracolumbar spine		
Flexion (80)		
Extension (25)		
Lateral flexion (35)		
Rotation (45)		
Lumbar spine		
Flexion		
Extension		

- *Sitting*:
  - Hip and knee flexion
  - Knee extension
  - Ankle dorsi flexion
  - Ankle eversion
- *Supine*:
  - Hip and knee flexion
  - Hip and knee extension
  - Hip abduction
  - Hip flexion with knee extension
  - Dorsiflexion with knee in extension
  - Ankle inversion
  - Toe flexion/extension
- *Prone/side lying*:
  - Knee flexion

Table 5.14: Range of motion—lower limb

Joint movements	*Active ROM*		*Passive ROM*	
	Right	*Left*	*Right*	*Left*
HIP				
Flexion (120)				
Extension (20)				
Abduction (45)				
Adduction (30)				
External rotation (45)				
Internal rotation (45)				
Knee				
Flexion (135)				
Extension (10)				
Ankle				
Plantar flexion (50)				
Dorsiflexion (20)				
Inversion (35)				
Eversion (15)				
Great toe				
MTP flexion (45)				
MTP extension (70)				
MTP abduction				
IP flexion				
Toes				
MTP flexion				
MTP extension				
MTP abduction				
PIP flexion				
DIP flexion				
DIP extension				

Muscle Length Assessment Technique

- Muscle length testing involves elongating the muscle in the direction opposite of its action while assessing its resistance to passive lengthening.
- Precise testing requires that one of the bony attachments of the muscle (usually the origin) be in a fixed position while the other bony attachment is moved passively in the direction of lengthening the muscle.

- In other words, muscle length testing assesses the resistance to passive movement. This is in contrast to typical flexibility or ROM testing.
- The actual ROM can be measured for documentation purposes, but it gives limited clinical information in muscle imbalance syndromes.
- The most valuable clinical information is the muscular end feel and the location of the ROM end feel. The elongation of the muscle should be performed slowly to avoid eliciting a quick stretch of the muscle spindle and subsequently inducing a twitch response and muscle contraction.
- In addition, for the best accuracy and precision, muscle length testing should be performed when the patient is not in acute pain in order to avoid pain inhibition and muscle guarding. In summary, there are four steps to assessing muscle length:
    1. Ensure maximal lengthening of the muscle from origin to insertion.
    2. Firmly stabilize one end (usually the origin).
    3. Slowly elongate the muscle.
    4. Assess the end feel.
- Clinicians do not have to perform muscle length testing on every muscle listed; instead, they should assess the muscles that the postural and movement pattern analysis indicate as being possibly tight. Once tight muscles have been identified, the clinician can establish a muscle imbalance pattern (if present) and begin to look for causes of the tightness.

Lower-Quarter Muscles

The muscles of the lower-quarter include those of the leg, pelvis, and lower back. The muscles prone to tightness are those involved in maintaining a single-leg stance. Tightness of the hip flexors and tightness of the thoracolumbar extensors are hallmark signs of Janda's LCS.

Modified Thomas Test for Hip Flexor

The modified Thomas test allows the clinician to assess four different muscles prone to tightness namely, the one-joint hip flexor, iliacus and psoas major, and the two-joint hip flexors, rectus femoris and TFL-ITB. Tightness of the hip flexors limits hip hyperextension in gait and may cause an anterior pelvic tilt. Weakness of the gluteus maximus often is due to facilitation of the hip flexors.

Patient Position

The patient is asked to sit on the edge of the table, with the coccyx and ischial tuberosities touching the table and one foot on the floor. Then, the patient is asked to flex the opposite hip and knee toward the chest and maintain the position with the hands **(Fig. 5.10)**.

Clinician Position

The clinician stands beside the leg not being tested, facing the patient. While supporting the patient by placing one hand on the midthoracic spine and the other on the knee, the clinician passively rolls the patient down to the table to the supine position. The clinician needs to ensure that the patient's knees are flexed, lumbar spine is flexed, and pelvis is in posterior rotation to fix the origin of the hip flexors.

Test

The clinician passively lowers the tested leg until resistance is felt or movement at the pelvis is detected. With the patient's thigh in the final resting position, the clinician observes whether it is in neutral and

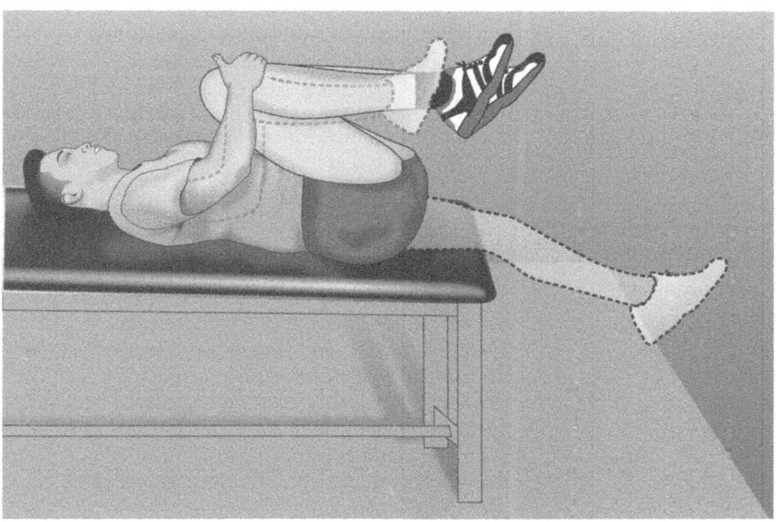

Fig. 5.10 Modified Thomas test for hip flexors

parallel to the table or abducted. A normal length of the one-joint hip flexors with the lumbar spine and sacrum flat on the table is indicated by the posterior thigh touching the table (0° of hip extension). With slight overpressure, the thigh should reach 10° to 15° of hyperextension. Prominence of a superior patellar groove suggests a short rectus femoris, while prominence of a lateral IT groove suggests a short IT band.

Major Postural Muscle Length and Strength Test Instructions (Table 5.15)

Assess the length of the major postural muscles as described below. Grade the strength of the muscles using the traditional five-grade

Table 5.15: Position for muscle length testing

Muscle	Normal ranges or end feel
Iliopsoas	0° hip extension, 10° with overpressure
Rectus femoris	90° knee extension, 125° with overpressure
TFL-IT band	0° hip abduction (neutral), 15–20° with overpressure
Adductors	0° hip abduction (neutral), 20–25° with overpressure in the modified Thomas test position 45° hip abduction in supine position
Hamstrings	80° hip flexion with contralateral leg extended 90° hip flexion with contralateral leg flexed
Triceps surae	0° ankle dorsiflexion
Quadratus lumborum	Thoracolumbar curve should be smooth and gradual
Piriformis	Gradual soft end feel
Upper trapezius	Gradual soft end feel
Levator scapulae	Gradual soft end feel
SCM	Gradual soft end feel
Pectoralis major	• *Sternal portion (lower fibers)*: With shoulder abducted at 150°, arm should be horizontal to table and 15–20° with overpressure • *Sternal portion (midfibers)*: With shoulder abducted to 90°, arm should be horizontal to table and 30° with overpressure • *Clavicular portion*: With shoulder abducted to 60°, arm should hang freely over table
Paraspinals	*Schober's test*: excursion of >2.4 in (6 cm)

classification. Record the results on the *Major postural muscle length and strength test results* form.

Sternocleidomastoid

- Place the patient in the supine position.
- Fix in place the muscle insertion at the sternum on the side to be tested.
- While stabilizing the head in a slightly tucked-in position, passively extend, contralaterally lateral flex, and ipsilaterally rotate the head **(Fig. 5.11)**
  - The muscle is short if the end feel is hard instead of soft.
- Repeat the above sequence on the opposite side and generally compare the muscle extensibility and end feel.

Upper Trapezius

- Place the patient in the supine position
- Passively flex and ipsilaterally rotate the head
- While stabilizing the head, depress the shoulder:
  - The muscle is short if the end feel is hard instead of soft
- Repeat the above sequence on the opposite side and generally compare the muscle extensibility and end feel.

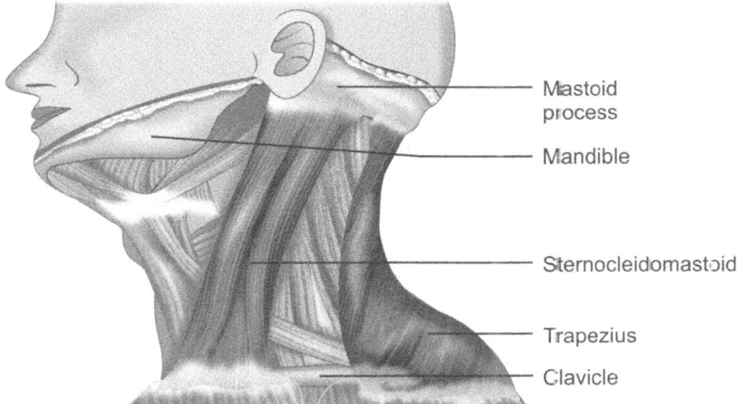

Fig. 5.11 Sternocleidomastoid and upper trapezius length testing (contralateral lateral flexion, ipsilateral rotation)

Levator Scapulae

- Place the patient in the supine position
- Passively flex and contralaterally rotate the head **(Fig. 5.12)**
- While stabilizing the head, depress the shoulder:
  - The muscle is short if the end feel is hard instead of soft.
- Repeat the above sequence on the opposite side and generally compare the muscle extensibility and end feel.

Pectoralis Major

- Place the patient in the supine position.
- Stabilize the trunk to prevent rotation.
- *Passively abduct the arms to 90°* **(Fig. 5.13)**:
  - The sternal portion of the muscles is short if the arms do not reach the table level.
  - The end feel should be soft on gentle overpressure.
- *Passively abduct the arms to 30°*:
  - The clavicular portion of the muscles is short if the arms do not reach at least 20° below the table level.
  - The end feel should be soft on gentle overpressure.
- Repeat the above sequence on the opposite side and generally compare the muscle extensibility and end feel.

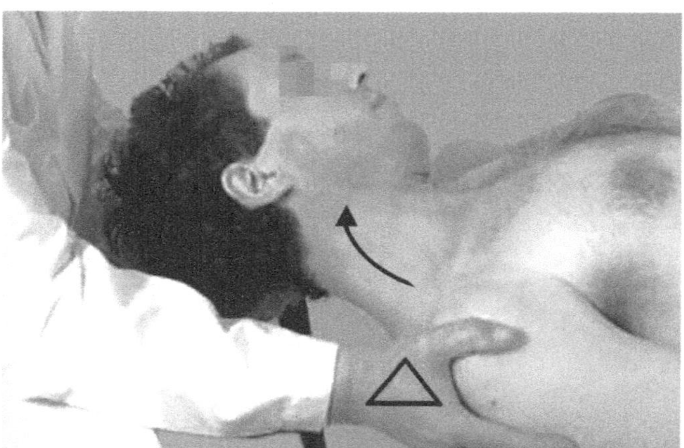

Fig. 5.12 Length testing of levator scapulae (passive flexion or contralateral rotation of head and depression of shoulder)

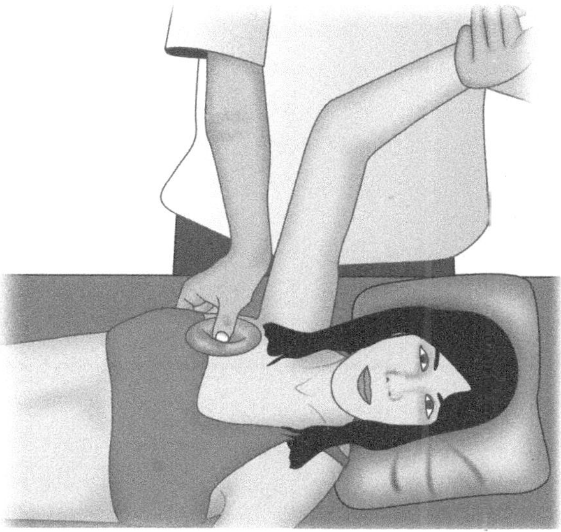

Fig. 5.13 Length testing of pectoralis major

Erector Spinae

- Sit the patient at the end of the table.
- *While stabilizing at the waist, have the patient bend forward*:
  - The erector spine are short if the lumbar curve does not reverse.

Quadratus Lumborum

- Place the patient in the side lying position.
- *Have the patient prop up on their elbow* **(Fig. 5.14A)**:
  - The ipsilateral muscle is short if the inferior angle of the scapula is not at least 2 in from the table.
- Repeat the above sequence on the opposite side and generally compare the muscle extensibility.

  Or
- Have the patient stand.
- *Have the patient perform a side bend* **(Fig. 5.14B)**:
  - The contralateral muscle is short if the lumbar curve is not smooth and convex upwardly.
- Repeat the above sequence on the opposite side and generally compare the muscle extensibility.

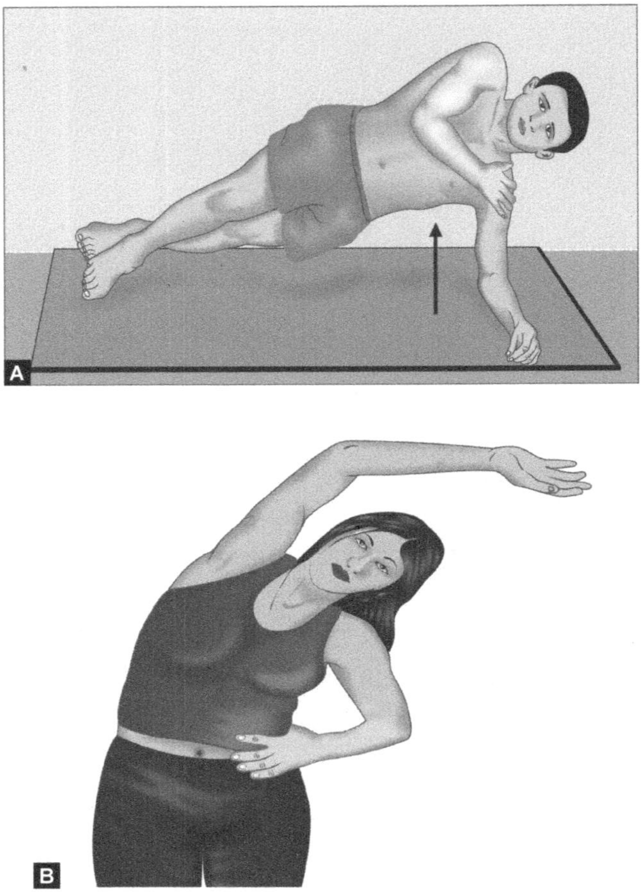

Figs 5.14A and B Length testing of quadratus lumborum: (A) in side lying; (B) in standing

Hip Abductors

- Place the patient in the modified Thomas position.
- *Passively adduct the test hip maximally* **(Fig. 5.15)**:
  - The TFL and ITB are short if adduction is <15–20°.
  - The groove in the ITB will deepen if it is short.
  - The end feel should be soft on gentle overpressure.

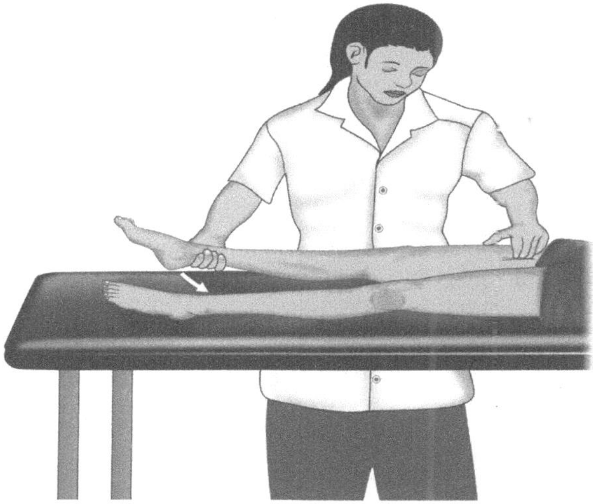

Fig. 5.15 Length testing of hip abductors

- Repeat the above sequence on the opposite side and generally compare the muscle extensibility and end feel.

Hip Adductors

The following tests evaluate and the two-joint long hip adductors the (gracilis, semimembranosus, semitendinosus) and the one-joint short hip adductors (pectineus; adductor magnus, brevis, and longus).

- Place the patient in the supine position (with the knees straight).
- *Passively abduct the test hip maximally* **(Fig. 5.16)**:
  - The long (two-joint) hip adductors are short if abduction is less than 40°.
  - The end feel should be soft on gentle overpressure.
  - Tight hamstrings may cause a false positive.
- *Bend the knee on the test hip side and then passively abduct the hip again*:
  - The short (one-joint) hip adductors are short if abduction does not increase from the first test.
  - The end feel should be soft on gentle overpressure.
- Repeat the above sequence on the opposite side and generally compare the muscle extensibility and end feel.

Hip Flexors

- Place the patient in the modified Thomas position with the test thigh off the side of the table **(Figs 5.16 and 5.17)**:
  - The iliopsoas is short if hip extension is <10–15°.
  - The rectus femoris is short if the knee compensatory extends with <100–105° of flexion.
  - The end feel should be soft on gentle overpressure.
- Repeat the above sequence on the opposite side and generally compare the muscle extensibility and end feel.

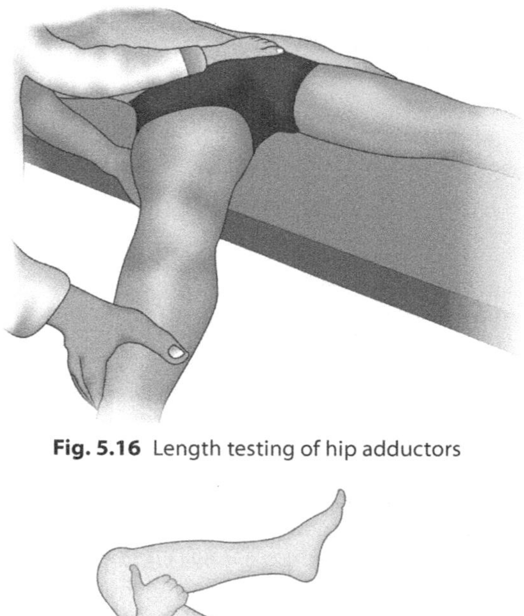

Fig. 5.16 Length testing of hip adductors

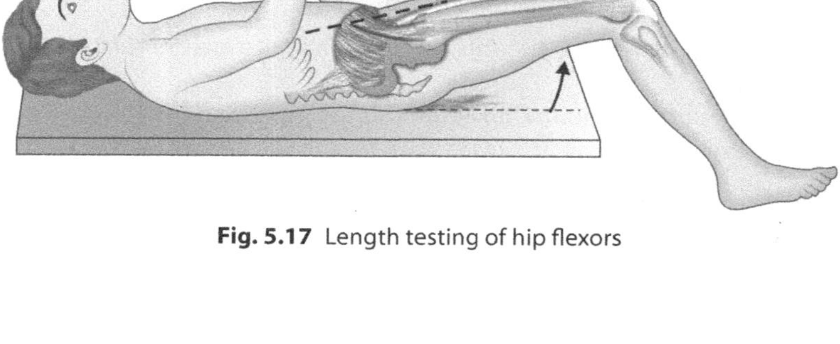

Fig. 5.17 Length testing of hip flexors

Hamstrings

- Place the patient in the supine position with the non-test hip and knee flexed.
- *Passively raise the test leg*:
  - The hamstring is short if the angle of rise is <80°.
- Repeat the above sequence on the opposite side and generally compare the muscle extensibility and end feel **(Fig. 5.18)**.

Hip External Rotators

- Place the patient in the supine position
- Passively flex the hip to <60° while fully adducting it
- Stabilize the pelvis (by pushing the knee upwards toward the hip along the long axis of the femur) and internally rotate the hip **(Fig. 5.19)**:
  - The muscle is short if the end feel is hard.
  - There may also be pain in the buttock.
- Repeat the above sequence on the opposite side and generally compare the muscle extensibility and end feel.

Foot Plantar Flexors

- Place the patient in the supine position with the knee flexed.
- *Passively dorsiflex the foot*:
  - The soleus (a one-joint muscle) is short if the foot does not dorsiflex to 90°.
  - The end feel should be soft on gentle overpressure.

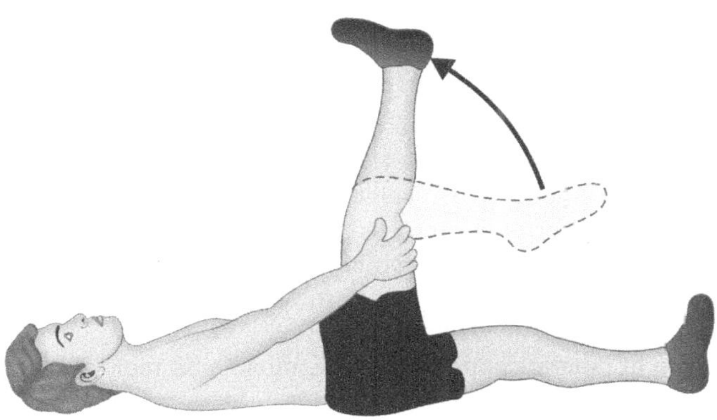

Fig. 5.18 Length testing of hamstrings

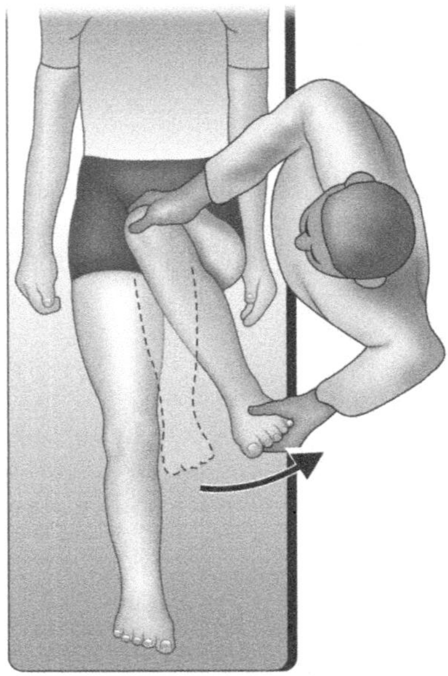

Fig. 5.19 Length testing of hip external rotators

- *Straighten the knee and then passively dorsiflex the foot again*:
  - The gastrocnemius (a two-joint muscle) is short if the foot does not dorsiflex to 90°.
  - The end feel should be soft on gentle overpressure.
- Repeat the above sequence on the opposite side and generally compare the muscle extensibility and end feel.

Measuring Limb Lengths (Figs 5.20A and B)

- Length of limb segments can be measured either directly between two skeletal landmarks or as vertical distance between a constant flat surface (as the floor) and a skeletal landmark.
- This latter is preferred as projected lengths, which through subtraction gives a number of derived segment lengths (e.g. trochanteric height minus total tibial height gives an estimate of the length of the femur or thigh; although not accurate).
- The use of tape measurement is the most valid tool for measuring limb length (long measurement).

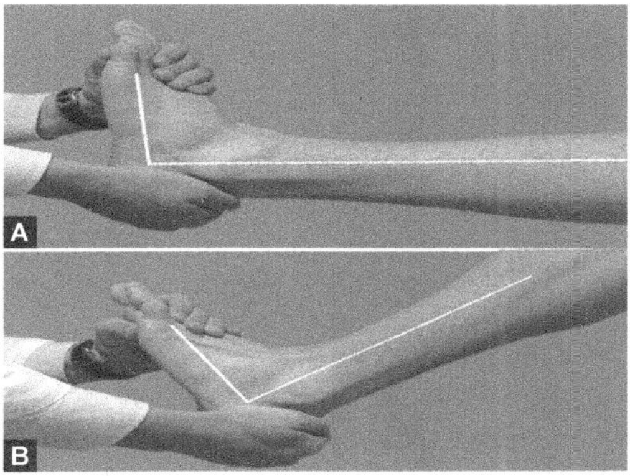

Figs 5.20A and B (A) Length testing of gastrocnemius; (B) Length testing of soleus

- Upper limb length discrepancy affects the cosmetic appearance, while lower limb length discrepancy affects both cosmetic appearance and function.

Inequality of lower limb length will:

- Affect gait pattern (function).
- Create degenerative changes in weight-bearing joints.
- Cause deformities, which may be non-structural at first, then become structural. Unilateral shortening of lower limb leads to pelvic tilt, scoliosis, dropping of shoulder and tilting of head.
- *Tape measurement is also used for round measurement or the contour of the*:
  - Muscle to detect atrophy or hypertrophy
  - Joint to determine swelling
  - Chest to determine its mobility.

Long Measurements

Upper Limb Length

- *Whole upper limb length*:
  - Measurement is taken from most superior lateral point of acromion process (acromial landmark) to the lower and lateral border of styloid process of radius (radial landmark). The arm is

positioned in the anatomical position, relaxed at the side of the subject **(Fig. 5.21)**.

- *Segmental measurement*:
  - *Upper arm length*: With arm flexed at 90º, so that ulnar surface of forearm and hand are horizontal and palms facing medially with fingers extended, measurement is taken from acromial landmark to the posterior surface of olecranon process of ulna **(Fig. 5.22A)**.
  - *Forearm length*: It is the distance from the head of radius (upper radial landmark) to the most distal point of the styloid process of radius (or styloin) **(Fig. 5.22B)**.
  - *Hand length*: With hand extended and the palm rested in the direction of the longitudinal axis of forearm, measurement is taken from styloid process at base of thumb to the tip of middle finger **(Fig. 5.22C)**.

Lower Limb Length

- *Whole lower limb length*:
  - To determine true leg length, first place the patient legs in precisely comparable positions and measure the distance from the anterior superior iliac spines (ASIS) to the medial malleoli of the ankles (from one fixed bony point to another). Begin measurement at

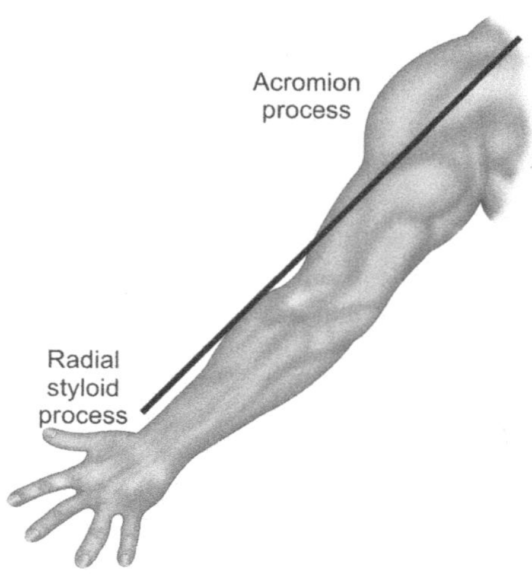

Fig. 5.21 Whole upper limb length measurement

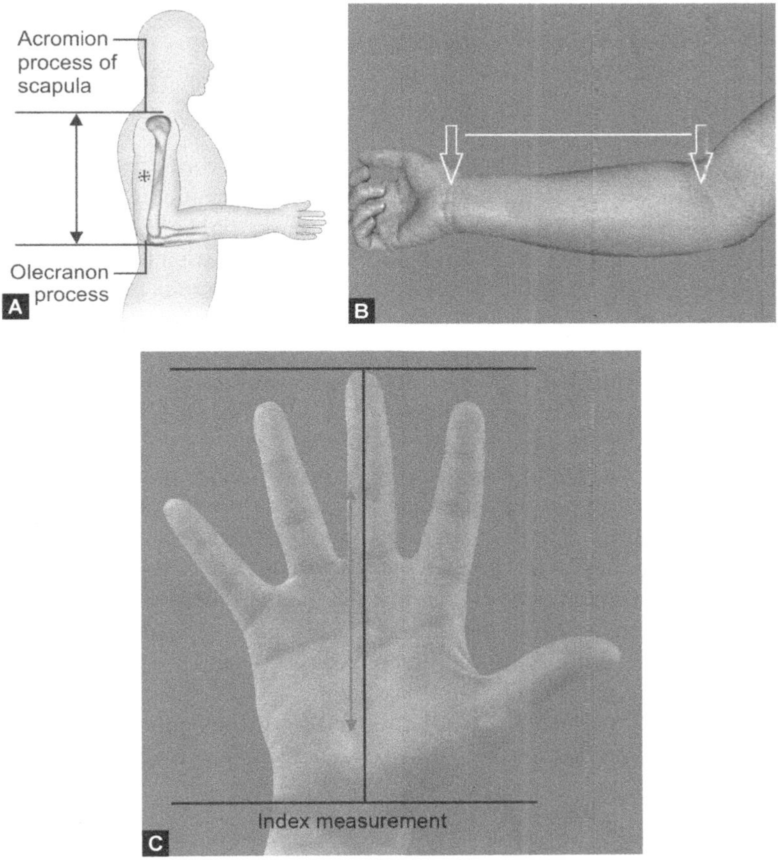

Figs 5.22A to C Segmental measurement: (A) Upper arm length measurement; (B) Forearm length measurement; (C) Hand length measurement

the slight concavity just below the ASIS, as the tape measure may slide if pressed directly onto the spine. If there is tilting of pelvis. Measurement will be taken from the umbilicus to the medial or lateral malleolus. If there is shifted umbilicus, measurement is then taken from xiphoid process to the medial or lateral malleolus. Apparent shortening (due to pelvic tilt) should be differentiated from true shortening (bony).

- *Segmental measurement*:
  - If during inspection, one of the patient's legs appears shorter than the other, the following procedures will assist in determining whether the discrepancy is true or only apparent.
- *True leg length discrepancy*:
  - Unequal distances between these fixed points verify that one lower extremity is shorter than the other. To determine in short order where the discrepancy lies (whether in the tibia or in the femur), ask the patient to lie supine, with his knees flexed to 90° and his feet flat on the table. If one knee appears higher than the other, the tibia of that extremity is longer; while if one knee projects furthers anteriorly than the other, the femur of that extremity is longer. A true shortening may be due to poliomyelitis or a fracture that crossed the epiphyseal plate during childhood **(Fig. 5.23)**.
- *Apparent leg length discrepancy*:
  - Before testing for apparent leg length discrepancy, no true leg length discrepancy should be confirmed (no true bony inequality). Apparent shortening may arise from pelvic obliquity, hip adduction or flexion deformity. During inspection, pelvic obliquity manifests itself as uneven ASIS or PSIS while the patient is standing. While the patient is in supine with his legs in the neutral position, measurement is taken from the umbilicus (or xiphisternal junction) to the medial malleolus (from a non-fixed point to a fixed bony point). Unequal distances signify an apparent leg length discrepancy, if the true leg length measurements are equal.

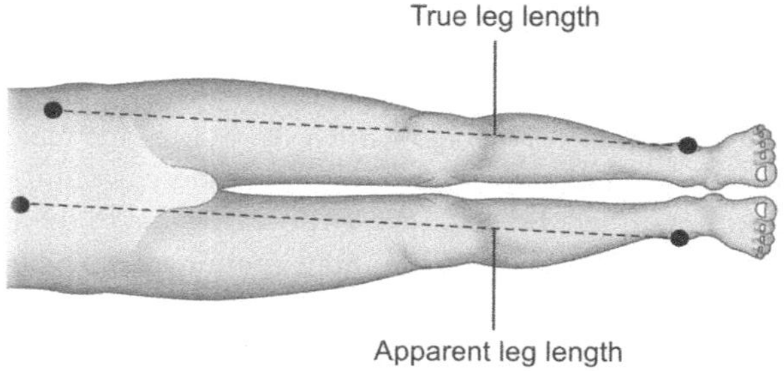

Fig. 5.23 Whole lower limb length measurement: (A) True leg length discrepancy; (B) Apparent leg length discrepancy

  - If there is an unequal limb length, the physical has to determine where the difference is via measuring from the anterior superior iliac spine to the greater trochanter of femur, then:
    - From the greater trochanter of femur to the lateral articulation of the knee joint (shortening of femur).
    - From the lateral articulation of knee joint to the medial malleolus (shortening of tibia).
- *Quick test for measuring lower limb length* **(Figs 5.24A and B)**:
  - From crook lying position, shortening or lengthening of femur can be detected via determining the height of both knee joints. Placing the two anterior superior iliac spines at the same level shows shortening or lengthening of the femur or tibia:
    - *From the lateral view*: A forward projection of knee denotes shortened tibia and lengthened femur.
    - *From the anterior view*: An upward projection of knee denotes shortened femur and lengthened tibia.
- *Other tibial length measurements*:
  - From the prone lying position with the knees flexed to 90°, relative heights are determined from the medial articulation of the knee joint to the most distal border of the medial malleolus (legs must be perpendicular to the plinth).
  - The subject is seated with the tested leg resting on opposite knee, so that the medial aspect of tibia faces upwards. With an anthropometer, measurement is taken from medial articulation of the knee joint to the medial malleolus.

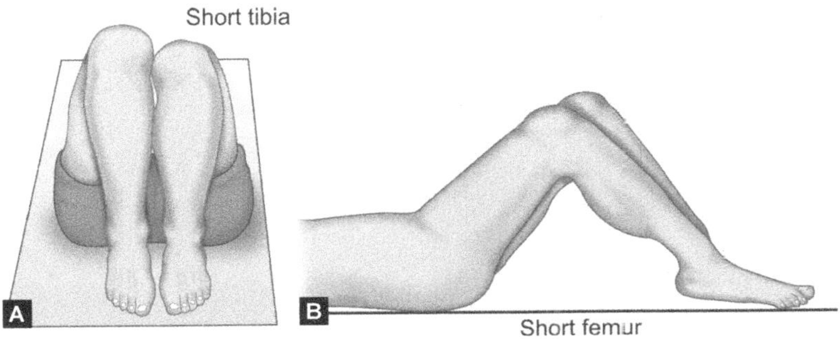

Figs 5.24A and B Quick test for measuring lower limb length: (A) Anterior view; (B) Lateral view

- *Foot length*:
  - It is the distance between the most posterior parts (center) of the heel to the most anterior part of the longest toe (2nd toe).

Round (Girth or Circumference) Measurement

This length is looped around the part to be measured and held so that the printed notches on the scale are next to each other (the stub end is pulled superior to the easing end). As the tension applied to the tape varies, skin surfaces should not be compressed or an observable space between the skin and the tape left. Tapes with spring easing are not recommended. Measurements should be recorded to the nearest 0.1 cm.

Head Girth

It is the maximum circumference of the head when the tape is located immediately superior to the eyebrows and positioned at the back of the head, so that the maximum parameter is measured **(Fig. 5.25A)**.

Neck Girth

The tape is located perpendicular to the long axis of the neck, slightly superior to the larynx **(Fig. 5.25B)**.

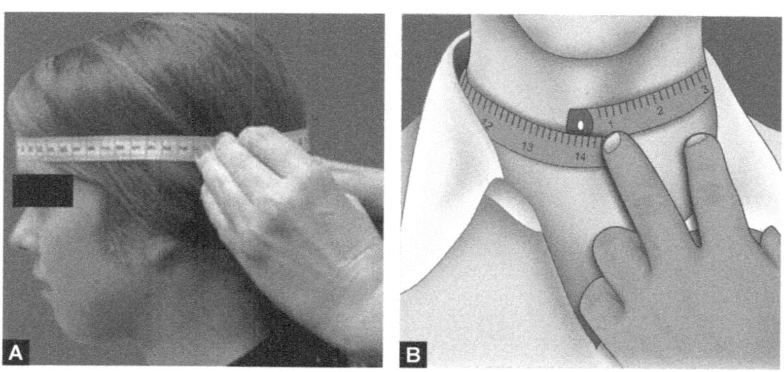

Figs 5.25A and B (A) Head girth measurement; (B) Neck girth measurements

Upper Limb Girth

- *Mid-arm girth*: It is also known as arm circumference, upper arm circumference, biceps circumference or relaxed arm girth. The tape is applied around the mid-upper arm **(Fig. 5.26A)**.
- *Forearm girth*: This measurement is the maximal girth of the forearm. It is taken around the upper third of forearm **(Fig. 5.26B)**.
- *Wrist girth*: It is the perimeter of the wrist taken distal to the styloid process of the radius and ulna **(Fig. 5.26C)**.

Trunk Girth

- *Chest girth*: The chest should be bare and the subject stands in a natural erect posture. Measurements are taken from under the axilla and around the chest, passing by the xiphoid process **(Fig. 5.27)**:
  - Just below the axillary fold.
  - At the level of the nipple.
  - At xiphoid process.

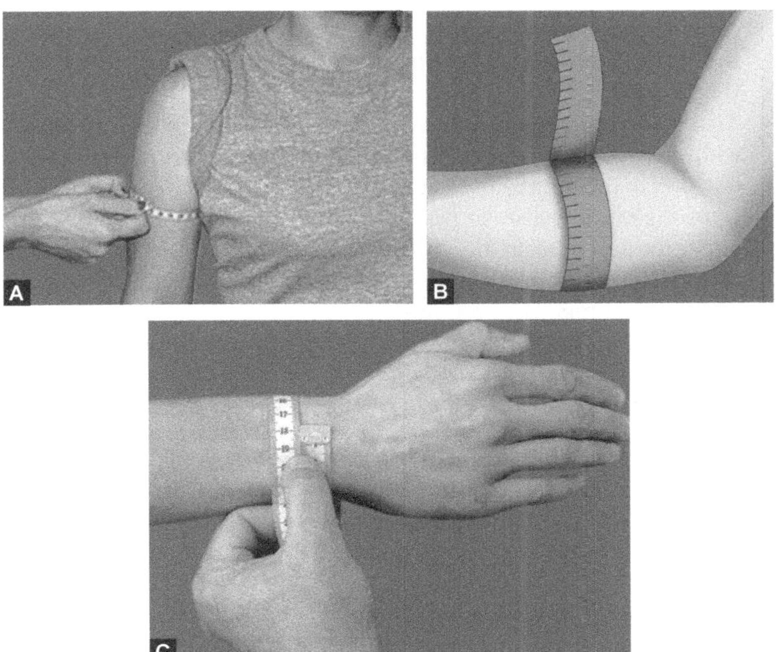

Figs 5.26A to C Upper limb girth measurements: (A) Mid arm girth; (B) Forearm girth; (C) Wrist girth

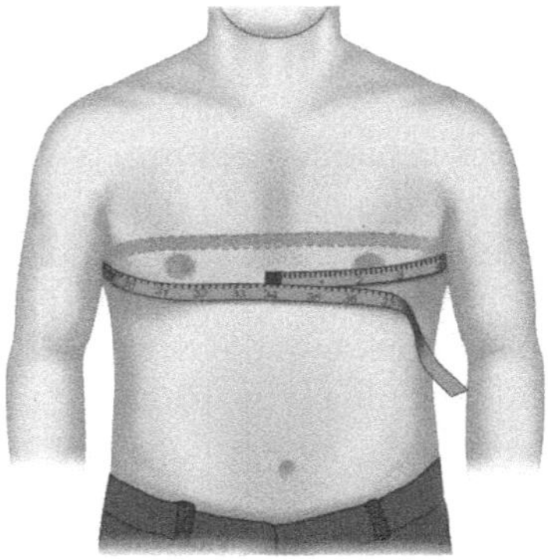

Fig. 5.27 Upper chest girth measurement

- *Waist girth*: It is measured at the narrowest part of the torso. The subject should be standing comfortably erect with hands by the side, neither intentionally contracting abdominal muscles nor breath-holding. The tape is placed around torso, so that it is snug but not compressing the skin and the underlying tissues. The measurements should be taken halfway between the ribs (12th rib) and the iliac crest **(Fig. 5.28A)**.
- *Abdominal circumference*: This measurement is sometimes confused with the waist girth. It is the perimeter distance around the torso at the level of the umbilicus **(Fig. 5.28B)**.
- *Gluteal girth*: It is also known as the buttocks or hip circumference. This is the perimeter at the level of the greatest posterior protuberance of the gluteals. The subject stands erect with minimal clothing, with the feet together and no intentional contraction of the gluteal muscles. The tape is placed compressing any overlying clothing but not the soft tissues **(Fig. 5.29)**.

Lower Limb Girth

- *Thigh girth*: It is the circumference of the thigh, which is measured when the subject stands erect with the legs slightly parted and his weight distributed equally on both feet. The tape is looped around the lower leg **(Fig. 5.30)**.
  - *Proximal or upper thigh girth*: About 1 cm below the gluteal fold, horizontal to the long axis of femur.

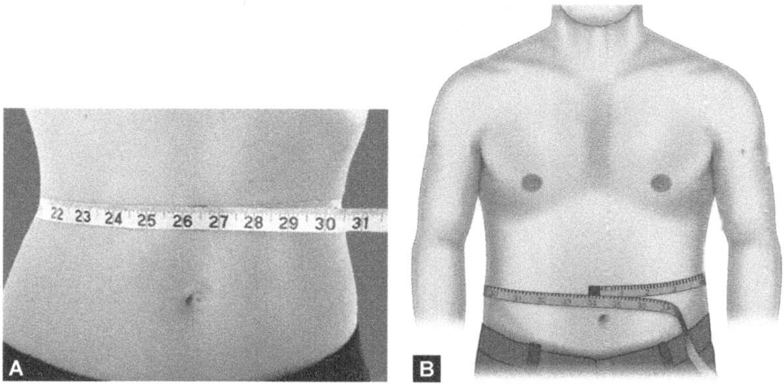

Figs 5.28A and B (A) Waist girth measurement; (B) Abdominal circumference measurement

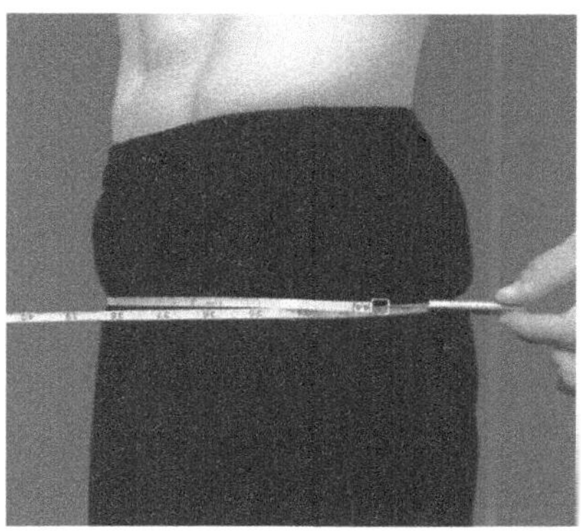

Fig. 5.29 Gluteal girth measurements

- *Mid-thigh*: It is the mid-distance between the inguinal crease and the proximal border of patella.
- *Distal thigh*: From just proximal to femoral epicondyles.

- *Knee girth*: It is taken around the knee at the level of mid-patella (for joint swelling) and 5 cm above the upper border of patella and 5 cm below the level of patella (for muscle wasting) **(Fig. 5.31A)**.
- *Calf girth*: It is the maximum circumference of the calf, when the subject is positioned as for the thigh circumference. Measurements are taken around the bulky area of the calf (two bellies of the gastrocnemius muscles) **(Fig. 5.31B)**.

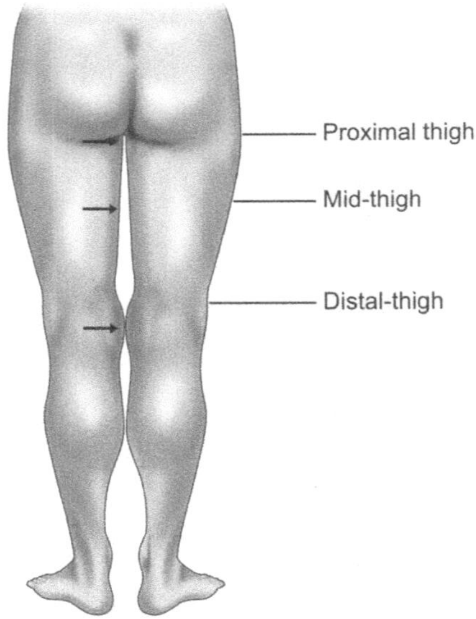

Fig. 5.30 Thigh girth measurements

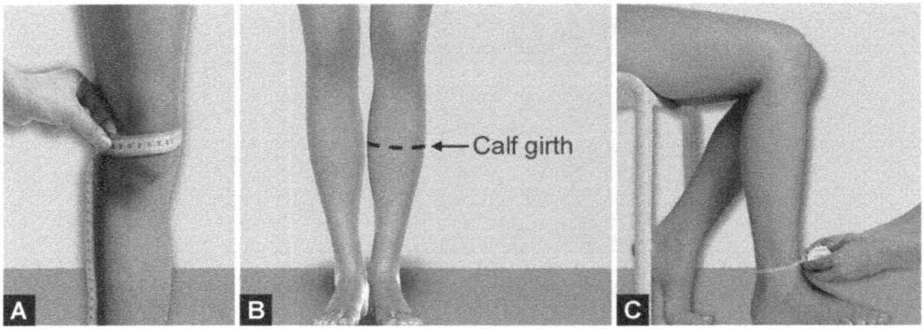

Figs 5.31A to C (A) Knee girth measurements; (B) Calf girth measurement; (C) Ankle girth measurement

- *Ankle girth*: It is the minimum circumference of the lower leg, just proximal to the malleoli **(Fig. 5.31C)**.

Upper Motor Neurone, Lower Motor Neurone and their Lesions (Fig. 5.32)

- All the neurons contributing to the pyramidal and extra-pyramidal systems should be called *upper motor neurons (UMN)*.

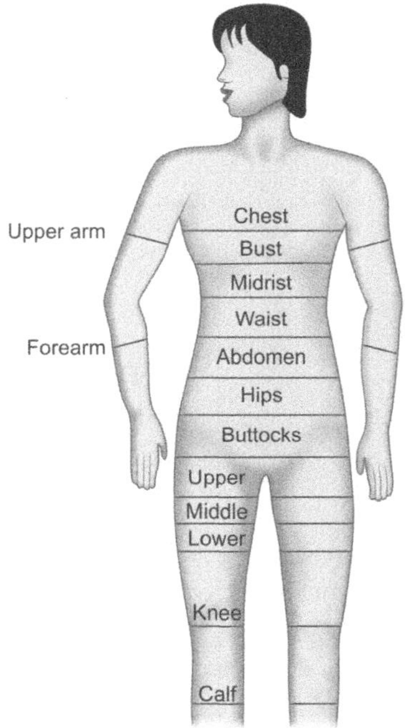

Fig. 5.32 Whole body girth measurement

- The anterior horn cells and the related neurons in the motor nuclei of some cranial nerves are called *lower motor neurons (LMN).*
- Axons of these cells give rise to the peripheral motor nerves. These are lowest in position in the motor system and receive all the inputs from higher centers like medulla, pons, mid-brain and cerebral cortex and transmit the same to the target organs.
- All impulses for motor activity are to be funnelled into them and these are also called *final common pathway.*

Signs of Upper Motor Neuron Lesions (Fig. 5.33)

- Paralysis or weakness of movements of the affected side but gross movements may be produced. No muscle atrophy is seen initially but later on some disuse atrophy may occur.
- *Babinski sign is present*: The great toe becomes dorsiflexed and the other toes fan outward in response to sensory stimulation along the

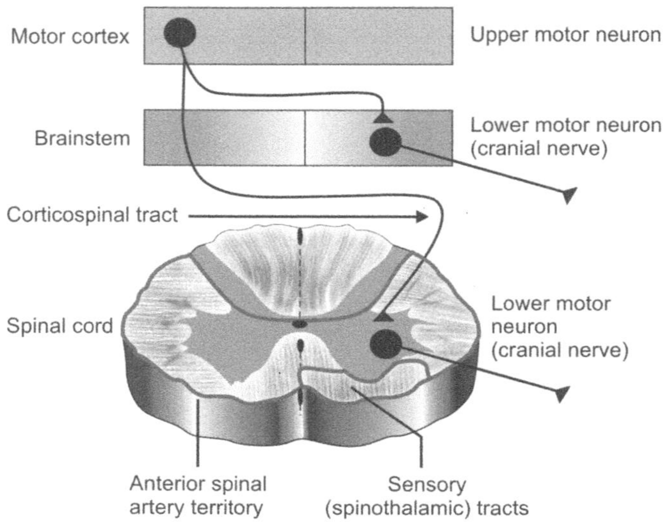

Fig. 5.33 Diagram for upper motor neuron and lower motor neuron

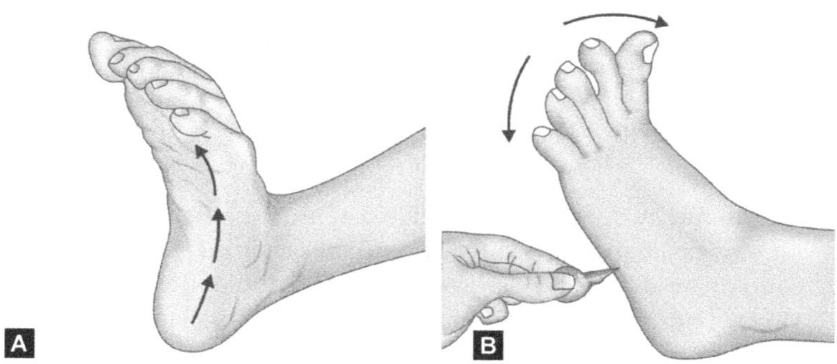

Figs 5.34A and B (A) Normal toe flexion; (B) Positive Babinski's reflex

lateral aspect of the sole of the foot. The normal response is plantar flexion of all the toes **(Figs 5.34A and B)**.

- Loss of performance of fine-skilled voluntary movements especially at the distal end of the limbs
- Superficial abdominal reflexes and cremasteric reflex are absent
- Spasticity or hypertonicity of the muscles
- *Clasp-knife reaction*: Initial higher resistance to movement is followed by a lesser resistance
- Exaggerated deep tendon reflexes and clonus may be present.

Signs of Lower Motor Neuron Lesions

- Flaccid paralysis of muscles supplied
- Atrophy of muscles supplied
- Loss of reflexes of muscles supplied
- Muscles fasciculation (contraction of a group of fibers) due to irritation of the motor neurons—seen with naked eye.
- Muscle fibrillation (contraction of individual fibers)—detected only by EMG
- Muscle contracture (shortening of paralyzed muscles)
- Presence of muscle wasting
- *Reaction of degeneration*: When the LMN is cut, a muscle will no longer respond to interrupted electrical stimulation 7 days after nerve section, although it will still respond to direct current. After 10 days, response to direct current also ceases.

Difference or Comparison between Upper Motor Neuron Lesion (UMNL) and Lower Motor Neuron Lesion (LMNL) (Table 5.16)

Table 5.16: Mnemonic for basis of difference: STORM baby

Basis of difference (STORM baby)	*UMNL*	*LMNL*
S = Strength	Lowers	Lowers
T = Tone	Increases (spastic)	Decreases (flaccid)
O = Others	• Superficial reflexes absent • Clonus	• Fasciculation • Fibrillations • Reaction of degeneration
R = Reflexes = DTR or deep tendon reflexes	Increased	Decreased
M = Muscle mass	Slight loss only	Decreases/atrophy
Baby = Babinski sign	Positive (toe up)	Negative (toe down)

Findings of Motor System Examination

- *Weakness in all four limbs*:
  1. With increase reflexes and extensor plantar response
     - Cervical cord lesion
     - Bilateral pyramidal lesions.

2. With absent reflexes
   - Polyradiculopathy
   - Peripheral neuropathy or myopathy
3. Mixed upper motor neurone and lower motor neurone weakness
   - MND
   - Mixed cervical myelopathy and radiculopathy.
4. Normal reflexes
   - Fatigable weakness, particularly with associated cranial nerve abnormality - myasthenia gravis.
   - Variable weakness, normal tone: consider hysterical weakness, if mental state appropriate.

- *Weakness in both the legs*:
  - Both increased reflexes and extensor plantar responses
    - Lesion in spinal cord. The lesion above the root level of highest moor abnormalities. A level may be ascertained with sensory signs.
  - With absent reflexes in the leg
    - Polyneuropathy, cauda equine lesion or peripheral neuropathy.
- *Unilateral arm and leg weakness*:
  - UMN with high cervical cord, brainstem or above
  - Contralateral sensory findings indicate lesion of half ipsilateral cervical cord lesion.
  - Contralateral cranial nerve lesions or brainstem signs indicate the level of brainstem affected.
  - Ipsilateral facial or tongue indicate lesion above brainstem.
- *Syndrome limited to a single limb*:
  - UMN sign limited to single limb can be caused by lesion in spinal cord, brainstem or cerebral hemisphere. Motor sign alone cannot distinguish between possibilities. This relies on other signs for example cranial nerve or sensory abnormality or diagnosis may not possible without further investigation.
  - If LMN common syndromes seen are as follows.
  - Upper limb
    - Hand

6 Sensory Assessment

DEFINITION

Sensory integrity is the ability to organize and use sensory information.

AGE RELATED SENSORY CHANGES

Alteration in sensory function occurs with normal aging.

- Decline in average weight of brain with aging
- Degeneration of neurons
- Depletion of neural dendrites
- Reduction in conduction velocity of sensory nerves
- Degeneration of some myelinated fibers of spinal cord
- Decrease in distance between node of ranvier in peripheral nerve

CLASSIFICATION OF SENSORY SYSTEM

- *Superficial sensation*:
  - Exteroceptor responsible
  - Responsible for perception of pain, temperature, light touches and pressure
  - Receive stimuli from external environment via skin and subcutaneous tissue.
- *Deep sensation*:
  - Proprioceptors responsible
  - Responsible for joint sense, joint position
  - Receive stimuli from muscle, tendon and ligament
- *Combined cortical sensation*:
  - Combination of both the superficial and deep sensory mechanism
  - It requires information from both proprioceptive and exteroceptive receptors as well as intact function of associated areas.

CLASSIFICATION OF SENSORY RECEPTOR

- *Mechanoreceptor*:
  - Cutaneous sensory **(Figs 6.1 and 6.2)**
  - Deep sensory **(Table 6.1)**
- *Thermoreceptors*:
  - Hot
  - Cold
- *Nociceptors*:
  - Pain
  - Free nerve ending
- *Chemoreceptors*:
  - Taste
  - Smell
  - Arterial O_2

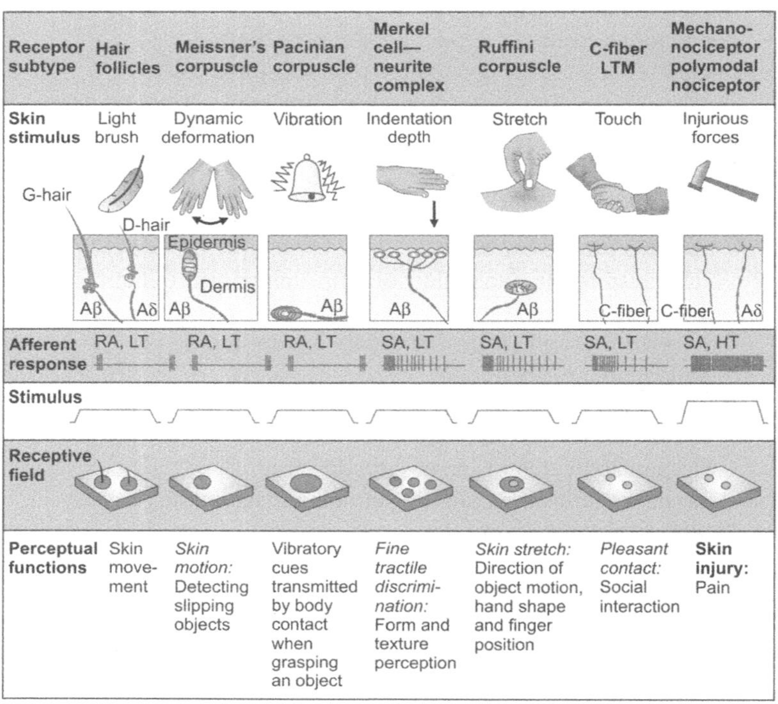

Fig. 6.1 Type of receptors and their functions

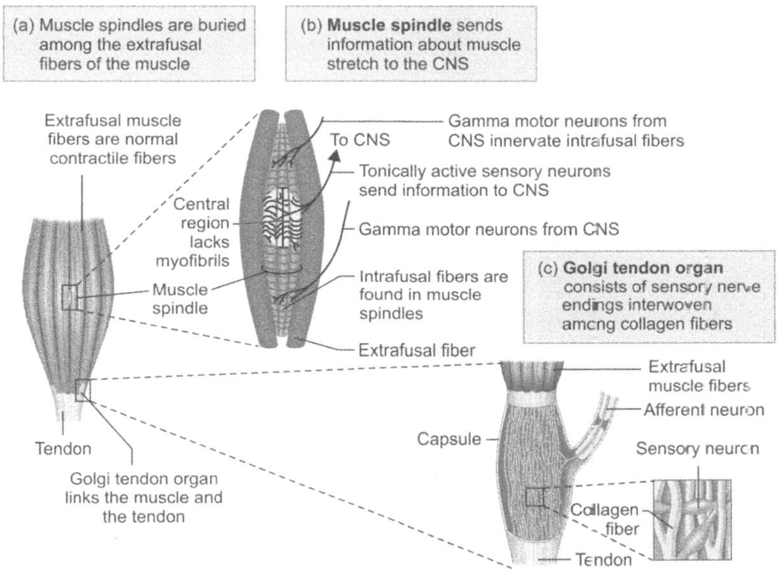

Fig. 6.2 Function of deep sensory receptors

Table 6.1: Deep sensory receptors	
Muscle receptor	*Joint receptor*
• *Muscle spindles*: – *Location*: Parallel to muscle fibers – *Function*: Position and movement sense	• *Ruffini endings*: – *Location*: Joint capsule and ligament – *Function*: Direction and velocity of joint movement
• *Golgi tendon organ*: – *Location*: Proximal and distal tendinous insertion. – *Function*: Monitor tension within the muscle, inhibition of contracting muscle and facilitation of antagonist	• *Golgi type ending*: – *Location*: Ligaments – *Function*: Detect rate of joint movement
• *Free nerve endings*: – *Location*: Fascia of muscle – *Function*: Pain and pressure	• *Free nerve endings*: – *Location*: Joint capsule and ligament – *Function*: Pain and crude joint movement
• *Pacinian corpuscle*: – *Location*: Fascia of muscle – *Function*: Vibration, deep pressure	• *Pacinian endings*: – *Location*: Joint capsule – *Function*: Monitor rapid joint movement

- Osmolarity
- Blood CO_2
- Blood glucose
- *Photo receptor*:
  - Rods
  - Cons.

Cutaneous Sensory Receptors

- *Free nerve ending*:
  - *Location*: Throughout body
  - *Sensation*: Touch, pressure, tickle, itch
- *Hair-follicle ending*:
  - *Location*: At base of each hair follicle.
  - *Function*: Sensitive to mechanical movement and touch.
- *Merkel's disks*:
  - *Location*: Below epidermis in hairy and glabrous skin.
  - *Function*: Low intensity touch, velocity of touch, tactile localization, two point discrimination.
- *Ruffini ending*:
  - *Location*: Deeper layer of dermis.
  - *Function*: Perception of touch and pressure.
- *Krause's end-bulb*:
  - *Location*: Dermis.
  - *Function*: Perception of touch and pressure.
- *Meissner's corpuscle*:
  - *Location*: In dermis. High in finger tips, lips and toes.
  - *Function*: Discriminative touch, recognition of texture.
- *Pacinian's corpuscles*:
  - *Location*: Subcutaneous tissue layer.
  - *Function*: Perception of deep touch and vibration.

Spinothalamic Tract (Table 6.2 and Fig. 6.3)

Leminiscal System (Fig. 6.4)

Diffusely terminate at all levels of lower brainstem and thalamus.

- Afferent fibers conveying the superficial sensations are small slow conducting.

Table 6.2: Transmission of sensory signals

System	*Type of sensation*	*Afferent fibers*	*Origin*	*Termination*
Spino-thalamic	Nondiscriminative Crude localization	Small Slowly conducting	Skin	From dorsal horn cross in SC, 2nd order project to lower brainstem and thalamus
Leminiscal	• Discriminative (stereognosis, two point discrimination) • Precise localization	Large rapidly conducting	• Skin • Joint • Tendon	• From dorsal column. 2nd order project to contralateral thalamus • 3rd order project to secondary cortex

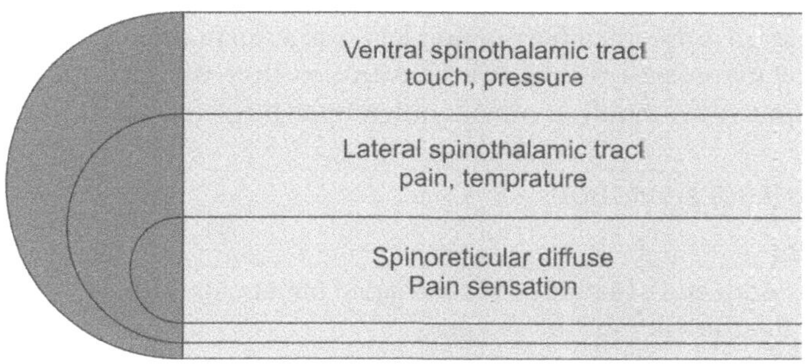

Fig. 6.3 Functions of anterior spinal tract

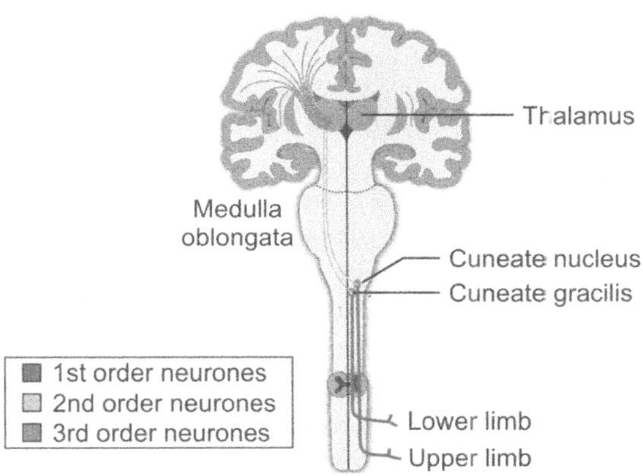

Fig. 6.4 Sensory pathway

- Afferent fibers conveying discriminative sensation are larger, faster and travel by dorsal leminiscus.
- First check superficial sensation then deep sensation and combine cortical sensation.
- If affection of superficial sensation some impairment of deep sensation may also be noticed.
- The dermatomes are cutaneous areas that correspond to the spinal segment providing their innervations **(Fig. 6.5)**.
- Sensory examination should perform in distal to proximal manner.
- If single extremity is affected then deficits tends to be more.
- Boundaries of impairment should be identified. This information is transferred to a sensory assessment form peripheral nerve involvement should also identified and this form then entered in medical record.
- During testing the application of stimuli should be applied in a random, unpredictable manner with variation in timing.
- Scar tissue area will be less sensitive so they will give diminished response to stimuli so consideration must be given to that.

Superficial Sensation

- *Pain*:
  - Sharp end of safety pin or reshaped paper clip is used
  - Instrument must be cleaned
  - To avoid summation of impulse stimuli should not be applied too close to each other.
  - The instrument must be sharp enough to deflect the skin but not puncture it.
    - *Response*: Patient is asked to verbally indicate when stimulus is felt. All areas of body should be tested.
- *Temperature*:
  - Test tube with 5–10°C and between 40–45°C taken
  - Test tubes are randomly placed in contact with skin areas to be tested. All surfaces should be tested.
    - *Response*: Patient is asked to indicate when stimulus is felt and to reply "warm", "cold" or "unable to tell".
      It is difficult to perform as the tubes are exposed to room air.
- *Light touch*:
  - Camel hair brush, piece of cotton or tissue is used. Areas to be tested is lightly touched or stroked.

  - *Response*: Patient is asked to indicate when he or she recognize stimulus by responding "Yes" or "No".
- *Pressure*:
  - Thumb or fingertip in use to apply firm pressure, pressure should be firm enough to indent the skin and stimulate deep receptors.
    - *Response*: Patient is asked to indicate when he or she recognize stimulus applied by responding "yes" or "no".

Deep Sensation

- *Kinesthesia*:
  - It examines awareness of movement.
  - The extremity to be assessed is moved passively through a relatively small range of motion.
  - Demonstration of the procedure should be performed prior to actual testing.
  - This will ensure that the patient and agree on term to describe the direction of movements.
  - *Response*:
    - Patient is asked to indicate direction of motion while extremity is in motion.
    - "Up, down, in, out"
    - Patient may respond simultaneously duplicating the movement with opposite extremity.
    - During testing movement of larger joint is usually discerned move quickly than that of smaller joint.
    - Therapist's grip should remain constant and minimal to reduce tactile stimulation.
    - Romberg's test should be performed for joint position sense.
- *Proprioception*:
  - It examines joint position sense and awareness joints at rest.
  - The extremity or joint to be assessed is moved through a range of motion and held in static position.
  - Small increment in range of motion are used.
  - "Initial, mid or terminal range"
  - As with kinesthesia caution should be used with hand placement to avoid excessive tactile stimulation.
  - *Response*:
    - Patient is asked to describe position verbally or to duplicate the position of the extremity or joint with contralateral extremity.

- *Vibration*:
  - *Test*: Requires tuning fork that vibrates at 128 Hz.
  - The ability to perceive a vibratory stimulus is tested by placing the box of a vibrating tuning fork on a bony prominence.
  - Intact patient will perceive vibration, if there is impairment patient will be unable to distinguish between vibrating and non-vibrating tuning fork.
  - Earphones may be used for this test procedure to reduce auditory cues from the vibrating fork.
  - Frequency of vibration cannot be held constant during the test procedure.
  - *Response*:
    - Patient is asked to respond by verbally identifying the stimulus as vibrating or nonvibrating each time fork is placed in contact with a bony prominence.

Combined Cortical Sensations

- *Tactile object recognition (stereognosis)*:
  - *Test*: Require use of items of different sizes and shapes
  - A variety of small, easily obtainable and culturally familiar objects can be used.
  - The object may include keys, coins, combs, safety pins and pencils.
  - The patient is given single object allowed to manipulate object and then ask to identify item verbally.
    - *Response*: Patient is asked to name object verbally.
- *Tactile localization*:
  - This test assesses ability to localize touch sensation on the skin.
  - Using a fingertip touches different skin surfaces. After each application of a stimulus the patient is given time to respond.
    - *Response*: Patient is asked to identify location of stimuli by pointing the area or by verbally description. Tactile localization may test separately or included with other tests.
    - Accuracy of localization over different parts of body may be compared to determine the relative sensitivity of different areas.

- *Two point discrimination*:
  - It assesses ability to perceive two points applied to the skin simultaneously.
  - It is measure of smallest distance between two stimuli that can still be perceived as two distinct stimuli.
  - Asthesiometer, paper clip, ECG or caliper can be used to check it.
  - During test procedure two tips of small instrument applied to skin simultaneously, two tips are gradually brought closer together until the stimuli are perceived as one.
  - The smallest distance between the stimuli that is still perceived as two distinct points is measured with a ruler and recorded.
  - It is important to consider that perception of two point discrimination varies considerably for different individuals and body parts, being most refined in distal upper extremity.
    - *Response*: Patient is asked to identify perception of "one" or "two" stimuli.

  Normal Values
  - *Fingers*: 2–3 mm
  - *Upper lip*: 4–5 mm
  - *Cheek*: 6 mm
  - *Nose*: 7 mm
  - *Palm*: 10 mm
  - *Forehead*: 35 mm
  - *Foot*: 20 mm
  - *Belly*: 30 mm
  - *Forearm*: 35 mm
  - *Upper arm*: 39 mm
  - *Shoulder*: 41 mm
  - *Thigh*: 42 mm
  - *Calf*: 45 mm.
- *Double simultaneous stimulation*:
  - Ability to perceive a simultaneous touch stimulus on opposite sides of the body, proximally and distally on a single extremity.
  - Proximally and distally on the one side of body.
  - Proximally and distally on opposite sides of body.

Extinction phenomena: Use to describe a situation in which only the proximal stimulus is perceived with extinction of the distal.

Response: Patient states when he or she perceive a touch stimulus and number of stimuli felt.

- *Recognition of weight (barognosis)*:
  - Series of small object of same size but of graduated weight is used.
  - Therapist places series of different weight in same hand one at a time or to place different weight in each hand simultaneously.
    - *Response*: The patient responds by indicating that the object is "heavier" or "lighter".
- *Traced figure identification (Graphesthesia)*:
  - Recognition of letters, numbers or designs traced on the skin is assessed by use of eraser end of a pencil.
  - Series or combination of letters, numbers or designs in traced on palm of patient's hand.
  - Between each separate drawing the palm should be gently wiped with soft cloth to clearly indicate a change in figures to the patient.
  - This test is also a useful substitute for stereognosis when paralysis prevents grasping an object.
    - *Response*: Patient is asked to identify verbally the figures drawn on the skin.
- *Recognition of texture*:
  - *Test*: It examines ability to differentiate among various textures. Suitable texture may include cotton, wool or silk.
  - The items are placed individually in patient's hand.
  - Patient is allowed to manipulate the simple texture.
  - Response
    - Patient is asked to identify the individual textures as they are placed in the hand.
    - They may be identified by name or by texture.

Common mistakes

- *Generally*: Starting proximally rather than distally.
- *Vibration sense and joint position sense*: Inadequate explanation, hurried testing without checking.
- *Pinprick*: Drawing blood because of nonplused needle, varied pressure or calloused skin.
- *Light touch*: Varied pressure.

Points to be remember

- The ankle, knee, groin and axilla are all areas of relatively heightened sensitivity.
- Test vibration sense first, then temperature then joint position sense, then pin prick. Test light touch last.
- Start distally than work proximally.
- Map any area of sensory loss starting in the area of abnormal sensation then moving towards the normal area.
- Keep a mental drawing of what you have found in mind.

To improve the ability of test:

- Use of consistent guidelines for completing the test.
- Administration of test by trained skillful examiner.
- Subsequent retest performed by the same individual.

Gradation of sensation

- *Grade 1*: Intact (normal accurate response)
- *Grade 2*: Decreased (delayed response)
- *Grade 3*: Exaggerated (increase sensitivity or awareness of stimulus after removed)
- *Grade 4*: Inaccurate (inappropriate perception of stimulus)
- *Grade 5*: Absent (no response)
- *Grade 6*: Inconsistent or ambiguous (Response inadequate to determine function accurately).

Dermatomes

A dermatome is an area of skin supplied by sensory neurons that arise from a spinal nerve ganglion. Symptoms that follow a dermatome (e.g. like pain or a rash) may indicate a pathology that involves the related nerve root. Examples include *somatic dysfunction* of the spine or viral infection. *Referred pain* usually involves a specific, "referred" location so is not associated with a dermatome **(Figs 6.5 to 6.7)**.

Viruses that lie dormant in nerve ganglia (e.g. *varicella zoster virus*, which causes both *chickenpox* and *herpes zoster* commonly *shingles*), often cause either pain, rash or both in a pattern defined by a dermatome. However, the symptoms may not appear across the entire dermatome.

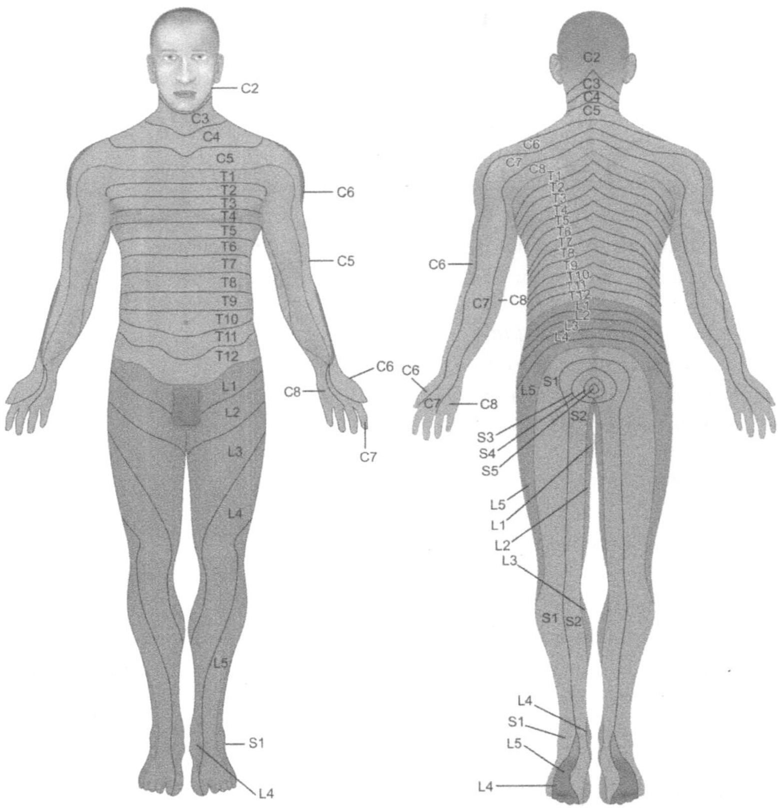

Map Key			
L1, 2, 3, 4	Anterior and inner surface of lower limbs	L4, 5, S1	Foot
L4	Medial side of great toe	S1, 2, L5	Posterior and outer surface of lower limbs
S1	Lateral margin of foot and little toe	S2,3,4	Perineum
T10	Level of umbilicus	T12	Inguinal or groin regions
C5	Clavicles	C5, 6, 7	Lateral parts of upper limbs
C8, T1	Medial sides of the upper limbs	C6	Thumb
C6, 7, 8	Hand	C8	Ring and little fingers
T4	Level of nipples		

Fig. 6.5 Dermatomal location

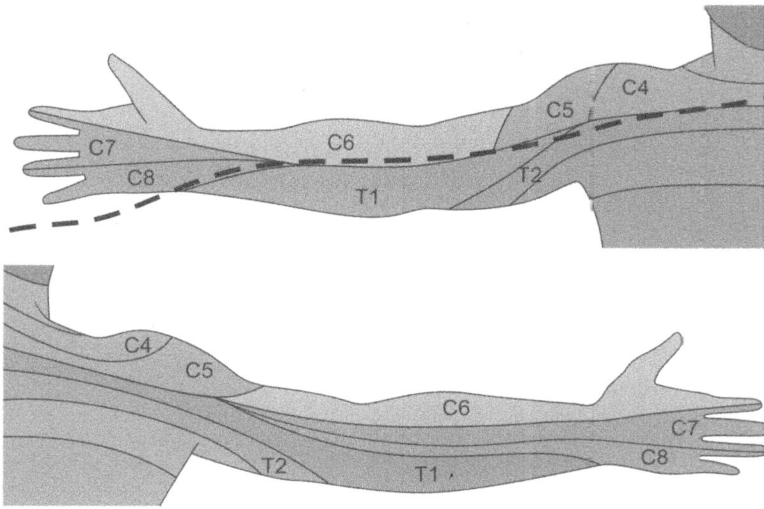

Fig. 6.6 Upper limb dermatomes

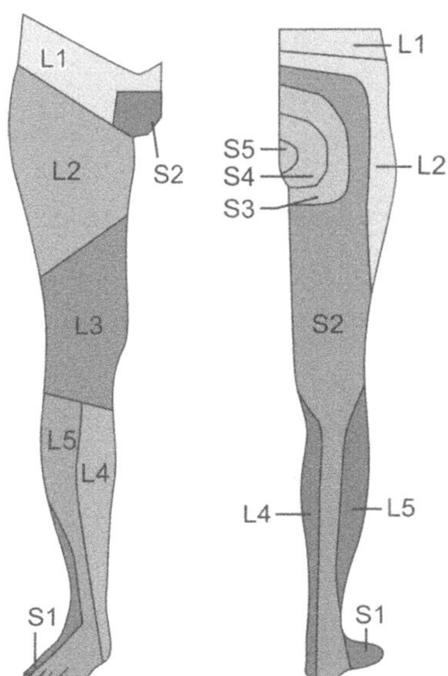

Fig. 6.7 Lower limb dermatomes

Dermatomal testing	*Dermatome*
Posterior aspect of head/occiput	C2
Lateral aspect of neck	C3
Acromioclavicular Joint	C4
Over deltoid	C5
Tip of thumb/radial side of wrist	C6
Tip of middle finger	C7
Tip of little finger/ulnar side of wrist	C8
Medial elbow	T1
Medial upper arm	T2
Segmental trunk	T3-T12
Groin (by report)	L1
Upper 1/3 of anterior thigh	L2
Medial knee	L3
Lateral knee to medial malleolus	L4
Lateral lower leg to dorsum of big toe	L5
Heel	S1
Medial aspect of posterior thigh	S2
Perianal area (by report)	S3,4,5

Patterns of Sensory Loss (Figs 6.8 to 6.11)

- *Single nerve*: Sensory loss within the distribution of a single, most commonly median, ulnar, personal, lateral cutaneous nerve to thigh. Causes
  - Diabetes mellitus
  - Rheumatoid arthritis
  - Hypothyroidism
  - Multiple single nerve lesions
  - Vacuities
- *Root or roots*: Sensory deficits confined to a single root or a number of roots in close proximity—common roots in the arm C5, C6 and C7 and in the leg L4, L5 and S1.
  Common causes: Compression by prolapsed intervertebral disc
  - *Rare causes*: Tumors

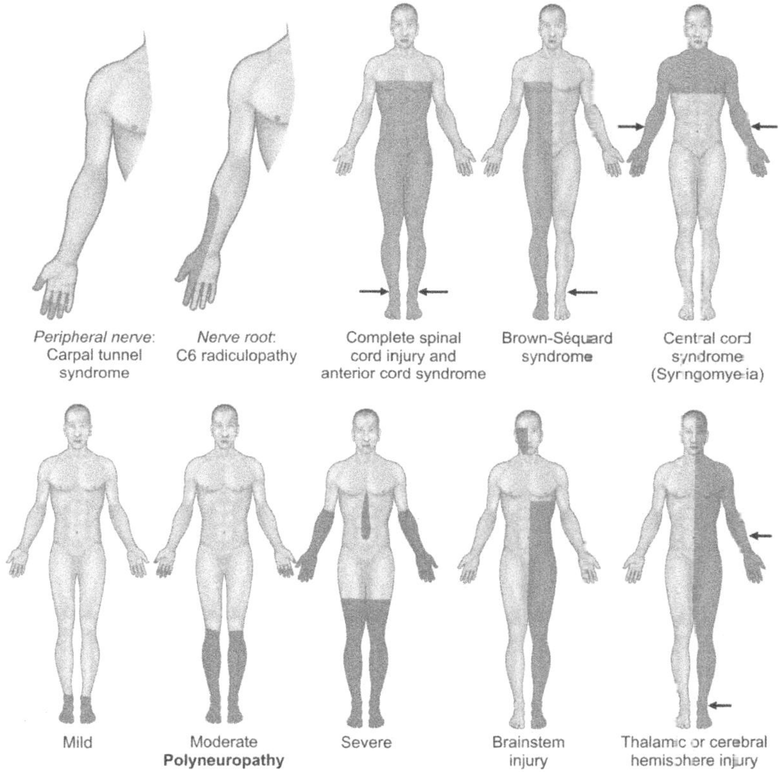

Fig. 6.8 Patterns of sensory loss in different conditions

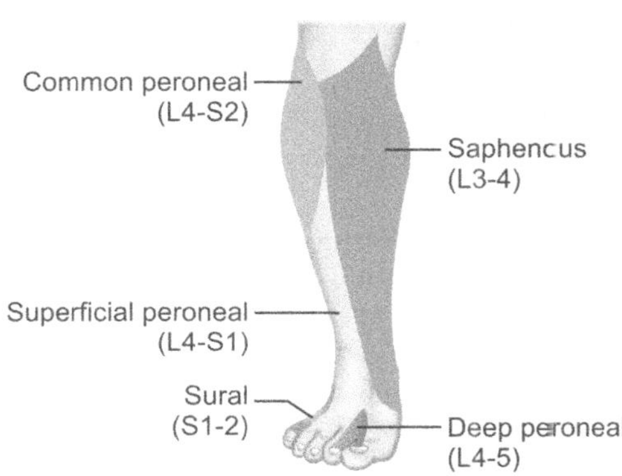

Fig. 6.9 Sensory distribution in leg

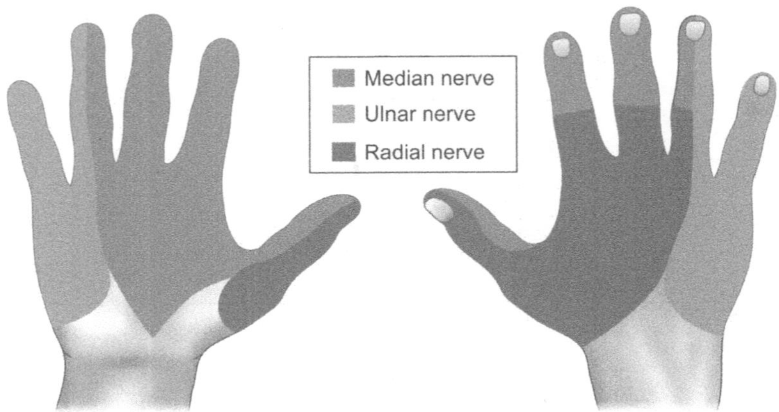

Fig. 6.10 Sensory distribution in hand

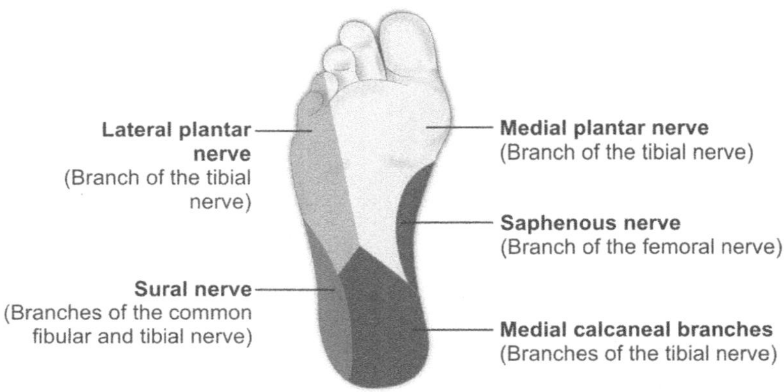

Fig. 6.11 Sensory distribution in foot

- *Peripheral nerve*: Distal glove and stoking deficit.
  Common causes: Diabetes mellitus, vitamin B_1 deficiency
  - *Rare causes*: Guillain-Barré syndrome (GBS), inherited neuropathy, vacuities, vitamin deficiencies.
- *Spinal cord*: Five patterns of loss can be recognized.

Complete transverse section: Hyperesthesia at the upper levels with loss of all modalities a few segments below the lesion.

Causes

- Transverse myelitis
- Cervical spondylysis
- Multiple sclerosis.

Rare cause: Intraspinal tumors, spinal abscess, postinfectious.

- *Hemisection of cord*: Loss of joint position sense and vibration sense on same side as the lesion and pain and temperature on opposite side a few level below the lesion.
  Causes: Same as transaction.
- *Central cord*: Loss of pain and temperature sensation at the level of the lesion, where the spinothalamic fibers cross in the cord, with other modality preserved-seen in syringomyelia.
  Causes: Syringomyelia
- *Posterior column loss*: Loss of joint position sense and vibration sense with intact pain and temperature.
  - *Anterior spinal syndrome*: Loss of pain and temperature below the level with preserved joint position sense and vibration sense.
- *Brainstem*: Loss of pain and temperature on the face and on the opposite side of the body.
  Common causes: Lateral medullary syndrome.
- *Thalamic sensory loss*: Hemisensory loss of all modalities.
- *Cortical loss*: Parital lobe—the patient is able to recognize all sensations but localizes them poorly—loss of two point discrimination, a stereognosis, sensory inattention.
- *Functional loss*: This diagnosis is suggested by a nonanatomical distribution of sensory deficit frequently with inconstant findings.

Terminologies for Abnormal Sensation

- *Abarognosis*: Inability to recognize weight.
- *Allesthesia*: Sensation perceived at a site remote from point of stimulation.
- *Allodynia*: Pain produce by non noxious stimulus.
- *Analgesia*: Complete loss of pain sensitivity.
- *Atopognosia*: Inability to localize sensation.
- *Causalgia*: Painful, burning sensation.
- *Dysesthesia*: Touch sensation experience as pain.
- *Hypoalgesia*: Decrease sensitivity to pain.
- *Hyperalgesia*: Increase sensitivity to pain.

- *Hypoesthesia*: Decrease sensitivity to sensory stimulus.
- *Pallanesthesia*: No sensitivity to vibration.
- *Paresthesia*: Abnormal sensation such as numbness, prickling or tingling without cause.
- *Thalamic syndrome*: Partial or complete paralysis of one side of body associated with severe pain, produce exaggerated, prolong or painful stimulus.
- *Thermalgesia*: Inability to perceive heat.
- *Thermanesthesia*: Inability to perceive sensation of heat and cold.
- *Thermhyperesthesia*: Increase sensitivity to temperature.
- *Thermhypesthesia*: Decrease temperature sensibility.
- *Therm anesthesia*: Loss of light touch sensibility.

PAIN (FLOW CHART 6.1)

The Interoceptive or Visceral Sensation

Somatic Pain

Somatic pain can be classified as either:

- *Cutaneous, superficial or peripheral pain*: Pain that arises from the skin and muscles or peripheral nerves themselves. In general, this pain has two components, the initial response:
  - Followed by later response

Flow chart 6.1 Classification of pain

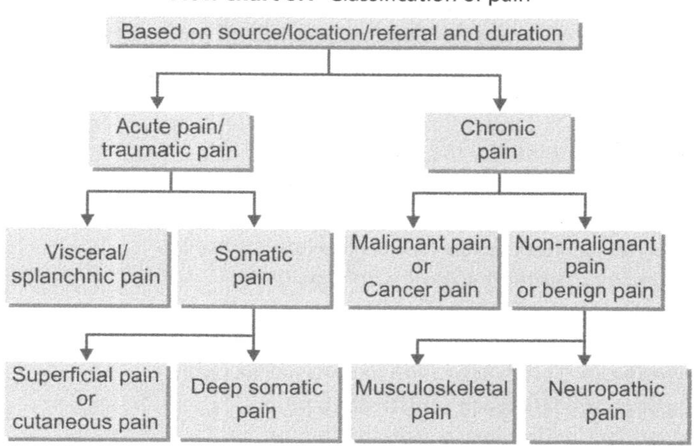

- These signals are transmitted via different pathway.
    - Pricking pain reaches the CNS via neospinothalamic tract (i.e. LST) to the VPL (or VPM) and to the SCI.
    - Burning and soreness pain resulting from tissue damage reaches the CNS via the paleospinothalamic tract (AST) and archispinothalamic tract to brain stem nuclei and to PF-CM complex, etc.
- *Deep pain*: This pain arises from joint receptors tendons and fascia (i.e. deep structures). The quality of deep pain is dull, aching or burning. Deep pain is accompanied by a definite autonomic response associated with sweating and nausea, changes in blood pressure and heart rate. Somatic deep pain reaches the CNS mainly via the paleospinothalamic and archispinothalamic tract.

Reaction to somatic pain: Sudden, unexpected damage to the skin is followed by three responses:

1. *Startle response*: This is a complex psychosomatic response to a sudden unexpected stimulus which includes: A flexion reflex, postural readjustment and orientation of the head and eyes to examine the damaged area.
2. *Autonomic response*: This response includes: NE and E release, ACTH and/or cortisol release, and vasoconstriction and piloerection.
3. *Behavioral response*: This response includes: Vocalization, rubbing designed to diminish pain, learning to respond to sudden pain and psychosomatic pain.

Visceral Pain

- In the visceral organs, nociceptors respond to mechanical stimulation such as pressure, tissue damage, and chemical stimulation.
- Most noxious information carried by visceral afferents does not give rise to conscious sensation. Visceral pain is diffuse, less precisely graded and typically accompanied by slowing of the heart, lowered blood pressure, cold sweats and nausea.
- It conveys also hunger, thirst, electrolyte balance, deregulation in the respiratory and circulatory systems.
- In the visceral organs, free nerve endings are scattered, and any stimulus that excites these nerve endings causes visceral pain. Such stimuli include spasm of the smooth muscle in a hollow viscus, or distention or stretching of the ligament, such as a stone blocking the ureter or the gall ducts.

- Stretching of the tissues such as intestinal obstruction can also provoke visceral pain.
- Visceral pain is also caused by chemical means as a result of gastrointestinal lesions, and tumors as well as thrombosis of an artery.
- In many cases, visceral pain is not localized to the site of its cause, rather in a distant site.

Thalamic Pain

- Stroke or occlusion in the thalamogeniculate artery (a branch of the posterior cerebral artery), which supplies the lateroposterior half of the thalamus, can result in a thalamic lesion, which is often accompanied by neurologic conditions several months after the initial event.
- The condition is associated with a devastating intracranial pain in the contralateral side of the thalamic lesion and sensory loss. In some cases, severe facial pain is experienced without any sensory loss. The pain resulting from an intracranial lesion is also termed "central pain".
- Lesions in the spinothalamic tract and its targets of termination as well as local manifestations of diencephalic lesions are usually complex.
- They can induce alteration of sensory, motor and endocrine components because of the functional diversity of the thalamus. Subjects with this syndrome experience spontaneous aching and burning pain in body regions where sensory stimuli normally do not lead to pain. Because the brain and the spinal cord do not contain nociceptors, the pathological process presumably directly stimulates nociceptive pathways, or it prevents the activation of the pain suppression pathways. This condition is also known as thalamic pain syndrome or Dejerine-Roussy syndrome.

Neuropathic Pain

- Neuropathic pain is a sharp, shooting and devastating pain. It is a persistent pain that arises from functional changes occurring in the CNS secondary to peripheral nerve injury.
- Once the nerve is damaged, the damaged nerve elicits sustained activation of nociceptors and/or nociceptive afferents.

- The neuropathic pain is due to an abnormal activation of the nociceptive system without specifically stimulating the nociceptors.
- Neuroplastic changes occurring in the CNS secondary to the afferent barrage are believed to culminate in CNS neuronal hyperexcitability.
- Many scientists suggest that "sensitization" of the nervous system following injury is a factor in neuropathic pain. Neuropathic pain can usually be controlled by anti-inflammatory drugs and opioids.
- In some cases, such as in diabetics, AIDS, cancer, etc. no treatment or relief is available to neuropathic pain.
- Neuropathic pain should not be confused with neurogenic pain, a term used to describe pain resulting from injury to a peripheral nerve but without necessarily implying any neuropathy.

Psychosomatic Pain

- Psychic reaction to pain includes all the well-known responses to pain such as anguish, anxiety, crying, depression, nausea and excess muscular excitability through the body.
- These reactions vary tremendously from one person to another following a comparable degree of pain stimuli. The sensation of pain can be influenced by emotions, past experiences and suggestions. The same stimulus can elicit different responses in different subjects under the same conditions.
- Recently, positron emission tomography (PET) has been used to study pain pathways and psychosomatic pain centers.
- For example, volunteers had their hands dipped in hot water (50°C) while they were conscious. They then dipped their hand again in hot water (50°C) after a post-hypnotic suggestion that the pain would be either more or less unpleasant than the first time.
- The PET scans of their brains showed that activity in the anterior cingulate cortex changed in accordance with how unpleasant they expected the pain to be. However, the intensity in the primary somatosensory cortex remained constant (i.e. the emotional component of pain is independent of its sensation).

Referred Pain

Referred pain is a painful sensation at a site other than the injured one. The pain is not localized to the site of its cause (visceral organ) but instead is localized to a distant site. One possible exception is that the axons carry pain information from the viscera enters into the spinal

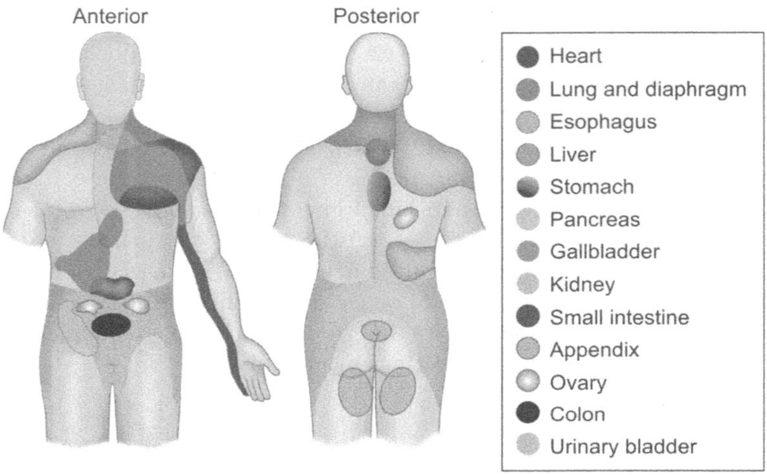

Fig. 6.12 Referred pain, the sites for referred pain from various organs are shown

cord by the same route as the cutaneous pain sensation axons. Within the spinal cord there is a convergence of the information on the same nocineurons. This convergence gives rise to the phenomenon of referred pain **(Fig. 6.12)**. For example, pain associated with angina pectoris, or myocardial infarction is referred to the left chest, left shoulder, and upper left arm. Pain resulting from distention of the colon is referred to the periumbilical area. The following are some hypothesis to explain referred pain:

- *Common dermatome hypothesis*: When pain is referred, it is usually to a structure that developed from the same embryonic segment or dermatome as the structure in which the pain originates. Radiating pain down the left arm is the result of a myocardial infarction, or pain originating from the shoulder (dermatomes 3-5).
- *Convergence and facilitation theories*: Inputs from visceral and skin receptors converge on the same spinal cord neuron (i.e. viscerosomatic neurons). Therefore, visceral pain is referred to skin area because the nociceptors' terminals from the viscera terminate in the spinal cord on the same neurons that receive input from the skin.
- *Facilitation or irritable focus*: Pain impulses from the viscera alone are unable to pass directly from spinal cord neurons to the brain, but create an "irritable focus". When visceral and skin impulses arrive together, the information transmitted to higher centers and the brain interprets the pain as being from the skin.

- *Learned phenomenon*: Visceral information arrives in the CNS. However, the brain interprets that the impulses originate from the site of a previous surgical operation, trauma or localized pathologic process.

Phantom (Illusory) Pain

- *Phantom* or *illusory pain* is the experience of pain without any signals from nociceptors. It occurs in a subject with previous injuries such as amputation in which the dorsal roots are literally absent from the cord.
- Even though no sensory signals can enter the cord, the subject often feels extreme pain in the denervated parts of the body. For example, an amputee will often apparently feel pain in a part of his body that has been removed.
- The phenomenon of phantom limb pain is a common experience after a limb has been amputated or its sensory roots have been destroyed in which the pain is felt in a part of the body that no longer exists. Pain from an amputated arm is referred to the viscera as a result of disruption to the "balance" between different peripheral inputs to the dorsal horn.
- A complete break of the spinal cord also often leads to a phantom body pain below the level of the break. The source of phantom pain is complex and not well understood. It has been suggested that there may be abnormal discharges:
  - From the remaining cut ends of nerves which grow into nodules called *neuromas*
  - From overactive spinal neurons
  - From abnormal flow of signals through the somatosensory cortex
  - From burst-firing neurons in the thalamus.

Acute Pain

Acute pain arises from activation of nociceptors for a limited time and is not associated with significant tissue damage (e.g. a pin prick).

Chronic Pain

- *Chronic pain* is prolonged pain lasting for months or longer that arises from tissue injury, inflammation, nerve damage, tumor growth, lesion or occlusion of blood vessels.

- Chronic or inflammatory pain can sensitize the nervous system, evoking chemical, functional, and even structural changes that serve to "prime the pain-processing pump".
- Chronic pain, such as lower back pain, rheumatoid and osteoarthritis, and headache (see "Headaches" below) may result from constant inflammatory activity which activates G proteins.
- In some cases, the pain persists long after the injury heals, but there is no treatment that will eliminate the pain.

Sensitization

- One possible explanation for chronic pain is a phénomenon called *sensitization*. Following continuation and prolong noxious stimulation, nearby silent nociceptive neurons that previously were unresponsive to stimulation, now become responsive.
- In addition, some of the chemicals produced and released at the injured site also alter the physiological properties of nociceptors. The nociceptors begin to initiate pain signals spontaneously, which cause chronic pain.
- In addition, weak stimuli, such as a light touch that previously had no effect on these nociceptors, will further activate the nociceptors which result in severe pain signals. This phenomenon is referred to as "peripheral sensitization".
- The outcome of peripheral sensitization results in a greater and more persistent barrage of nerve impulses firing in the CNS. The persistent barrage of nerve impulses results in long-term changes in nerve cell activity at the level of the spinal cord and higher centers in the brain. This phenomena is referred to as "central sensitization".
- It appears that peripheral and central sensitization persists after the injury apparently has healed. The sensitization of nociceptive neurons after injury results from the release of different chemicals from the damaged area.
- It is known that substance P and calcitonin gene-related peptides are released from peripheral nerve ending which stimulate most cells to release algesic substances which further potentiates the pain from the injury.
- In contrast, central sensitization resulting from severe and persistent injury which cause prolonged release of glutamate on

nociceptive dorsal horn cells, this constant glutamate release via G protein dependent phosphorylation cascades results in opening of postsynaptic ion channels gated by the NMDA receptors.
- This phenomenon is also termed "wind up". This activation produces hyperexcitability of the dorsal horn cells and causes "central sensitization". Pain experts now agree that treating chronic pain early and aggressively yields the best results and prevents patients from developing physical and psychological conditions that could worsen the pain.

Fibromyalgia

Fibromyalgia is characterized by widespread chronic pain throughout the body, including fatigue, anxiety and depression. It is now believed that it has a genetic component which tends to run in families.

Headaches

A *headache* is a poorly understood type of pain that can be either acute or chronic. There are about 300 different types and causes of headaches. The following are some categories of disorders associated with headaches:
- Intracranial structural disease
- Infectious disease
- Cerebrovascular ischemia
- Cerebral vein thrombosis
- Metabolic disease
- Toxic exposures
- Medications
- Extracranial pressure disorders
- Sinusitis
- Vasculitis and collagen vascular disease
- Hemorrhage (parenchymal and subarachnoid)
- Trauma
- Withdrawal syndromes
- Severe hypertension
- Dental, cranial vault, TMJ, and myofascial disorders
- Cervical spine and occipitocervical junction disorders.

Pain Assessment

Pain History

- Pain characteristics
- Onset—Sudden, gradual, traumatic
- Duration
- Location
  - Focal/Multifocal
  - Generalized/referred
  - Superficial/deep
- Quality
- Intensity
- Associated symptoms
- Exacerbating and relieving factors:
  - Circumstances in which pain is provoked or exacerbated
  - Specific activity or posture and any avoidance measure that can be taken to prevent onset.
  - Effect of medication and alternative medical approach.
- Past and current management therapies
- Relevant medical and family history
- Psychosocial history
- Impact of pain on daily life—work, daily activities, personal relationships, sleep, appetite, emotional state
- Patient (and family's) expected goals for treatment
- Ask the patient = even persons with moderate impairment (e.g. MMSE = 12) can still reliably report pain with good test-retest reliability.
- Preferred pain terminology is very important as the word for "pain" varies from person to person. Some people think of "pain" to be different from an intense ache or hurt. At bedside we should ask a variety of these qualifiers "Are you aching? Hurting? Having discomfort?" to illicit the best response
- Use a pain scale that works for that particular individual and remain consistent throughout subsequent interviews with the same patient
- *Use*: Simplest, clear explanation, give examples **(Fig. 6.13)**
  - Give time to grasp task and respond
  - Repetition KEY
- It is important to use a pain scale whenever possible as it can help guide you in terms of treatment efficacy. Studies have shown that

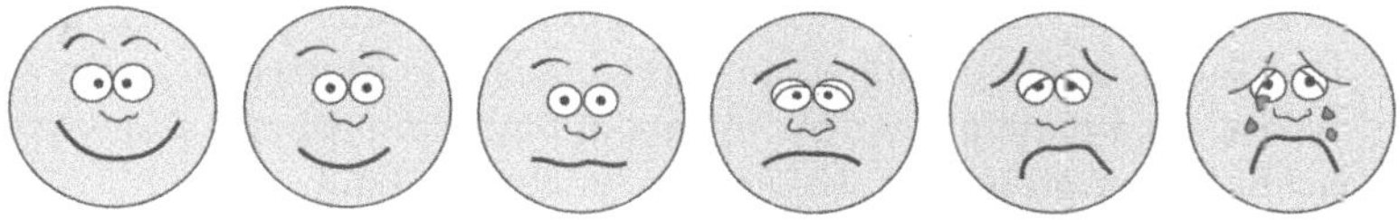
0
No hurt
1
Hurts
little bit
2
Hurts
little more
3
Hurts
even more
4
Hurts
whole lot
5
Hurts
worst

Fig. 6.13 Facial pain rating scale

more than 80% of cognitively impaired persons are able to reliably complete a pain scale. The importance is in finding one that works for the individual. I will give you some examples in the next few slides. When describing the tool to a cognitively impaired individual you want to be patient and give simple and clear explanations, providing examples whenever possible. You need to give the patient time to process the information and formulate a response. You may have to repeat the instructions a few times before they get it. Keep in mind that these patients are often hard of hearing and have poor vision so you need to make sure they are wearing their glasses and hearing aids.

- High rate of completion of tools even with low MMSE <12.

Technique

Pain must be assessed using a multidimensional approach, with determination of the following:

- Chronicity
- Severity
- Quality
- Contributing/associated factors
- Location/distribution or etiology of pain, if identifiable
- Mechanism of injury, if applicable
- Barriers to pain assessment.

Pain Scales

Pain measures fall into two categories:

1. *Single-dimensional scales*: These scales assess a single dimension of pain and, through patient self-reporting, measure only pain intensity; these scales are useful in acute pain when the etiology is clear.

2. *Multidimensional scales*: These measure the intensity, nature, and location of pain, as well as, in some cases, the impact that pain is having on a patient's activity or mood; multidimensional scales are useful in complex or persistent acute or chronic pain.

Pain Assessment in the Elderly

Pain assessment can be particularly difficult in elderly patients for the following reasons:

- Underreporting of discomfort because the patient does not want to complain
- Use of pain to mask other newly developing physical or cognitive disabilities
- Decreases in hearing and visual acuity, so that pain assessment tools that require extensive explanation or visualization to perform will be more difficult and possibly less reliable.

The verbal descriptor scale may be the easiest tool for the elderly to use. It allows patients to use common words to describe what they are feeling.

Pain Assessment in Infants

The following tools use a combination of behavioral and physiologic measurements to assess pain in infants:

- *CRIES*: Uses 5 variables (i.e. crying, requires oxygen, increased vital signs, expression, sleeplessness) on a scale of 0–2 points to assess neonatal postoperative pain.
- *Modified behavioral pain scale*: Uses 3 factors (facial expression, cry, movements); has been validated for children aged 2–6 months.

Core Principles of Pain Assessment

- Every older adult has the right to appropriate assessment and management of pain. Pain should be assessed in all individuals living in nursing homes.
- Pain is always subjective. Therefore, the individual's self-report of pain is the single most reliable indicator of pain. The therapist needs to accept and respect this self-report.
- Physiological and behavioral (objective) signs of pain (e.g. tachycardia, grimacing) are neither sensitive nor specific for pain. Such observations should not replace individual self-report unless the individual is unable to communicate.

- Assessment approaches, including tools, must be appropriate for the individual. Special considerations are needed for those with difficulty communicating. Family members should be included in the assessment process, when possible.
- Pain can exist even when no physical cause can be found. Thus, pain without an identifiable cause should not be routinely attributed to psychological causes or discounted.
- Different levels of pain in response to the same stimulus may be experienced by individuals; that is, a uniform pain threshold does not exist.
- Pain tolerance varies among and within individuals depending on factors including heredity, energy level, coping skills, and prior experiences with pain.
- Individuals with chronic pain may be more sensitive to pain and other stimuli.
- Unrelieved pain has adverse physical and psychological consequences. Therefore, clinicians should encourage the reporting of pain by individuals who are reluctant to discuss pain, deny pain when it is likely present, or fail to follow through on prescribed treatments.
- Pain is an unpleasant sensory and emotional experience, so assessment should address both physical and psychological aspects of pain.

7 Motor-sensory Link

REFLEX INTEGRITY

A reflex is an involuntary, predictable, and specific response to a stimulus dependent on an intact reflex arc (sensory receptor, afferent neuron(s), efferent neuron(s), and responding muscle(s) or gland).

SUPERFICIAL CUTANEOUS REFLEXES

- Superficial cutaneous reflexes are elicited with a light stroke applied to the skin.
- The expected response is brief contraction of muscles innervated by the same spinal segments receiving the afferent inputs from the cutaneous receptors.
- A stimulus that is strong may produce irradiation of cutaneous signals with activation of protective withdrawal reflexes.
- Cutaneous reflexes include the plantar reflex, confirming toe signs (Chaddock), and abdominal reflexes.

THE SUPERFICIAL REFLEXES OF THE UPPER EXTREMITIES

The Palmar Reflex

- *Stimulus*: Gentle stroking across the palm of hand.
- *Response*: Flexion of the fingers or a closing of the hand.
- *Abnormality*: The response is minimal or absent in normal individuals beyond the first few months of life. When exaggerated this response is referred to as a grasp reflex.
- *Reflex center*: Sensory and motor innervation is C6-T1 via the median and ulnar nerves.

The Scapular or Interscapular Reflex

- *Stimulus*: Scratching the skin over the scapula or in the interscapular space.

- *Response*: Contraction of the scapular muscles with retraction and sometimes elevation of the scapula; there may be associated adduction and external rotation of the arm.
- The reflex is related to the deep scapulohumeral reflex, and the innervation is similar.

The Superficial Abdominal Reflexes

- *Patient's position*: Supine.
- *Stimulus*: Brisk stroke over each quadrant of abdominals from periphery to umbilicus **(Fig. 7.1)**.
- *Response*: The response is a quick, flicking contraction followed by immediate relaxation.
- *Abnormality*: They may be sluggish or absent in normal individuals with lax abdominal tone, in those who are obese, or in women who have borne children.
- *Reflex center:*
  - *Upper abdominals*: T8-T9 spinal segment.
  - *Mid abdominal*: T10 spinal segment.
  - *Lower abdominals*: T11-T12 spinal segment.
- The epigastric reflex is similar, but elicited by a stimulus moving from the xiphoid toward the umbilicus, there is usually no retraction or movement of the umbilicus.

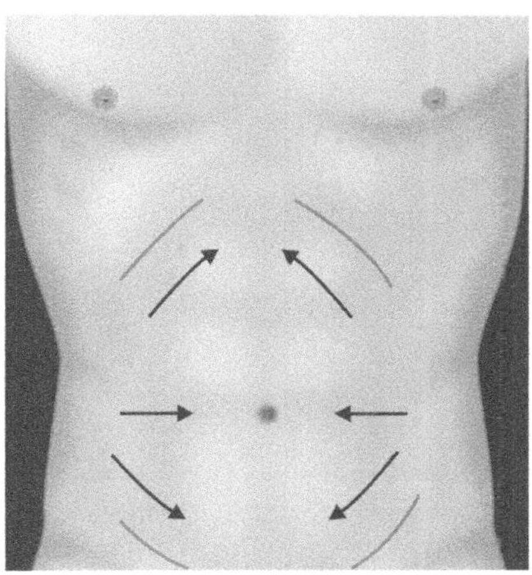

Fig. 7.1 Direction of stroking to elicit abdominal reflex

THE SUPERFICIAL REFLEXES OF THE LOWER EXTREMITIES

The Cremasteric Reflex

- *Stimulus*: This reflex is elicited by stroking or lightly scratching or pinching the skin on the upper, inner aspect of the thigh.
- *Response*: The response consists of a contraction of the cremasteric muscle with a quick elevation of the homolateral testicle **(Fig. 7.2)**.
- *Abnormality*: The cremasteric reflex may be absent in elderly males, in individuals who have a hydrocele or varicocele, and in those who have had orchitis or epididymitis.
- *Reflex center*: The innervations is through the ilioinguinal and genitofemoral nerves (L1-L2).
- The cremesteric reflex must not be confused with the scrotal, or dartos, reflex, which produces a slow, writhing, vermicular contraction of the scrotal skin on stroking the perineum or thigh or applying a cold object to the scrotum.

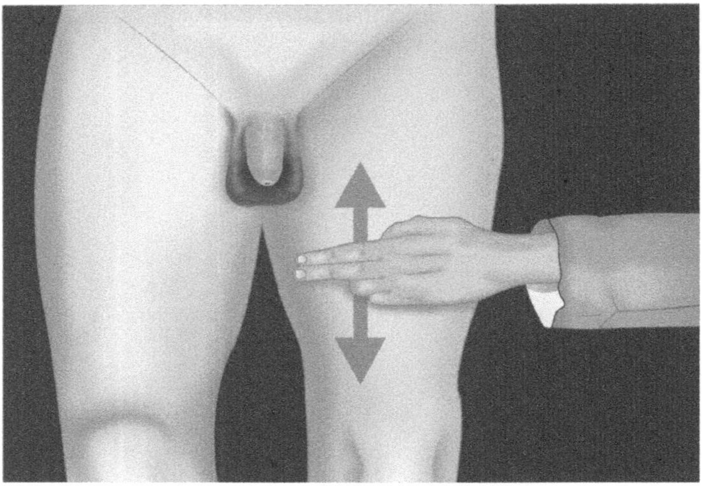

Fig. 7.2 Area of stroking for cremasteric reflex

The Gluteal Reflex

- *Stimulus*: Stroking the skin over the buttocks.
- *Response*: A contraction of the gluteal muscles may follow.
- *Reflex center*: The gluteus maximus is innervated by the inferior gluteal nerve (L4-S2), and the skin of this area is innervated by the cutaneous branches of the posterior rami of the lumbar and sacral nerves.

The Plantar Reflex

- *Stimulus*: Stroking the plantar surface of the foot from the heel forward is normally followed by plantar flexion of the foot and toes.
- *Response*: There is individual variation in the response, and some variability dependent upon the site of maximal stimulation. Flexion is the normal response after the first 12–18 months of life **(Fig. 7.3A)**.
- *Abnormality*: The pathologic variation of the plantar reflex is the Babinski sign. A tonic plantar reflex with slow, prolonged contraction has been described as a sign of frontal lobe and extrapyramidal disease **(Fig. 7.3B)**.
- *Reflex center*: This reflex is innervated by the tibial nerve (L4-S2).

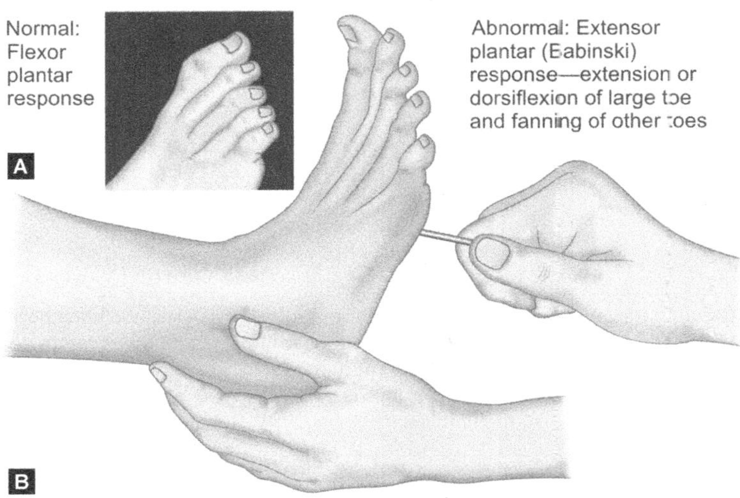

Figs 7.3A and B (A) Normal plantar response; (B) Abnormal plantar response (positive Babinski sign)

The Superficial Anal Reflex (Table 7.1)

- *Stimulus*: Stroking or pricking the skin or mucous membrane in the perianal region.
- *Response*: Contraction of the external sphincter.
- *Reflex center*: The reflex is mediated by the inferior hemorrhoidal nerve (S2-S5).
- Assessment of the superficial anal reflex is particularly important when a cauda equina or conus medullaris lesion is suspected.

Table 7.1: Examination of superficial reflexes

Superficial reflexes (Cutaneous)	*Stimulus*	*Response*
Plantar (S1,S2)	With blunt object (key or wooden end of applicator stick), stroke the lateral aspect of the sole, moving from the heel to the ball of the foot, curving medially across the ball of the foot Alternate stimuli for plantar (for sensitive feet): • *Chaddock*: Stroke lateral ankle and lateral aspect of foot • *Oppenheim*: Stroke down tibial crest	Normal response is flexion (plantar flexion) of the great toe, and sometimes the other toes (negative Babinski sign) Abnormal response, termed as positive Babinski sign, is extension (dorsiflexion) of the great toe with fanning of the four other toes (indicates UMN lesions) Same as for plantar
Abdominal reflexes Above umbilicus = T8-T10 Below umbilicus = T10-T12	Position patient in supine, relaxed. Make brisk, light stroke over each quadrant of the abdominals from the periphery to the umbilicus	Localized contraction under the stimulus, causing the umbilicus to move toward the stimulus Masked by obesity Can be absent in both UMN and LMN disorders

Clinical Importance of Superficial Reflexes

- In peripheral nerve disorder superficial reflexes are normal.
- In neuromuscular junction disorder superficial reflexes are normal.
- In muscle disorder superficial reflexes are normal, decrease or absent in involve nerve.
- In UMN disorder superficial reflexes are decrease or absent.
- In extrapyramidal disorder superficial reflexes are normal or slightly increase.
- In cerebellar disorder superficial reflexes are normal.
- In psychogenic disorder superficial reflexes are normal.

DEEP TENDON REFLEXES

- The deep tendon reflex (DTR) results from stimulation of the stretch-sensitive IA afferents of the neuromuscular spindle producing muscle contraction via a monosynaptic pathway.
- It is tested by tapping sharply over the muscle tendon with a standard reflex hammer or with the tips of therapist's fingers.
- To ensure adequate response, the muscle is positioned in midrange and the patient is instructed to relax.
- Stimulation can result in observable movement of the joint (brisk or strong responses). Weak responses may be evident only with palpation (slight or sluggish responses with little or no joint movement).
- Reflexes are graded on a 0 to 4+ scale:
  - 0 No response
  - 1 + present but depressed, low normal
  - 2 + Average, normal
  - 3 + increased, brisker than average; possibly but not necessarily abnormal
  - 4 + very brisk, hyperactive, with clonus; abnormal.

Technique

- The primary problem areas in eliciting DTRs are poor tools and poor technique. These reflexes are best tested using a high-quality rubber percussion hammer.
- To properly obtain a reflex, a crisp blow must be delivered to quickly stretch the tendon. It can be substituted by fingers, the edge of

a stethoscope or anything else handy, sometimes to the point of absurdity.

- A soft rubber hammer is most desirable. A blow with an ancient, desiccated, stony hard hammer may cause pain for the patient and interfere with the response.
- The hammer should never leave bruises on either the patient or the examiner.
- Proper technique is much more difficult to describe than to demonstrate. The hammer strike should be quick, direct, crisp and forceful, but no greater than necessary.
- The most effective blow is delivered quickly with a flick of the wrist, holding the handle of the hammer near its end and letting it spin through loosely held fingertips. Putting the index finger on top of the handle and using primarily elbow motion, common faults, make it much harder to achieve adequate velocity at the hammer head. Another common mistake is "pecking": striking the tendon with a timid, decelerating blow, pulling back at the last instant.
- The patient should be comfortable, relaxed, and properly positioned. It may help relaxation to divert the patient's attention with light conversation.
- The optimal position is usually about midway in the range of motion of the muscle to be tested. Sometimes, as in the ankle reflex, positioning includes passively stretching the muscle slightly.
- An adequate stimulus must be delivered to the proper spot. Reinforcement methods are necessary if the reflex is not obtainable in the usual way.
- The part of the body to be tested should be in an optimal position for the response. In order to compare the reflexes on the two sides of the body, the position of the extremities should be symmetric.
- During the reflex examination, the patient should keep the head straight, since looking to one side, as is the temptation, may alter reflex tone, especially in the arms (tonic neck reflex).
- The DTRs may be influenced to some degree by voluntary mental effort. Merely by concentrating some individuals are able to somehow alter reflex excitability. Mentally induced reflex asymmetry is possible and may be clinically relevant in some cases.
- The examiner can feel as well as see the contraction. Placing one hand over the muscle is often useful, especially when responses are

sluggish. A reflex quadriceps contraction can sometimes be felt even when insufficient to produce visible contraction or knee movement.

- The activity of a reflex is judged by the speed and vigor of the response, the range of movement, and the duration of the contraction. An absent reflex often makes a dull, thudding sound when the tendon is struck.
- The DTRs usually examined include the biceps, triceps, brachioradialis, knee (quadriceps), and ankle (Achilles) tendon reflexes.
  - If DTRs are difficult to elicit, the responses can be enhanced by specific reinforcement maneuvers.
  - Jendrassik maneuver
    - The patient hooks together the fingers of hands and attempts to pull them apart. While this pressure is maintained, lower extremity reflexes are tested.
    - Maneuvers that can be used to reinforce responses in the upper extremities include squeezing the knees together, clenching the teeth, or making a fist with the contralateral extremity.

The Biceps Reflex

- *Position of limb*: With the arm relaxed and the forearm slight pronated and midway between flexion and extension.
- *Therapist's grasping and taping*: Therapist places the palmar surface of her extended thumb or finger on the patient's biceps tendon, and then strikes the extensor surface with the reflex hammer. Pressure on the tendon should be light; too much pressure exerted with the thumb or finger against the tendon makes the reflex much harder to obtain. The examiner may hold the patient's arm with the elbow resting in her hand **(Fig. 7.4)**.
- *Response*: Contraction of the biceps muscle with flexion of the elbow. Since the biceps is also a supinator, there is often a certain amount of supination.

Exaggerated reflex: If the reflex is exaggerated, the reflexogenic zone is increased and the reflex may even be obtained by tapping the clavicle.

Reflex spread: There may be abnormal spread with accompanying flexion of the wrist and fingers and adduction of the thumb.

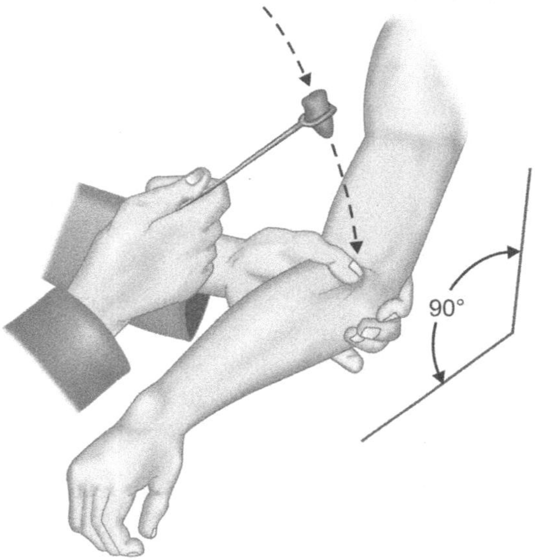

Fig. 7.4 Biceps reflex

The Triceps Reflex

- *Position of limb*: The arm is placed midway between flexion and extension, and may be rested in the patient's lap, on her thigh or hip, or on the therapist hand.
- *Tapping*: This reflex is elicited by tapping the triceps tendon just above its insertion on the olecranon process of the ulna **(Fig. 7.5)**.
- *Response*: The response is contraction of the triceps muscle with extension of the elbow.
- *Paradoxical or inverted triceps jerk*: It consists of flexion of the elbow with percussion of the triceps tendon. This response appears when the afferent arc of the triceps reflex is damaged, as in lesions of the seventh and eighth cervical segments, particularly when there is an element of spasticity, as in cervical spondylosis with radiculomyelopathy.

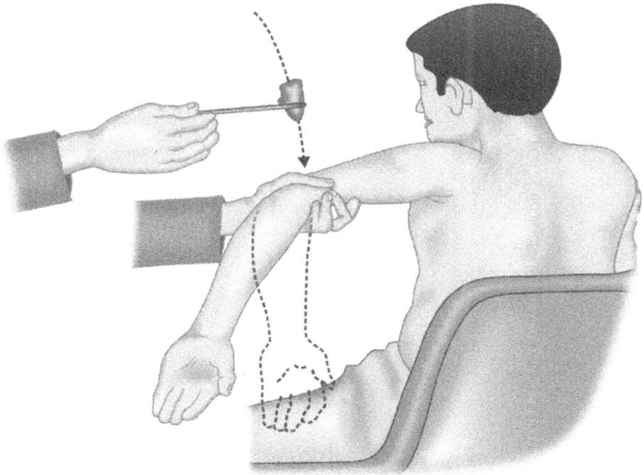

Fig. 7.5 Triceps reflex

The Brachioradialis (Radial Periosteal or Supinator) Reflex

- *Position of limb*: The forearm in semi flexion and semipronation causes flexion of the elbow, with variable supination. The supination is more marked with the forearm extended and pronated, but there is less flexion.
- *Tapping*: Tapping just above the styloid process of the radius **(Fig. 7.6)**.
- *Response*: A local contraction can be elicited from any muscle by directly striking the muscle belly.
- *Exaggerated reflex*: If the reflex is exaggerated, there is associated flexion of the wrist and fingers, with adduction of the forearm. When the afferent limb of the reflex is impaired, there may be a twitch of the flexors of the hand and fingers without flexion and supination of the elbow; this is termed inversion of the reflex.

The following upper-extremity reflexes may be elicited only to a slight extent in normal persons. They may become conspicuous when there is hyperreflexia.

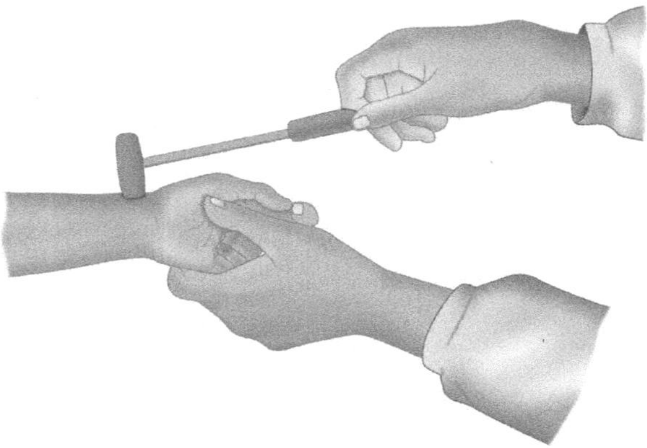

Fig. 7.6 Brachioradialis reflex

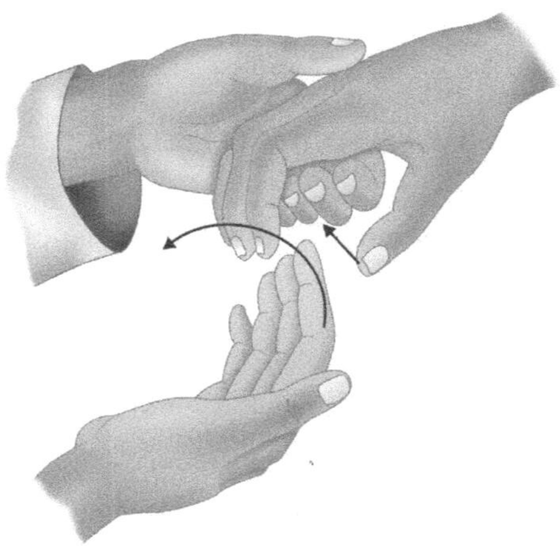

Fig. 7.7 The finger flexor reflex (Wartenberg's sign)

This is one of several signs attributed to Robert Wartenberg.

- *Position of limb*: To elicit the finger flexor reflex, the patient's hand is in supination, resting on a table or a solid surface, with the fingers slightly flexed.
- *Therapist grasping*: The examiner places her fingers against the patient's fingers, and taps the backs of her own fingers lightly with the reflex hammer **(Fig. 7.7)**.

- *Response*: The response is flexion of the patient's fingers and the distal phalanx of the thumb. The reflex may be reinforced by having the patient flex her fingers slightly as the blow is delivered.
- *Alternate technique*: An alternate technique is for the patient to hold the hand in the air, palm down, the examiner touching fingers with palm up, with the blow delivered in an upward direction from below. The nerve supply, as in the wrist flexion reflex, is through the median and ulnar nerves (C8-T1). This reflex is difficult for the inexperienced examiner to elicit, and it is often absent in normals.

The Scapulohumeral Reflex

- *Stimulus*: Tapping over the vertebral border of the scapula, either at the tip of its spine or at its base near the inferior angle **(Fig. 7.8)**.
- *Response*: Causes retraction of the scapula through action of the rhomboid muscles reflex center—dorsal scapular nerve, C4-C5.

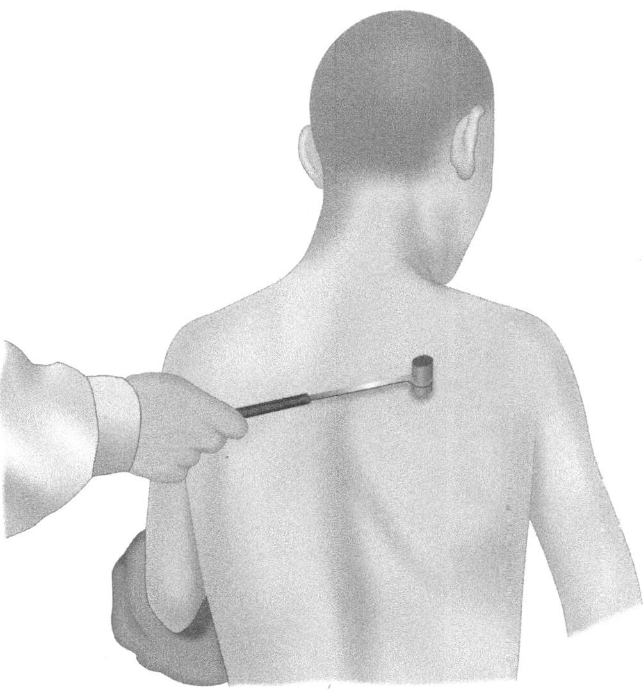

Fig. 7.8 Scapulohumeral reflex

- There may be associated elevation of the scapula and adduction and external rotation of the humerus through the trapezius, latissimus dorsi, infraspinatus, and teres minor.

The Deltoid Reflex

- *Stimulus*: Tapping over the insertion of the deltoid muscle at the junction of the upper and middle third of the lateral aspect of the humerus.
- *Response*: Slight abduction of the upper arm.
- *Reflex center*: Axillary nerve, C5-C6.

The Pectoralis Reflex

- *Position of limb*: With the patient's arm in midposition between abduction and adduction.
- *Therapist's grasping*: The examiner places her finger as nearly as possible on the tendon of the pectoralis major muscle near its insertion on the greater tuberosity of the humerus **(Fig. 7.9)**.
- *Stimulus*: Tapping the finger causes adduction and slight internal rotation of the arm at the shoulder.
- *Response*: The contraction of the muscle may be felt but usually not seen in the normal individual.

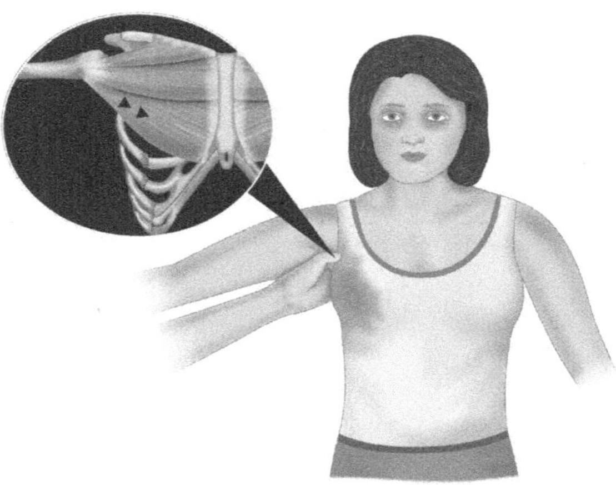

Fig. 7.9 Pectoralis reflex

- *Abnormality*: In patients with cervical spondylotic myelopathy, a hyperactive pectoralis reflex indicates spinal cord compression at the C2-C3 and/or C3-C4 levels.
- *Reflex center*: This reflex is mediated by the medial and lateral pectoral (anterior thoracic) nerves (C5-T1).

The Latissimus Dorsi Reflex

- *Position of limb*: With the patient prone and her arm abducted and in slight external rotation.
- *Therapist's grasping*: The examiner places her fingers on the tendon of the Lattisimus dorsi near its insertion in the intertubercular groove of the humerus.
- *Stimulus*: Tapping her finger with the reflex hammer.
- *Response*: This produces abduction and slight internal rotation of the shoulder.
- *Reflex center*: This reflex is mediated by the thoracodorsal (long sub scapular) nerve (C6-C8).

The Clavicle Reflex

- *Stimulus*: A tap over the lateral aspect of the clavicle.
- *Response*: Extensive contraction of various muscle groups in the upper limb.
- There are individual variations, but normally the response should be the same on each side.
- This is not a specific reflex, but an indication of spread of the reflex response.
- It is useful in comparing the reflex activity of the two upper limbs.

The Pronator Reflex

- *Position of limb*: With the elbow in semiflexion and the forearm semipronated.
- *Stimulus*: Tapping over either the volar surface of the distal radius or the dorsal aspect of the styloid process of the ulna.
- *Response*: Produce brief supination followed by pronation of the forearm. There may also be flexion of the wrist and fingers.
- The major muscles participating in this response are the pronator teres and pronator quadratus.

- *Abnormality*: This reflex may be exaggerated early when corticospinal tract lesions develop.

The Wrist Extension Reflex

- *Position of limb*: With the forearm pronated and the wrist hanging down.
- *Stimulus*: Tapping the extensor tendons of the wrist.
- *Response*: Contraction of the extensor muscles and extension at the wrist.
- *Abnormality*: Under certain circumstances there may be flexion of the wrist and fingers on tapping the dorsum of the carpometacarpal area.
- *Reflex center*: This reflex is mediated by the radial nerve (C6-C8).

The Wrist Flexion Reflex

- *Position of limb*: With the hand supinated and the fingers slightly flexed.
- *Stimulus*: Tapping the flexor tendons of the wrist on the volar surface of the forearm at or above the transverse carpal ligament.
- *Response*: Contraction of the flexor muscles of the hand and fingers.
- *Reflex center*: This reflex is innervated by the median and ulnar nerves (C6-T1).
- This is also known as the hand flexor reflex.

The Thumb Reflex

Tapping the flexor pollicis longus tendon just above the pronator quadratus is followed by flexion of the distal phalanx of the thumb.

The Patellar Reflex (Quadriceps Reflex, Knee Jerk)

- *Stimulus*: A firm tap on the tendon draws the patella down, stretching the quadriceps, provoking reflex contraction.
- *Therapist grasping*: If the examiner places one hand over the muscle, and with the other hand taps the patellar tendon just below the patella, she can palpate the contraction as well as observe the rapidity and range of response. Palpation helps in judging the latency between the time of the stimulus and the resulting response.

- *Position of patient*: The patient may sit in a chair with the knees slightly extended and the heels resting on the floor, or sit on an examination table with the legs dangling. If the patient is lying in bed, the examiner should partially flex the knee by placing one hand beneath it and then tap the tendon **(Fig. 7.10)**.
- *Response*: Slight contraction of knee extensors.
- The responses on the two sides can be compared by lifting both knees simultaneously, supporting them on one forearm as the patient's heels rest lightly on the bed, before tapping the tendons.

Another Technique

Position of limb: Patient sit with one leg crossed over the other and tapping the patellar tendon of the uppermost leg, but this method does not facilitate side-to-side comparison.

- *Reflex center*: The patellar reflex is mediated by the femoral nerve (L2-L4).
- *Reflex spread*: If there is reflex spread, extension of the knee may be accompanied by adduction of the hip, which on occasion is bilateral, or there may be bilateral knee extension.
- *Abnormality*:
  - If the reflex is brisk, the contraction is strong and the amplitude of the movement is large.

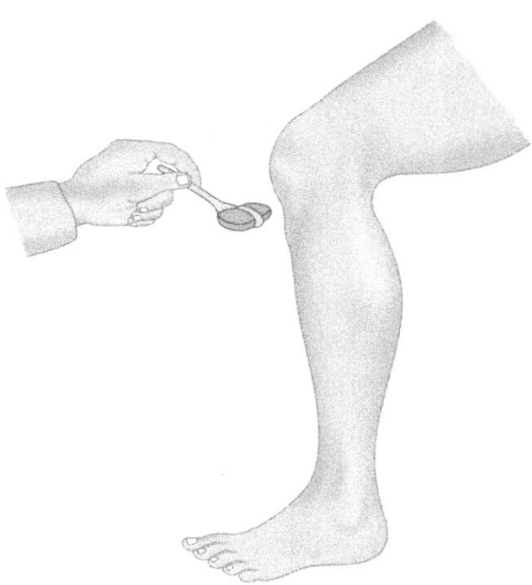

Fig. 7.10 Patellar reflex

- *Exaggerated reflex*: If the reflex is exaggerated, the response may be obtained not only by tapping the tendon in the usual spot, but also just above the patella (suprapatellar or epipatellar reflex); the tendon can be tapped directly, or, with the patient recumbent, the examiner can place her index finger on the upper border of the patella and tap the finger to push down the patella.
- Marked exaggeration of the patellar reflex may be accompanied by patellar clonus.
- Absence of the patellar reflex is known as Westphal's sign.
- An inverted patellar reflex may be seen with lesions of the nerve or nerve roots supplying the quadriceps—tapping the patellar tendon results in contraction of the hamstrings and flexion of the knee.

The Achilles Reflex (Ankle Jerk, Triceps Surae Reflex)

The ankle jerk is obtained by striking the Achilles tendon just above its insertion on the calcaneus. The resulting contraction of the posterior crural muscles, the gastrocnemius, soleus, and plantaris, causes plantar flexion of the foot at the ankle.

- *Position of patient*: If the patient is seated or lying in bed, the thigh should be held in moderate abduction and external rotation and the knee flexed **(Fig. 7.11)**.
- *Alternate method*: If the patient is supine, access to the tendon requires placing the legs into a frog-leg position with the knees apart and the ankles close together. Some prefer to have the patient cross the leg to be examined atop the other shin or ankle ("figure four position", as the legs form a 4). The examiner should place one hand under the foot and pull upward slightly to passively dorsiflex the ankle to about a right angle.
- *Reflex center*: The Achilles reflex is mediated by the tibial nerve (S1).
- The ankle jerk is by far the most difficult reflex to master.
- *There are two critical variables*: Proper stretch and efficient striking.
- Too much passive dorsiflexion makes the tendon too taut and unable to be stretched.
- *Abnormality*:
  - *Hyperactive ankle jerk*: If the ankle jerk is hyperactive, it may be elicited by tapping other areas of the sole of the foot, the medioplantar reflex, or by tapping the anterior aspect of the ankle, the paradoxical ankle reflex.

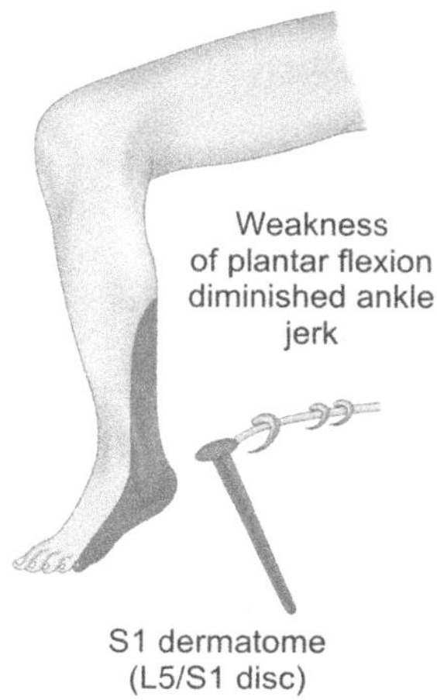

Fig. 7.11 Ankle jerk

- A hyperactive reflex may also result in extra beats or even clonus when the tendon is percussed.
- *Reflex spread*: When there is reflex spread, striking the achilles tendon may cause flexion of the knee. Although the achilles reflex, when carefully elicited, should be present in normal individuals, it tends to diminish with age and its bilateral absence in elderly individuals is not necessarily of clinical significance.

The knee and ankle reflexes are the most important DTRs in the lower extremities. The following reflexes are less significant. The response may be minimal or even absent in normal individuals. Because the responses may be difficult to elicit even in normal subjects, side-to-side comparison is critical. To be significant, absence must be unilateral exaggeration of these difficult-to-obtain reflexes suggests the presence of corticospinal tract disease.

The Adductor Reflex (Obturator Nerve, L2-L4)

- *Position of limb*: With the thigh in slight abduction.
- *Stimulus*: Tapping over either the medial epicondyle of the femur in the vicinity of the adductor tubercle, or the medial condyle of the tibia.

- *Response*: Contraction of the adductor muscles of the thigh and inward movement of the extremity.
- *Abnormality*:
  - *Exaggerated reflex*: If the reflex is exaggerated, there may be crossed, or bilateral, adduction. A slight crossed adductor response is not necessarily abnormal, but strong crossed adduction, or adduction of the opposite leg when obtaining the knee jerk, suggests corticospinal tract disease.
  - *Hyperreflexia*: When there is hyperreflexia, an adductor response may also be obtained while the patient is seated by tapping the spinous processes of the sacral or lumbar vertebrae (the spinal adductor reflex) or by tapping the crest or the superior spines of the ilium.
  - *Absent reflex*: An absent adductor reflex with a normal patellar reflex has been described as a sign of strangulated obturator hernia (Hannington-Kiff sign).

The Internal Hamstring (Semimembranosus and Semitendinosus, or Posterior Tibiofemoral) Reflex

This reflex is elicited by striking the semitendinosus and semimembranosus tendons just above their insertions on the tibia.

- *Patient's position*: This may be done with the patient seated or recumbent, with the leg abducted and slightly rotated externally and the knee flexed.
- *Stimulus*: The therapist fingers are placed over the tendons on the medial posterior aspect of the knee, and the fingers tapped with the reflex hammer.
- *Response*: The response is knee flexion.
- *Reflex center*: This reflex is mediated by tibial portion of the sciatic nerve, primarily by the L5 nerve root. It is the only DTR useful in the evaluation of suspected L5 radiculopathy.

The External Hamstring (Biceps Femoris, or Posterior Peroneo-femoral) Reflex

- This reflex is elicited by striking the biceps femoris tendon just above its insertion.
- *Patient's position*: With the patient sitting, recumbent or lying on the opposite side, and the knee moderately flexed.

- *Stimulus*: The therapist fingers are placed over the tendon on the lateral posterior aspect of the knee and tapped.
- *Response*: The response is knee flexion. The reflex may also be elicited by tapping the head of the fibula (fibular reflex).
- *Reflex center*: This reflex is mediated by tibial portion of the sciatic nerve, primarily by the S1 nerve root.
- The external hamstring reflex is sometimes helpful in sorting out whether an absent ankle jerk is due to peripheral neuropathy or radiculopathy. If due to neuropathy, the external hamstring will usually be preserved, but in radiculopathy it may be depressed in concert with the ankle reflex.

The Tensor Fascia Lata Reflex (Superior Gluteal Nerve, L4-S1)

This reflex is tested by tapping over the origin of the tensor fascia lata near the anterior superior iliac spine, with the patient recumbent. The response consists of slight abduction of the thigh.

The Gluteal Reflexes

- *Stimulus*: Tapping the lower portion of the sacrum or the posterior aspect of the ilium near the origin of the gluteus maximus muscle.
- *Response*: Contraction of the muscle and extension of the thigh.
- This reflex is best tested with the patient recumbent, with her weight on the opposite side so there is moderate flexion of the ipsilateral thigh; it may also be elicited with the patient prone.
- *Reflex center*: The reflex is mediated by the inferior gluteal nerve (L5-S2).

A gluteus medius reflex may on occasion be elicited by striking the anterior iliac crest near the site of origin of the muscle. The response is slight abduction and medial rotation of the hip. The innervation is the same as for the tensor fascia.

The Extensor Hallucis Longus Reflex

- *Stimulus*: Using a finger, the examiner pushes down on the dorsal surface of the great toe; tapping the finger.
- *Response*: Extension of the toe that may be felt more than seen.

- *Reflex center*: This reflex is mediated by the deep peroneal nerve, primarily by the L5 nerve root. The response may be absent in L5 radiculopathy.

The Tibialis Posterior Reflex (Tibial Nerve, L5-S1)

- *Stimulus*: Tapping the tendon of the tibialis posterior just above and behind the medial malleolus.
- *Response*: Inversion of the foot.
- This reflex is best examined with the patient prone and the foot, in a neutral position or in slight eversion, extended beyond the edge of the bed. The leg should be supported by the examiner and slightly flexed at the knee. It may be absent in L5 or S1 radiculopathy.

The Peroneal (Tibialis Anterior) Reflex

- *Position of limb*: With the patient's foot plantar flexed and inverted.
- *Stimulus*: The examiner presses a finger firmly over the distal ends of the first and second metatarsal bones.
- *Response*: A brisk tap to the finger is followed by eversion and dorsiflexion of the foot.
- The reflex is due to contraction of muscles supplied by the deep and superficial peroneal nerves (L4-S1).

The Plantar Muscle Reflexes

There are numerous reflexes in which the response is flexion of the toes. These are difficult to elicit in normal individuals, of limited clinical significance, and of importance only when exaggerated.

ABNORMALITIES OF THE DEEP TENDON (MUSCLE STRETCH) REFLEXES (TABLE 7.2)

Abnormal DTRs are either hypoactive or hyperactive.

- When hypoactive, the response varies from diminished or sluggish to complete absence of the reflex.
- Hyperactive reflexes are characterized by varying degrees of decreased latency, increased speed and vigor of response, increased range of movement, decrease in threshold, extension of the reflexogenic zone, and prolongation of the muscular contraction.

Table 7.2: Examination of deep tendon reflexes

Myotactic reflexes (stretch)	*Nerve*	*Root*	*Stimulus*	*Response*
Jaw	Cranial nerve V		Patient is sitting, with jaw relaxed and slightly open. Place finger on top of chin; tap downward on top of finger in a direction which causes the jaw to open	Jaw rebounds and closes
Biceps	Musculocutaneous nerve	C5, C6	Patient is sitting with arm flexed and supported. Place thumb over the biceps tendon in the cubital fossa, stretching it slightly. Tap thumb or directly on tendon	Slight contraction of elbow flexors
Brachioradialis (supinator)	Radial nerve	C5, C6	Patient is sitting with arm flexed onto the abdomen. Place finger on the radial tuberosity and tap finger with hammer	Slight contraction of elbow flexors, slight wrist extension or radial deviation
Triceps	Radial nerve	C6, C7	Patient is sitting with arm supported in abduction, elbow flexed. Palpate triceps tendon just above olecranon. Tap directly on tendon	Slight contraction of elbow extensors
Finger flexors	Median nerve	C6-T1	Hold hand in neutral position. Place fingers across palmar surface of distal phalanges of four fingers and tap	Slight contraction of finger flexors

Contd...

Contd...

Myotactic reflexes (stretch)	*Nerve*	*Root*	*Stimulus*	*Response*
Hamstrings	Tibial branch, sciatic nerve	L5, S1, S2	Patient is prone with knee semi flexed and supported. Palpate tendon at the knee. Tap on finger or directly on tendon	Slight contraction of knee flexors
Quadriceps (patellar, knee jerk)	Femoral nerve	L2,L3,L4	Patient is sitting with knee flexed, foot unsupported. Tap tendon of quadriceps muscle between the patella and tibial tuberosity	Slight contraction of knee extensors
Achilles (ankle jerk)	Tibial	S1-S2	Patient is prone with foot over end of the plinth or sitting with knee flexed and foot held in slight dorsiflexion. Tap tendon just above its insertion on the calcaneus. Maintaining slight tension on the gastrocnemius-soleus group improves the response	Slight contraction of plantar flexors

- The reflexes should be compared on the two sides of the body, the arms to the legs, and the knees to the ankles.
- The DTRs are normally symmetric, and reflexes otherwise normal may be abnormal if different from expected. For example, a 1+ biceps jerk in a patient with suspected cervical radiculopathy, while "normal", may be judged abnormal if the opposite biceps jerk is 2+.
- The DTRs are usually comparable in the upper and lower extremities. Slight differences are permissible but a pronounced difference may be significant (e.g. in thoracic myelopathy the DTRs in the legs may be much brisker than in the arms, even though not clearly pathologic).

- A proximal to distal gradient may also be significant. Symmetric 1+ ankle jerks when all of the other reflexes are 2+ may signal mild peripheral neuropathy. When asymmetry is the main finding, it is sometimes difficult to tell whether one side is increased or the other side decreased.

Hypoactive Reflexes

- When a reflex is hypoactive, there is a sluggish response and/or a diminution in the range of response.
- An increase in stimulus intensity may be necessary to elicit the reflex, or repeated blows may be necessary, for a single stimulus may be subliminal. A DTR is absent if it is not obtained even with reinforcement.
- A depressed or absent reflex results from dysfunction of some component of the reflex arc. Interference with the afferent limb may be caused by lesions involving the sensory nerve, posterior root, dorsal root ganglion, or intramedullary pathways between the dorsal root entry zone and the anterior horn (e.g. syringomyelia).
- Abnormalities of the motor unit and final common pathway that make up the efferent limb of the reflex arc occur in many conditions, but particularly with radiculopathy and peripheral nerve lesions. In neurogenic processes, DTRs are lost out of proportion to atrophy and weakness.
  - With a *peripheral nerve lesion*, a reflex may not return until much of the motor function has recovered. Sometimes there is persistent areflexia following lesions of the nerve root or peripheral nerve, even after complete return of both motor and sensory functions. In myasthenia gravis the reflexes are affected only when there is severe and extensive involvement, but in Lambert-Eaton syndrome depressed reflexes are common.
  - In *periodic paralysis*, DTRs may be temporarily absent during attacks.
  - In *myopathy*, reflexes are lost in proportion to the atrophy and weakness.
  - When *atrophy* and weakness are severe, reflexes may disappear. In many forms of muscular dystrophy, the proximal reflexes disappear early, while the distal reflexes may persist until the later stages of the disease.

The DTRs may also be decreased or absent in various other conditions.

- They are often absent in *deep coma, narcosis, heavy sedation,* and *deep sleep.* They are characteristically absent during nerve block, caudal anesthesia, and spinal anesthesia.
- They are absent in spinal shock following a sudden transverse lesion of the spinal cord, but reappear below the level of the lesion after a period of 3–4 weeks, and usually become hyperactive.
- In Adie's syndrome, the tonic pupils are accompanied by depressed or absent reflexes.
- *Delayed relaxation* may also occur in *myotonic disorders.*
- In *diabetic neuropathy,* there may be either prolongation of the reflex time or decrease or absence of the reflexes before there is other evidence of nervous system involvement.
- The reflexes may appear to be decreased or absent in neurologic disorders in which there is marked spasticity or rigidity with contractures and in diseases of the joints characterized by inflammation, contractures, and ankylosis.
- The apparent hyporeflexia is due to lack of motility at the joint or pain on moving the joint; careful observation may disclose a muscle contraction even though there is no movement at the joint.

Hyperactive Reflexes

- *Reflex hyperactivity is characterized by the following*: A decrease in reflex threshold; a decrease in the latency, the time between tendon percussion and the reflex contraction; an exaggeration of the power and range of movement; prolongation of the reflex contraction; extension of the reflexogenic zone (or zone of provocation); and spread of the reflex response.
- When the reflex threshold is decreased, a minimal stimulus may evoke the reflex, and reflexes that are not normally obtained may be elicited with ease.
- Very hyperactive DTRs may sometimes be elicited with extremely slight percussion.
- Another manifestation of decreased reflex threshold may be a widening of the area from which the reflex may be elicited, and application of the stimulus to sites at some distance from the usual one may evoke the response; the patellar reflex may be elicited by tapping the tibia or dorsum of the foot, and the biceps and other arm reflexes by tapping the scapula.

- There may also be abnormal spread of the response.
- One stimulus may provoke repetitive responses and sometimes elicit sustained clonus.
- The DTRs become hyperactive with *lesions of the corticospinal or pyramidal* system. Spasticity and hyperreflexia are likely related to involvement of a variety of structures in the descending motor pathways at cortical, subcortical, midbrain, and brainstem levels.
- Hyperreflexia results from a lowering of the reflex threshold due to increased excitability of the lower motor neuron pool related to dysfunction of some or all of these structures. From a clinical point of view, the terms pyramidal, corticospinal, or upper motor neuron are used to encompass these changes.
- A lesion at any level of the corticospinal system or other related upper motor neuron components, from the motor cortex to just above the segment of origin of a reflex arc, will be accompanied by spasticity and hyperreflexia. The characteristic posture in hemiplegia is flexion of the upper extremities, with more marked weakness of the extensors; and extension of the lower extremities, with more marked weakness of the flexors. Consequently, the flexor reflexes are exaggerated to a greater degree in the upper extremities, and the extensor reflexes in the lower.
- The reflexes may be present in spinal cord lesions in spite of the absence of sensation. A reflex may be increased if the tone of the antagonist muscle is diminished (e.g. an increased knee jerk may occur if there is weakness of the hamstrings).
  - Exaggeration of the DTRs may occur in *psychogenic disorders, and in anxiety,* the reflexes vary in these conditions; they may be normal, or they may be decreased owing to voluntary or involuntary tension of the antagonistic muscle, but they are most frequently increased.
  - There is no increase in the reflexogenic zone in *psychogenic lesions,* and although there may be irregular repeated jerky movements (spurious clonus), no true clonus is present. Furthermore, there are no other signs of organic disease of the corticospinal system.
  - *In lesions of the extra pyramidal system* there are no consistent reflex changes. The activity of the response depends on the level of muscle tone, and the amount of rigidity that is present. Usually the reflexes are slightly exaggerated, owing to increased muscle tone, but this is not a consistent finding. Rigidity may cause depression or absence of the reflexes.

- In *diseases of the cerebellum* the reflexes may be diminished and pendular: Eliciting the patellar reflex while the foot is hanging free, may elicit a series of to-and-fro pendular movements of the foot and leg before the limb finally comes to rest. The increased swinging may result from hypotonia of the extensor and flexor muscles and a lack of the restraining influence they normally exert on each other.
- The *pendular response* may also be observed in chorea, but there is more frequently a "hung" reflex: If the patellar tendon is tapped while the foot is hanging free, the knee may be held in extension for a few seconds before relaxing, because of prolonged contraction of the quadriceps. In chorea, the response may not be obtained until the stimulus has been applied a number of times.
- Inverted and perverted reflexes occasionally, percussion of a tendon produce unexpected results.

Clinical importance of deep reflexes:
- In peripheral nerve disorder DTR is decrease or absent.
- In neuromuscular junction disorder DTR is normal or decrease.
- In muscle disorder DTR is normal, decrease in proportion to muscle weakness.
- In UMN disorder DTR is exaggerated.
- In extrapyramidal disorder DTR is normal or slightly increase or decrease.
- In cerebellar disorder DTR is pendular.
- In psychogenic disorder DTR is normal or increased.

Primitive and Tonic Reflexes (Table 7.3)

- Primitive and tonic reflexes are normally present during infancy and become integrated by the CNS at an early age. Once integrated, these reflexes are not generally recognizable in adults in their pure form. They may continue, however, as adaptive fragments of behavior, underlying normal motor control.
- Adult patients with brain injury (e.g. stroke, traumatic brain injury) may exhibit primitive and tonic reflexes affecting voluntary movement control and posture.
- Patients who exhibit these reflexes typically present with extensive brain damage and other UMN signs.

- Obligatory and sustained responses that dominate motor behavior are always considered pathological in the adult.
- Reflexes important to examine in the patient suspected of abnormal reflex activity include flexor withdrawal, traction, grasp, tonic neck, tonic labyrinthine, positive support and associated reactions.

Table 7.3: Examination of primitive reflexes

Primitive/spinal reflexes	*Stimulus*	*Response*
Flexor withdrawal **(Fig. 7.12)**	Noxious stimulus (pinprick) to sole of foot. Tested in supine or sitting position	Toes extend, foot dorsiflexes, entire LE flexes uncontrollably *Onset*: 28 weeks gestation *Integrated*: 1–2 months
Extensor thrust **(Fig. 7.12)**	Noxious stimuli to ball of one foot, knee is held straight	
Crossed extension	Noxious stimulus to ball of foot of LE fixed in extension; tested in supine position	Opposite LE flexes, then adducts and extends. *Onset*: 28 weeks gestation *Integrated*: 1–2 months
Traction **(Fig. 7.13)**	Grasp forearm and pull up from supine into sitting position	Grasp and total flexion of the UE *Onset*: 28 weeks gestation *Integrated*: 2–5 months
Moro	Sudden change in position of head in relation to trunk; drop patient backwards from sitting position	Extension, abduction of UEs, hand opening, and crying followed by flexion, adduction of arms across chest. *Onset*: 28 weeks gestation *Integrated*: 5–6 months
Startle	Sudden loud or harsh noise	Sudden extension or abduction of UEs, crying *Onset*: Birth *Integrated*: Persists
Grasp **(Figs 7.14A and B)**	Maintained pressure to palm of hand (palmar grasp) or to ball of foot under toes (plantar grasp)	Maintained flexion of fingers or toes. *Onset*: Palmar, birth, plantar, 28 weeks gestation *Integrated*: Palmar, 4–6 months; plantar, 9 months

- To obtain an accurate examination, the must be concerned with several factors.
  - The patient must be positioned appropriately to allow for the expected response.
  - An adequate test stimulus is essential, including both an adequate magnitude and duration of stimulation.
  - Keen observation skills are needed to detect what may be subtle movement changes and abnormal responses.
  - Palpation skills can assist in identifying tonal changes not readily apparent to eye.
  - Objective scoring of responses is essential.

A reflex scoring key:

- 0+ absent
- 1+ tone change: Slight, transient with no movement of extremities
- 2+ visible movement of extremities
- 3+ exaggerated, full movements of extremities
- 4+ obligatory and sustained movement, lasting for more than 30 seconds.

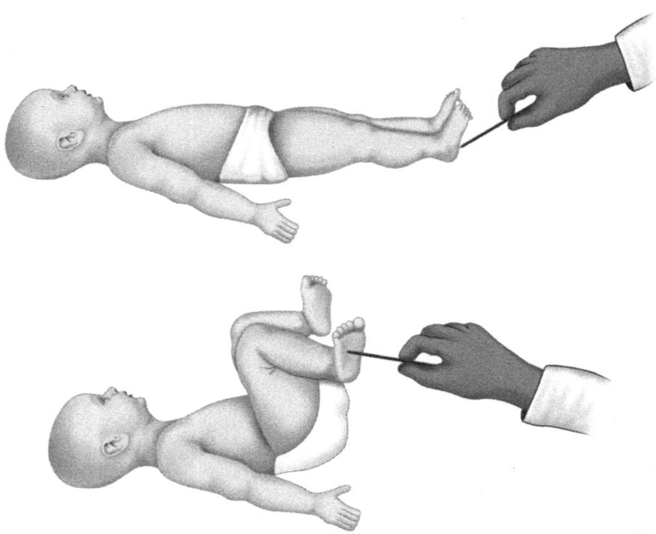

Fig. 7.12 Extensor thrust and flexor withdrawal

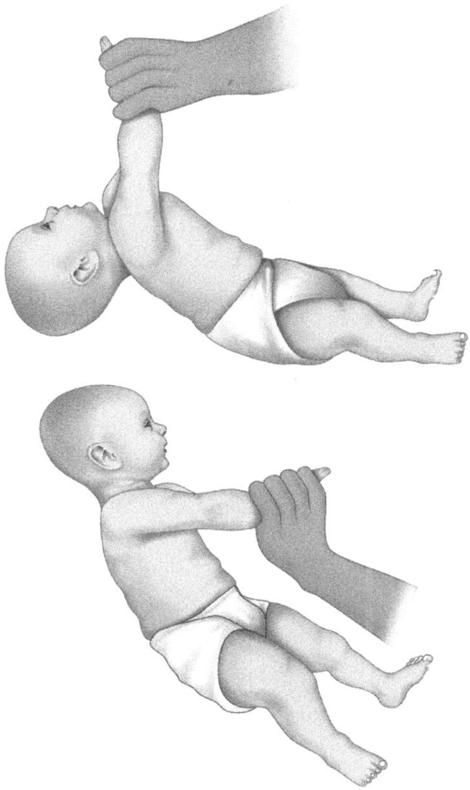

Fig. 7.13 Traction reflex

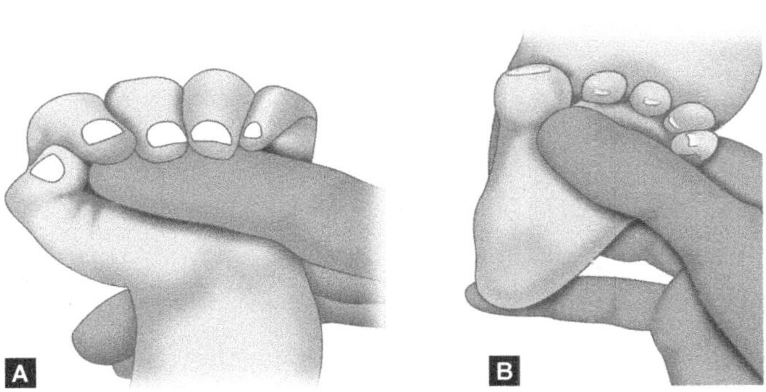

Figs 7.14A and B Grasp: (A) Palmar grasp; (B) Plantar grasp

EXAMINATION OF PRIMITIVE AND TONIC REFLEXES (TABLE 7.4)

Table 7.4: Examination of tonic reflexes

Tonic/Brainstem reflexes	*Stimulus*	*Response*
Asymmetrical tonic neck (ATNR)	Rotation of the head to one side	Flexion of skull limbs, extension of the jaw limbs, "bow and arrow" or "fencing" posture *Onset*: Birth *Integrated*: 4–6 months
Symmetrical tonic neck (STNR)	Flexion or extension of the head	*With head flexion*: Flexion of UEs, extension of LEs *With head extension*: Extension of UEs, flexion of LEs *Onset*: 4–6 months *Integrated*: 8–12 months
Symmetrical tonic labyrinthine (TLR or STLR)	Prone or supine position	*With prone position*: Increased flexor tone/flexion of all limbs; with supine: increased extensor tone/extension of all limbs. *Onset*: Birth *Integrated*: 6 months
Positive supporting **(Fig. 7.15)**		Rigid extension (co-contraction) of the LEs. *Onset*: Birth *Integrated*: 6 months
Associated reactions	Resisted voluntary movement in any part of the body	Involuntary movement in the resting extremity *Onset*: Birth: 3 months *Integrated*: 8–9 years

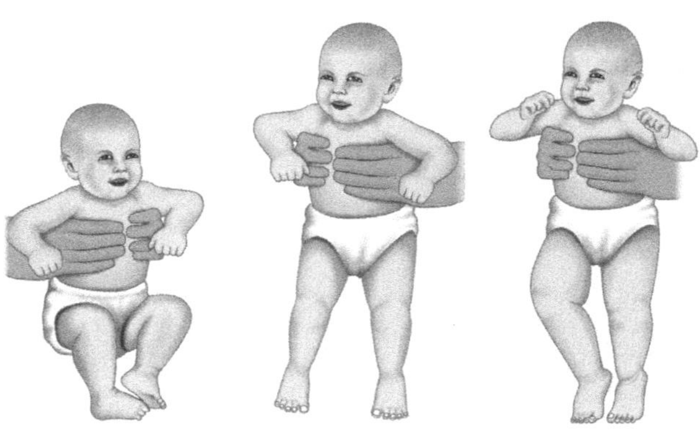

Fig. 7.15 Positive supporting

Findings

Increased Reflex

Causes: UMN lesion.

Absent Reflexes

- *Generalized indicates*: Peripheral neuropathy
- *Isolated indicates*: Peripheral nerve or a root lesion
- *Bilateral absent reflexes*: Indicates peripheral neuropathy
- Bilateral sciatic nerve lesion.

Reduced Reflex

- Occurs in peripheral neuropathy
- Muscle disease
- Cerebellar syndrome
- Reflexes can be absent in early stages of severe upper motor neurone lesion spinal shock.

Reflex Spread

The reflex tested is present but this response goes beyond the muscle normally seen to contract, e.g. fingers are seen to be flexing when supinator reflex is tested or hip adductors are seen to contract when testing knee reflex.

It indicates UMN occurring above the level of innervations of muscle to which the reflex spread.

Inverted Reflex

A combination of loss of reflex tested with reflex spread to muscle at lower level. The level of absent reflex indicates the level of lesion, for example, biceps reflex is absent but produce triceps response. It indicates lower motor neurone lesion at the level of absent reflex with upper motor neuron lesion below indicating spinal cord involvement at the level of absent reflex.

Pendular Reflex

It is usually best seen in the knee jerk where the reflex continues to swing for several beats. This is associated with cerebellar disease.

Slow Relaxing Reflex

This is especially seen at the ankle reflex and may be difficult to note. It is associated with hypothyroidism.

PATHOLOGIC REFLEXES

- Pathologic reflexes are responses not generally found in the normal individual.
- Some are responses that are minimally present and elicited with difficulty in normal but become prominent and active in disease, while others are not seen in normal at all.
- Some are related to postural reflexes or primitive defense reflexes that are normally suppressed by cerebral inhibition but become enhanced when the lower motor neuron is separated from the influence of the higher centers. Others are responses normally seen in the immature nervous system of infancy, then disappear only to reemerge later in the presence of disease.
- A decrease in threshold or an extension of the reflexogenic zone plays a role in many pathologic reflexes.
- Descending motor influences normally control and modulate the activity at the local, segmental spinal cord level to insure efficient muscle contraction and proper coordination of agonists, antagonists, and synergists.
- Disease of the *descending motor pathways* causes loss of this normal control so that activity spills from the motor neuron pool responsible for a certain movement to adjacent areas, resulting in the recruitment into the movement of muscles not normally involved.
- Some pathologic reflexes may also be classified as "associated movements," related to such spread of motor activity. Whether a certain abnormal response would be best classified as a reflex or an associated movement is not always clear.
- Most pathologic reflexes are related to disease involving the corticospinal tract and associated pathways. They also occur with frontal lobe disease and occasionally with disorders of the extra pyramidal system.

- The typical reflex pattern with lesions involving the corticospinal tract, the upper motor neuron syndrome, is exaggeration of deep tendon reflexes (DTRs), disappearance of superficial reflexes, and emergence of pathologic reflexes.

Frontal Release Signs

- While normal in infants and children, when present in an older individual they may be evidence of neurological disease, although some may reappear in normal senescence. Many of these are exaggerations of normal reflex responses.
- Responses often included as frontal release sign (FRS) include the palmomental reflex (PMR), grasp, snout, suck, and others.
- Frontal release signs occur most often in patients with
  - Severe dementias
  - Diffuse encephalopathy (metabolic, toxic, post anoxic)
  - After head injury
  - Other state in which the pathology is usually diffuse but involves particularly the frontal lobes or the frontal association areas.
- The Hoffman finger flexor reflex and its variants, which are sometimes classified as FRS and sometimes as corticospinal signs, are similarly present in a significant proportion of normal individuals.
- Clearly, these reflexes are a normal phenomenon in a significant proportion of the healthy population. They must be interpreted with caution and kept in clinical context.

Frontal Release Signs in Upper Extremity

- *Palmar grasp*:
  - *Stimulus*: Maintain pressure to palm of hand.
  - *Response*: Maintained flexion of fingers.
  - Forced grasping is an involuntary flexor response of the fingers and hand following stimulation of the skin of the palmar surface of the fingers or hand. The patient is instructed not to hold onto the therapist hand **(Fig. 7.16)**.

There are four variations and modifications:

1. If the therapist fingers are placed in the patient's hand, especially between the thumb and forefinger, or if the palmar skin is stimulated gently, there is slow flexion of the digits. The patient's fingers may close around the therapist fingers in a gentle grasp that can be relaxed

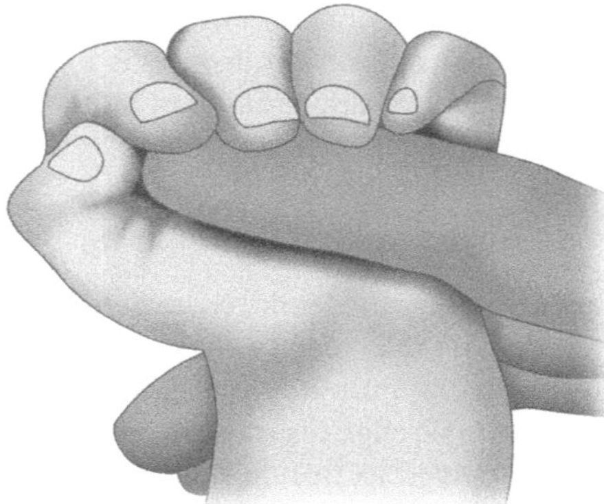

Fig. 7.16 Palmar grasp

on command. This is the simple grasp reflex, an exaggeration of the normal palmar reflex.

2. If the patient's flexed fingers are gently extended by the fingers of the examiner, they will flex against the therapist fingers in a "hooking" or traction response.
3. With a more marked grasp response, the strength of the grasp increases with attempts to withdraw the therapist hand or to extend the patient's fingers passively and there is loss of ability to relax the grasp voluntarily or on command. The grip may be so firm that the patient can be lifted from the bed by the examiner.
4. The sight of the observer's hand near but not touching the patient's hand, or even a very light touch on the patient's hand between the thumb and forefinger while her eyes are closed, leads to groping movements, termed the groping response. Other things may be substituted for the therapist fingers to elicit the grasp response (e.g. the handle of the reflex hammer).
   - The palmar grasp is normally present at birth and may be strong enough to suspend the infant by her own grasp.
   - The response begins to diminish at the age of 2–4 months.
   - It reappears primarily in association with extensive neoplastic or vascular lesions of the frontal lobes or with cerebral degenerative processes, usually contralaterally but occasionally ipsilaterally.
   - Although the grasp reflex is usually classified as an FRS or primitive reflex, it may also occur as evidence of corticospinal tract dysfunction in spastic hemiplegia.

- The grasping responses are exaggerations of normal reactions and occur as release phenomena, the groping response is a more complicated reaction that is modified by visual and tactile integration at the cortical level.
- Some patients who have bilateral grasp responses exhibit the phenomenon of self-grasping, with one hand grasping the contralateral forearm. When this sign is present unilaterally it suggests a contralateral frontal or parietal lobe lesion. When it occurs bilaterally, there is no localizing value.

- Palmomental reflex/palm chin reflex:
  - *Stimulus*: Scratching or stroking the palm of ipsilateral hand.
  - *Response*: Contraction of mentalis or orbicularis oris muscle causing wrinkling of skin of chin with slight retraction and sometimes elevation of angle of mouth **(Fig. 7.17)**.
  - It is contraction of the mentalis and orbicularis oris muscles causing wrinkling of the skin of the chin with slight retraction and sometimes elevation of the angle of the mouth in response to scratching or stroking the palm of the ipsilateral hand.
  - The reflex is best elicited by stroking a blunt point over the thenar eminence, either from wrist toward thumb or vice versa, or by tapping this area.
  - The PMR is so frequently present in normal persons that significance can only be attached to a marked exaggeration of the response or a conspicuous asymmetry between the two sides.
  - If the response is marked, the reflexogenic zone may be wide, including the hypothenar area. A trigger area outside the palm

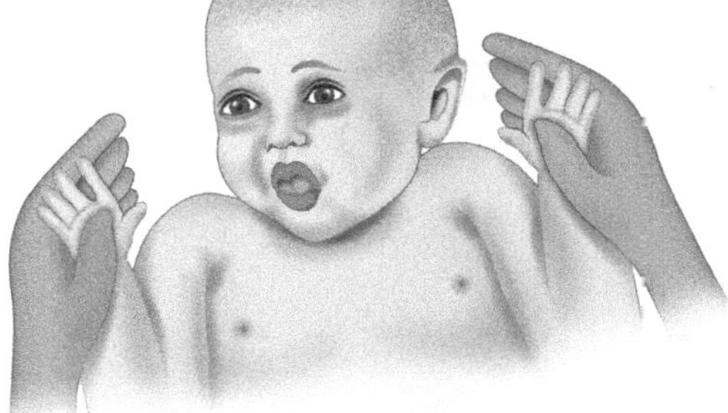

Fig. 7.17 Palmomental reflex

probably does not occur in healthy people. In neurological patients, the reflex can sometimes be elicited by stimulation of the forearm, chest, abdomen, or even the sole; and changing the name to "mentalis reflex" has been suggested.
- The reflex is weak and fatigable in normals, stronger and more persistent in disease.
- The PMR can help in the differential diagnosis of facial palsy—it is absent in peripheral facial palsy and may be exaggerated in central facial paresis.
- The pollicomental reflex is the same response to stroking the palmar surface of the thumb. The localizing value and clinical significance of these reflexes are limited. A unilateral PMR may occur with bilateral, contralateral, or ipsilateral lesions.

Other frontal release signs:
- *Orbicularis oculi reflex*:
  - *Stimulus*: Best elicited by pulling back, between thumb and index finger, a fold of skin on temple lateral to outer canthus, then briskly tapping the thumb or finger **(Fig. 7.18)**.
  - *Response*: Sudden stretch of muscle causes contraction of orbicularis oculi with closing of eye.
- *Glabellar tap*:
  - It is a primitive reflex
  - *Stimulus*: Tap lightly between the eyebrows **(Fig. 7.19)**.

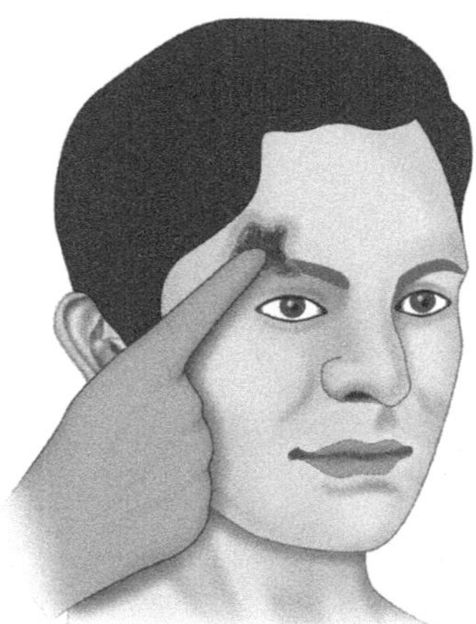

Fig. 7.18 Orbicularis occuli reflex

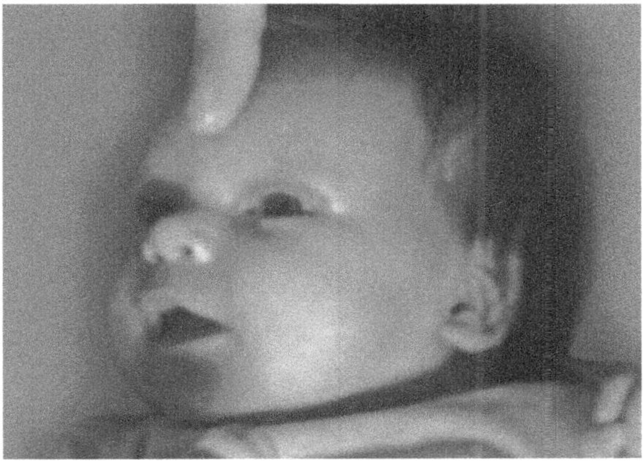

Fig. 7.19 Glabellar tap

- *Response*: The eyes shut.
- This reflex may normally be overcome rapidly, i.e. the individual soon fails to blink, usually less than five taps.
- In a patient with frontal release signs the reflex cannot be overcome, and they continue to blink for as long as the examiner cares to keep tapping.
- A similar response is seen with late parkinsonism.

• *Suck*:
  - *Stimulus*: Stroking, striking or touching the lips, stroking the tongue or stimulating palate **(Fig. 7.20)**.
  - *Response*: Sucking movements of lips tongue and jaw.
• *Snout*:
  - *Stimulus*: The snout reflex involves puckering or protrusion of the lips with percussion **(Fig. 7.21)**.
  - *Response*: The muscles around the mouth and base of the nose contract.
  - The snout reflex is brought about by tapping the upper lip lightly.
  - The contraction of the muscles causes the mouth to resemble a snout.
• *Head retraction*:
  - *Stimulus*: Sharp tap with reflex hammer just below nose with the head bent slightly forward.

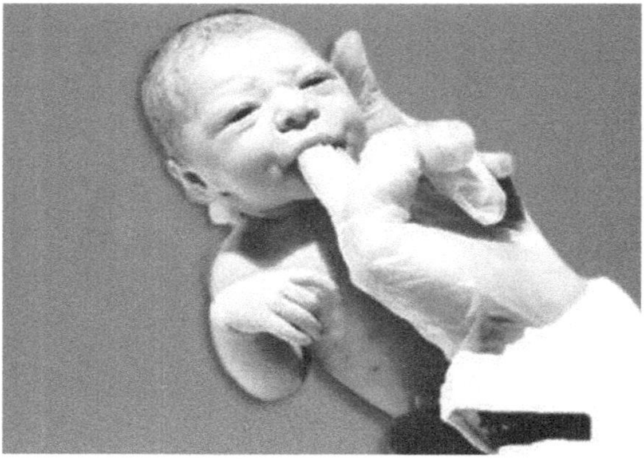

Fig. 7.20 Suck

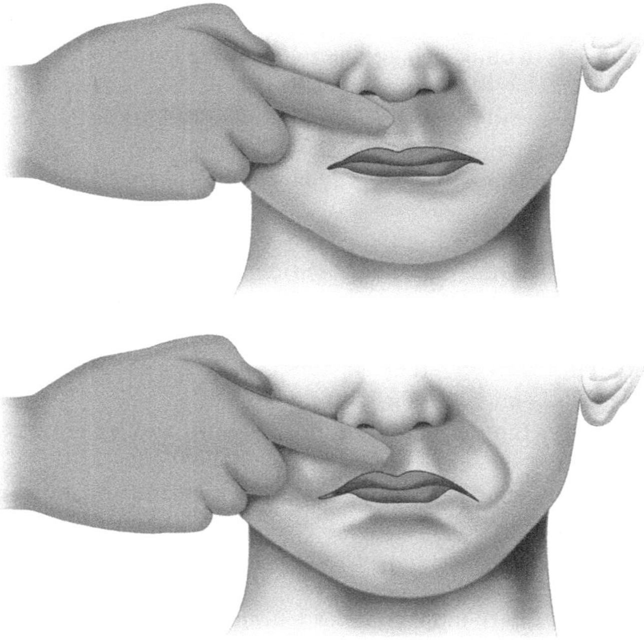

Fig. 7.21 Snout

- *Response*: Quick, involuntary backward jerk of head.
- Present in bilateral corticospinal lesion rostral to cervical spine, e.g. in amyotrophic lateral sclerosis.

- *Corneomandibular reflex*:
  - *Stimulus*: Stimulation of cornea **(Figs 7.22A to C)**
  - *Response*: Contralateral movement of mandible.
  - May be associated movement rather than a true reflex. Indicate supranuclear interruption of ipsilateral corticotrigeminal tract.

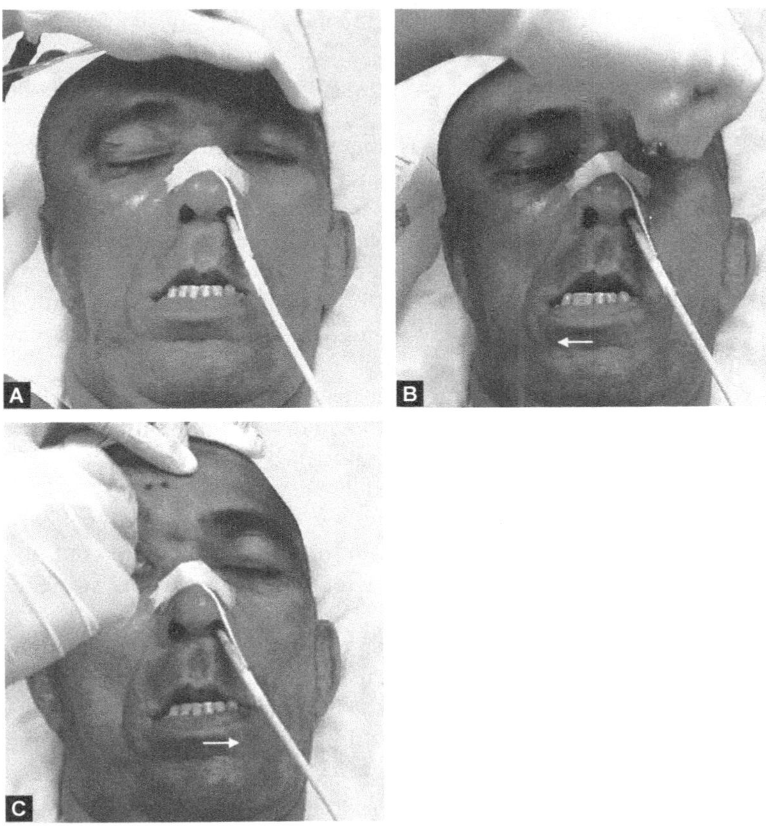

Figs 7.22A to C Corneomandibular response: (A) Normal; (B) Stimulation of left cornea produce movement of mandible towards right; (C) Stimulation of right cornea produce movement of mandible towards left

PATHOLOGIC REFLEXES IN THE LOWER EXTREMITIES

- Pathologic reflexes in the lower extremities are more constant, more easily elicited, more reliable, and more clinically relevant than those in the upper limbs.
- The most important of these responses may be classified as:
  - Those characterized in the main by dorsiflexion of the toes, and
  - Those characterized by plantar flexion of the toes.

Babinski's Sign

- The Babinski sign has been called the most important sign in clinical neurology. It is one of the most significant indications of disease of the corticospinal system at any level from the motor cortex through the descending pathways.
- *Stimulus*: The Babinski's sign is obtained by stimulating the plantar surface of the foot with a blunt point **(Fig. 7.23A)**.
- It is not true that the stimulus must necessarily be deliberately "noxious", although most patients find it at least somewhat uncomfortable even if the examiner is trying to be considerate.
- Some patients are very sensitive to plantar stimulation and only a slight stimulus will elicit a consistent response, stronger stimuli may produce confusing withdrawal.
- The stimulus should begin near the heel and be carried up the side of the foot at a deliberate pace, not too quickly, usually stopping at the metatarsophalangeal joints.
- The response has usually occurred by the time the stimulus reaches the midportion of the foot.
- If the response is difficult to obtain, the stimulus should continue along the metatarsal pad from the little toe medially, but stopping short of the base of the great toe.
- The most common mistakes are insufficiently firm stimulation, placement of the stimulus too medially and moving the stimulus too quickly, so that the response does not have time to develop.
- The only movements of significance are those of the great toe. Fanning of the lateral toes without an abnormal movement of the great toe is seldom of any clinical significance, and an absence of fanning does not negate the significance of great toe extension.

- The patient should be relaxed and forewarned of the potential discomfort. The knee must be extended; an up going toe may be abolished by flexion of the knee.
- The best position is supine, with hips and knees in extension and heels resting on the bed. Some neurologists will only check the plantar responses with the patient recumbent. If the patient is seated, the knee should be extended, with the foot held either in the therapist hand or on her knee.
- The response may sometimes be reinforced by rotating the patient's head to the opposite side. It may be inhibited when the foot is cold and increased when the foot is warm.
- Usually, the upward movement of the great toe is a quick, flicking motion sometimes mistaken for withdrawal by the inexperienced. The response may be a slow, tonic, sometimes clonic, dorsiflexion of the great toe and the small toes with fanning, or separation, of the toes. The slow great toe movement has been described as a "majestic rise".
- The Babinski sign is a part of the primitive flexion reflex. The central nervous system is organized according to movement patterns, and one of the most basic patterns is avoidance or withdrawal from a noxious stimulus.
- In higher vertebrates, the flexion response includes flexion of the hip and knee, and dorsiflexion of the ankle and toes, all serving to remove the threatened part from danger. Although the relevant muscles are anatomical extensors, and have extensor names (e.g. extensor hallucis longus), physiologically flexors serve to shorten a limb, so toe "extension" is in fact part of the flexion response. In human infants, the primitive flexion response persists, and an extensor plantar response is normal in infancy.
- Maturation of the descending motor systems suppresses the primitive flexion response. This may be necessary for normal ambulation, or else our legs and feet might be whipping into flexion unexpectedly, just from stepping on a pebble.
- The corticospinal tract is myelinated by about the end of the first year of life, about the time babies begin to walk. When there is disease involving the corticospinal tract, the primitive flexion response may reappear, and the first clinical evidence of this is the Babinski sign.
- With more severe and extensive disease the entire flexion response emerges, so that stimulation of the sole causes dorsiflexion not only

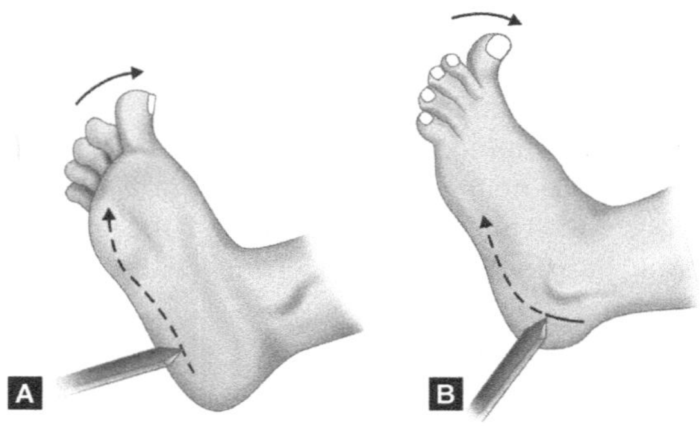

Figs 7.23A and B (A) Babinski's sign; (B) Chaddock sign

of the toe, but also the ankle, as well as flexion of the hip and knee (the "triple flexion" response, which for some perplexing reason has four parts). In addition, there is often contraction of the tensor fascia lata causing slight internal rotation at the hip and more rarely abduction of the hip (Brissaud reflex).

There are many other corticospinal tract responses in the lower extremities characterized by dorsiflexion of the toes.

Chaddock Sign

- *Stimulus*: Stimulating the lateral aspect of the foot, not the sole, beginning about under the lateral malleolus near the junction of the dorsal and plantar skin, drawing the stimulus from the heel forward to the small toe **(Fig. 7.23B)**.
- *Response*: It produces less withdrawal than plantar stimulation.
- The response is slow and often occurs toward the end of stimulation.
- There may even be contralateral or bilateral responses.
- The response may occur with passive extension of the knee or passive flexion of the hip and knee. Sometimes the toes are held in a tonic position of dorsiflexion and fanning.
- Such a tonic toe may become problematic, causing skin breakdown on the dorsum of the great toe from friction against the shoe.

Postural and Righting Reflexes

- The postural and righting reflexes are a complex group of reactions that are relevant primarily in pediatric neurology.

- Posture is largely reflex in origin, with involuntary muscle contraction creating the necessary tone, especially in the antigravity muscles, to maintain the erect posture and normal position.
- The vestibular nuclei, especially the lateral, are particularly important for maintaining contraction in the antigravity muscles.
- Standing may be thought of as a postural reflex, and any interference with the mechanisms mediating postural reflexes may interfere with the act of normal standing.
- Maintaining the orientation of the head to the body and of the head and body in space are basic functions. The complex reflex mechanisms of standing and righting involve the vestibular system, principally the utricle; proprioceptive impulses from muscles, tendons, and joints; exteroceptive impulses from the body surface; and visual stimuli.

Righting reactions involve at least five separate types of reflexes:

1. Labyrinthine righting reflexes acting on the neck muscles.
2. Neck righting reflexes acting upon the body.
3. Body righting reflexes acting upon the head.
4. Body righting reflexes acting upon the body.
5. Visual righting reflexes acting upon the head and body.
   - The proprioceptive stimuli involved in neck righting reflexes originate in the muscles, tendons, and other deep structures of the neck and are mediated through the upper two or three cervical nerves and segments, and possibly through the spinal accessory nerve.
   - They act principally on the head, but through the head act on the body as a whole. Afferents subserving body righting reflexes are analogous and arise from tissues in the trunk and extremities.
   - The visual righting reflexes are probably integrated in the cerebral cortex, but the impulses are mediated by the midbrain and the vestibular centers. When the eyes turn toward an object, the head and body follow.
   - Although vision plays a role in posture, lack of vision does not impair postural or righting reflexes if the other mechanisms are intact.
   - Conversely, loss of proprioception, as in posterior column disease, can be compensated for in part by visual input. Abnormalities of the postural and righting reflexes are clinically relevant in pediatric patients; in certain adult patients, particularly those with extrapyramidal disorders, disturbances of gait and balance, and

vestibular disorders; and in the aged. Loss of postural reflexes is an important feature of Parkinson's disease, and similar impairment is likely related to the tendency of the elderly to fall.

POSTURAL AND RIGHTING REFLEXES IN INFANCY AND CHILDHOOD

- Myelination of the nervous system begins during the second trimester and continues for a long period of time, well after birth and perhaps into adolescence. The most rapid phase of myelination occurs during the first 6 months after birth. Different systems myelinate at different times, and the order of myelination is related to the appearance and disappearance of the postural and righting reflexes seen in pediatric patients.
- Demonstration of these reflexes helps to establish gestational age and assess the function of the immature nervous system.
- Reflexes that are usually demonstrable in the normal neonate include the moro, tonic neck reflex, rooting and sucking, grasp, placing, stepping, and trunk incurvation.

The Moro Reflex

- This is the body startle reflex.
- *Stimulus*: Loud noise, quick movement directed toward the body, blow on the bed close to the body, tap on the abdomen, or sudden bright light.
- *Response*: Abduction and extension of all four extremities, extension of the spine, extension and fanning of the digits except for flexion of the distal phalanges of the index finger and thumb; followed in turn by flexion and adduction of the extremities **(Fig. 7.24)**.
- The reflex is present during the first 3 months of life; during the next 2 months there may be only extension and abduction of the arms and jerking of the knees; then the response gradually disappears, probably with the development of myelination.
- Children with motor deficits of cerebral origin may show the reflex in a fully developed form for years; the response may be unilateral if only one side is affected.

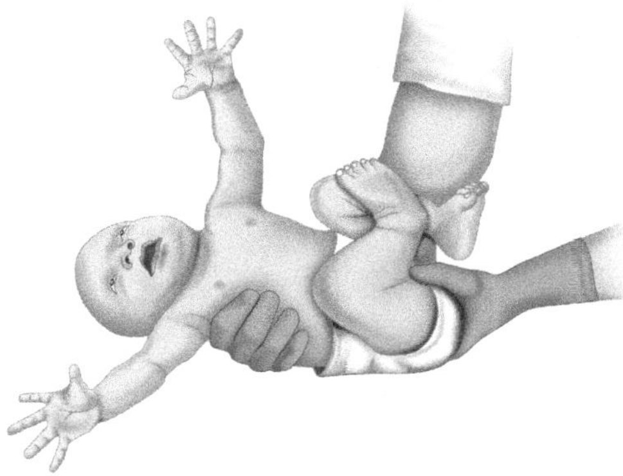

Fig. 7.24 Moro reflex

Landau Reflex

- This is present in normal infants during the first 1–2 years of life.
- *Position of infant*: An infant is held prone in the therapist hand with the body parallel with the floor.
- *Response*: There is extension of the head and spine so that the body forms an arc with the convexity downward. With the body in this position, passive flexion of the head causes flexion of the vertebral column, arms and legs, and the body forms an arc with the convexity upward. If the child is placed supine, there is flexion of the neck, spine, arms, and legs. This posture is probably a combination of otolith and tonic neck reflexes **(Fig. 7.25)**.

Tonic Neck Reflexes

- *Stimulus*: Passively turning the head toward one shoulder.
- *Response*: Causes increased extensor tonus on that side and increased flexor tonus on the opposite side the arm on the side toward which the head is turned goes into extension, and the leg may go into extension as well. On the opposite side the arm flexes and the leg may also flex.
- The posture has been likened to that of a fencing thrust. The extension is usually accompanied by supination, the flexion by pronation. If the head and neck are flexed, the arms flex and the legs go into extension. If the head and neck are extended, the arms extend and the legs go into flexion.

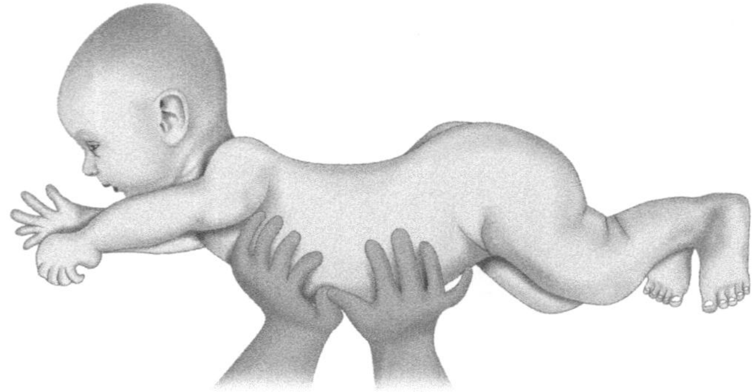

Fig. 7.25 Landau reflex

- Pressure over the vertebral prominance results in relaxation of all four limbs. Reflexes of this type are often found in an incomplete form in normal infants, but disappear by the age of 4–6 months.
- In later life, they may be demonstrable in patients who have "high" decerebration, or decortication, due to disease involving the upper brainstem or thalamodiencephalic level.
- The patient lies with the arms semi flexed over the chest and the legs in extension, but turning, flexion, or extension of the head causes the responses just described. These reflexes may contribute to the associated movements found in spastic hemiplegia and cerebral diplegia.

Asymmetric tonic neck reflex (ATNR):
- *Stimulus*: Rotation of head towards one side.
- *Response*: Flexion of one side and extension of other side **(Fig. 7.26)**.
- Retention of this reflex lead to:
  - Balance affection due to head movement to either side
  - Homolateral instead of normal cross pattern movement
  - Difficulty in midline activity
  - Poor ocular pursuit movement
  - Poor handwriting and poor expression of ideas
  - Visual perceptual difficulties, particularly in symmetrical representation of figures.

Symmetrical tonic neck reflex (STNR):
- *Stimulus*: Flexion/Extension of head
- *Response*: With head flexion: flexion of UE, extension of LE **(Fig. 7.27)**
- *With head extension*: Extension of UE, flexion of LE.

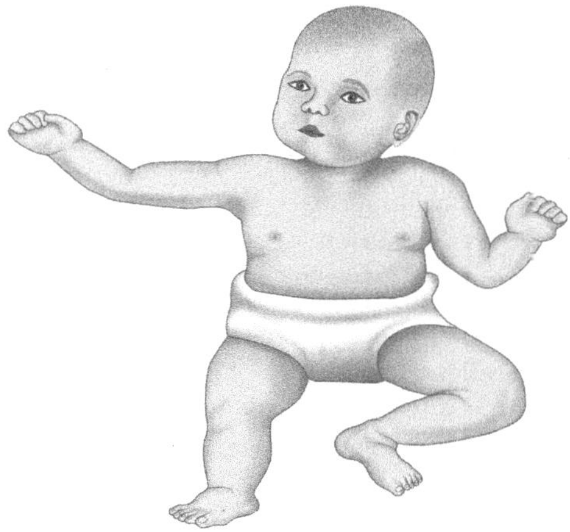

Fig. 7.26 Asymmetrical tonic neck reflex

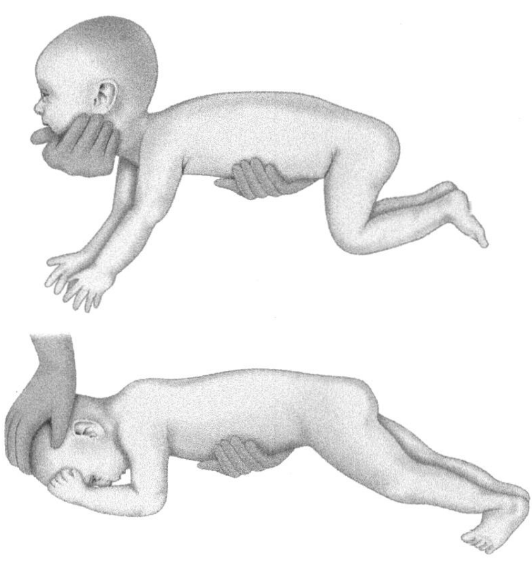

Fig. 7.27 Symmetrical tonic neck reflex

- Retention of this reflex lead to:
  - Poor posture
  - Tendency to slump when sitting, particularly at a desk or table
  - Simian walk
  - "W" leg position when sitting on floor
  - Poor eye hand coordination
  - Difficulty with readjustment of binocular vision
  - Slowness at copying task
  - Poor swimming skills.

Tonic labyrinthine reflex:

- *Stimulus*: Prone/supine position
- *Response*: With prone position—Flexion of all limbs **(Figs 7.28A and B)**
- *With supine position*: Extension of all limbs.
- Strongly residual TLR forwards
  - Poor posture stoop
  - Hypo tonus weak muscle tone
  - Vestibular related problem
  - Disliking of sporting activity, physical education, running
  - Oculomotor dysfunction

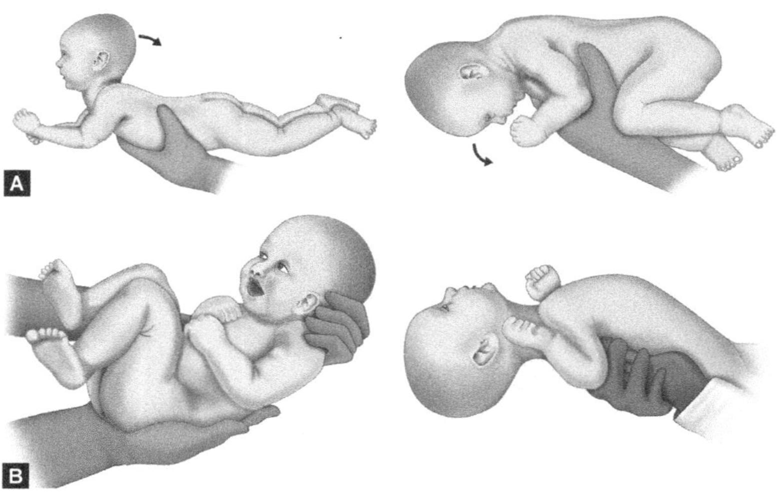

Figs 7.28A and B (A) Tonic labyrinthine prone reflex; (B) Tonic labyrinthine supine reflex

- Poor sequencing skills
- Poor sense of time
- Strongly residual TLR reflex backwards:
  - Poor posture—tendency to walk on toes
  - Poor balance and coordination
  - Hyper tonus—stiff jerky movements
  - Vestibular related problems (poor balance sense, motion sickness)
  - Oculomotor dysfunction
  - Poor sequencing skills
  - Poor organization skill.

The Neck Righting Response

- This is a variation of the tonic neck reflex.
- *Stimulus*: With the infant supine, its head is turned toward one side.
- *Response*: A positive response results in rotation of the shoulder, trunk, and pelvis toward that side, occasionally followed by a turn of the entire body. The response should be approximately equal on each side.
- The reflex appears at about the time the tonic neck reflexes disappear and can be obtained in nearly all infants by the age of 10 months; it disappears at about the time the child can arise directly without first turning on his abdomen.

Optical Righting Reaction

- *Stimulus*: Hold child from armpit in a suspended position then change position of head from side to side **(Fig. 7.29)**.
- *Response*: Eyes will move in the direction of head.

Body on Neck

- *Stimulus*: Supine rotate body to one side.
- *Response*: Head turns in line of body **(Fig. 7.30)**.
- Prolongation delays segmental rolling.

Body on Body

- *Stimulus*: Rotation of pelvis to one side.
- *Response*: Trunk and shoulder follow direction of pelvis **(Fig. 7.31)**.
- Prolongation delays segmental rolling.

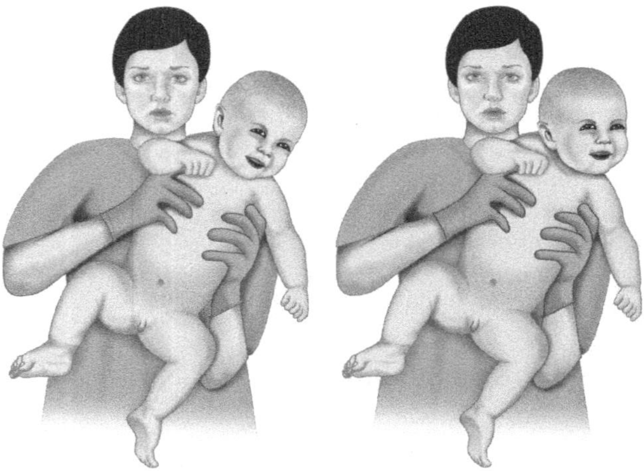

Fig. 7.29 Optical rightning reaction

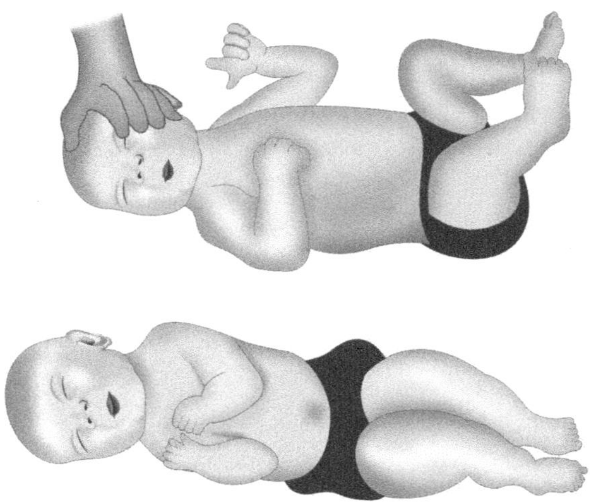

Fig. 7.30 Body on neck

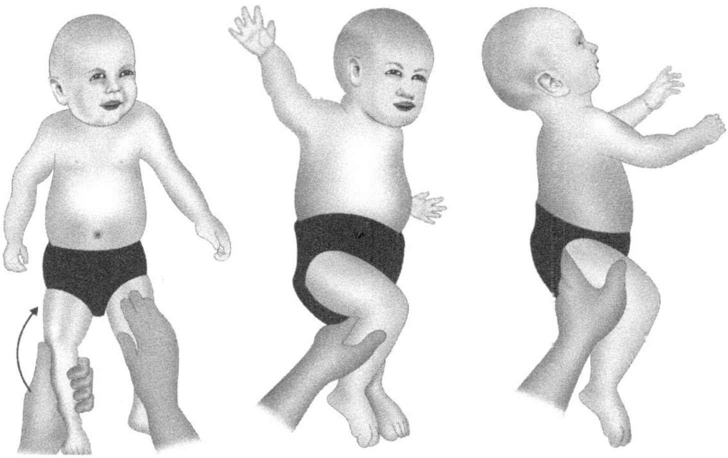

Fig. 7.31 Body on body

The Parachute Response

- The parachute response appears at the age of 8–9 months and persists.
- *Stimulus*: To elicit it, the infant is held prone in the air and then suddenly thrust head-first toward the examining table or floor **(Fig. 7.32)**.
- *Response*: When the response is present the arms immediately extend and abduct slightly and the fingers spread as if to attempt to break the fall.
- Asymmetry of the response indicates unilateral upper-extremity weakness or spasticity.
- Absence of the response is seen in severe motor disorders and dementia. The response does not depend upon vision and may be obtained in blindfolded children.

The Hand-Mouth Reflex of Babkin

- *Stimulus*: Pressure on the palm of the hand in premature and newborn infants.
- *Response*: Opening of the mouth, flexion of the neck, and sometimes closing of the eyes and flexion of the forearm **(Fig. 7.33)**.

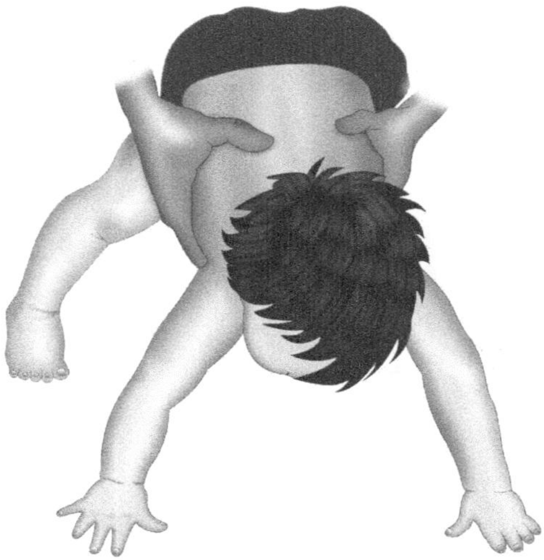

Fig. 7.32 The Parachute response

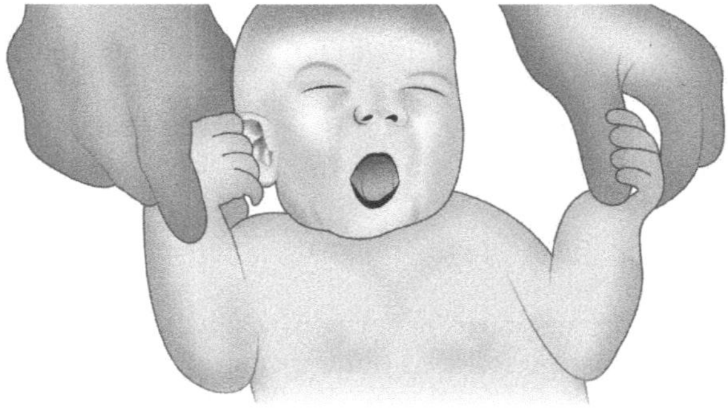

Fig. 7.33 Babkin response

- The response is easier to elicit and more pronounced if the stimulus is bilateral. Except in infants with retarded development this reflex disappears by the third or fourth month of life.

The Placing Reaction

- *Stimulus*: With the infant held vertically, touching the dorsum of each foot to the side of the examining table.
- *Response*: Causes placement of the foot on top of the table **(Fig. 7.34)**.
- The response usually disappears by the end of the first year of life, when voluntary movements make it difficult to interpret.
- It persists in children with motor deficits, and in them may be related to the reflexes of spinal automatism.

Supporting and Stepping Reactions

- *Stimulus*: Holding the infant vertically and allowing its feet to make firm contact with the top of the examining table.
- *Response*: It produces contraction of the lower extremities as if to support the weight. This is usually followed by automatic stepping or walking movements **(Figs 7.35A and B)**.
- These responses are usually present at birth and gradually disappear.

Associated Movements

- An associated movement (AM) is an unintentional, involuntary, spontaneous, automatic movement that accompanies some other voluntary (or involuntary) movement.
- The associated, or synkinetic, movement is often one that serves to fix a part of the body as another part is voluntarily activated.

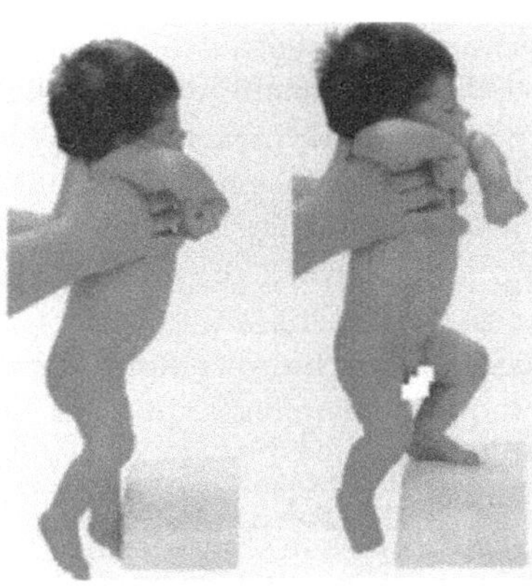

Fig. 7.34 Placing reaction

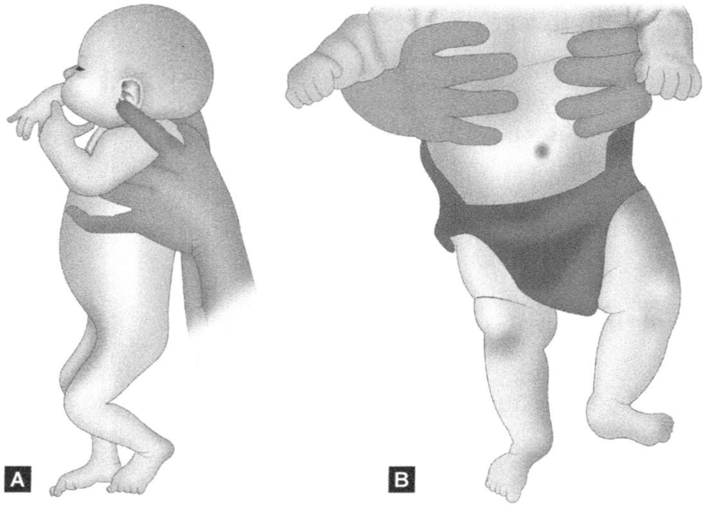

Figs 7.35A and B (A) Supporting reaction; (B) Stepping reaction

- Associated movements often occur because of activation of the synergistic and fixation muscles involved in a particular motion, or spread of the activation to nearby motor neuron pools.
- This activity is normally suppressed by the descending motor pathways, but in the face of disease becomes clinically apparent.
- The corticospinal pathways are concerned primarily with fine, fractionated, discrete movements of the distal extremities.
- Disease in the corticospinal pathways may eliminate discrete distal movement but not affect mass movements of the proximal muscles.
- The mass movements usually play a secondary, supportive role, particularly in fixation of the part to be moved. However, when the distal movements are paralyzed, the primary movement left may be the associated mass movement.
- Associated movements are more complex manifestations of motor function than the simple reflexes, but are more primitive than voluntary movements.
- They are probably initiated and largely controlled by the extrapyramidal system and its connections, although the corticospinal system also plays a role.

PHYSIOLOGIC ASSOCIATED MOVEMENTS

- Many associated movements are present physiologically; in fact they play a part in all normal motor activity.
- The activity of the antagonists, synergists, and muscles of fixation in any motor response may be considered associated movements. Generally, the term is used for more widespread responses.
- *Common examples of normal associated movements include the following*: Pendular swinging of the arms when walking; the play of the muscles of facial expression when talking; facial contortions or grimaces with violent exertion; movements of the head and neck with movements of the eyes; contraction of the frontalis muscle with elevation of the eyes; turning of the eyes, head, or body in response to vestibular or auditory stimulation; normal extension of the wrist with flexion of the fingers; generalized bodily accompaniments of yawning, stretching, coughing, and mental efforts. In some disease states, normal associated movements may decrease or disappear.
- The normal associated movements are lost in diseases of the extrapyramidal system, especially in the parkinsonian syndromes, where masking of facial expression and absence of arm swing when walking are prominent manifestations.
- In other conditions, normal associated movements may be exaggerated, and abnormal associated movements may be present.
- With lesions of the corticospinal system, a number of associated movements may appear that are not present normally.

PATHOLOGIC ASSOCIATED MOVEMENTS

- Abnormal or pathologic associated movements (AMs) are usually activity in paretic muscle groups that are brought out by active movement of other groups, and seen predominantly in disease of the corticospinal pathways.
- They may be present at all times, be brought out by special examinations, or become evident only during physical activity or periods of emotional stress.
- They usually accompany vigorous voluntary movements of another part, and occur on the hemiplegic side.
- Associated movements are slow, forceful movements of the already spastic parts that lead to the adoption of new postures.

- They have a longer latent period than primary movements. The greater the spasticity, the greater the extent and duration of the AMs.

Generalized Associated Movements

- *Generalized* associated movements occur in hemiplegia, where they tend to emphasize or enhance the characteristic hemiplegic posture.
- The associated movements often occur *with exertion, straining and attempts to grip with the paretic hand.* It may cause an increase in the spasticity, with increased flexion of the wrist, elbow, and shoulder; this is sometimes accompanied by associated facial movements on the involved side.The new posture may be maintained until the grip is relaxed.
- An involuntary, automatic movement such as a *yawn* may cause the affected arm to *extend at the elbow, wrist,* and *fingers,* remaining rigidly in this new attitude until the yawn passes off.
- Movements such as *coughing or stretching* may cause similar reactions.
- *Tonic neck reflexes* may also influence these generalized associated movements.
- *Turning the head toward the hemiplegic side* may cause increased extensor tonus on that side, and turning it to the normal side may be followed by either increased flexor tonus on the paretic side or flexion of the arm and extension of the leg.

Symmetric (Imitative or Contralateral) Associated Movements (Mirror Movements)

- In the normal infant there is a tendency for movements of one limb to be accompanied by similar involuntary movements of the opposite limb; this disappears as coordination and muscle power are acquired.
- These movements may persist to a certain extent in children, most frequently in the form of transient mirror movements, or involuntary imitative movements of the contralateral portions of the body; they may be present only as mirror writing. Similar movements are sometimes observed in adults who are in the process of acquiring new patterns of movement or who are exerting excessive physical or mental effort.
- Mirror movements usually disappear or become inconspicuous at adolescence, their persistence to any marked degree should be considered pathologic.

- They may occur in patients with brain injuries, disturbances of cerebral development, and dysplasias of the upper portion of the spinal cord; under such circumstances there are usually associated abnormalities of motor function, tone, and reflexes.
- Occasionally, persisting mirror movements are familial, and not accompanied by other signs of neurologic disease.
- In certain neurologic disorders, forceful voluntary movements of one limb may be accompanied by identical involuntary movements of the same limb on the other side. They are usually seen in the paretic limb when the opposite healthy one is forcefully moved, although occasionally such movements may appear in the healthy limb on extreme attempts to move the affected extremity (especially in extrapyramidal disease).
- They appear particularly during exertion to carry out a quick or strenuous movement. When squeezing the therapist hand with the healthy hand, the paretic hand may flex. Any forceful movement on the normal side may be followed by a similar but slow tonic duplication of the movement on the paretic side.
- There may be a spreading of the response, evolving into a generalized associated movement with assumption of the characteristic positions. If the patient clenches the normal hand while the head is straight, flexion of the paretic hand may be accompanied by flexion and adduction of the paretic arm.
- If the head is turned to the paretic side, flexion may be replaced by extension, and if the head is turned to the normal side, flexion and adduction of the paretic arm may be increased.
- Imitation synkinesias by themselves have little localizing significance, occurring with lesions in various portions of the neuraxis. Their value in neurologic assessment is in conjunction with other findings.

Coordinated Associated Movements

Coordinated associated movements are involuntary movements of synergistic muscle groups that accompany a voluntary movement of a paretic limb. They are exaggerations or perversions of ordinary synergistic and cooperative movements, and may be classified into three groups:

1. Movements, not present normally, which accompany movements of a paretic limb.
2. Contralateral coordinated associated movements.

3. Associated movements, normally present, which are abolished in cerebral hemiplegia. These responses may be useful in the differentiation between organic and nonorganic deficits.

Coordinated Associated Movements in the Paretic Limb

- Coordinated AMs that accompany voluntary motion of involved extremities in patients with hemiparesis are characterized by a spread of movement from one muscle or group of muscles to others.
- They alter the position of the part and lead to the adoption of new postures. They do not appear in the normal individual or in nonorganic weakness.

Wartenberg's Sign

- Active flexion of the terminal phalanges of the four fingers of a paretic hand about a firm object, or against resistance offered by the therapist fingers similarly flexed, is followed by adduction, flexion, and opposition of the thumb.
- In a normal extremity the thumb remains in abduction and extension.
- The patient, lying supine with legs abducted, attempts to sit up while holding the arms crossed on the chest. Normally, the legs remain motionless and the heels down. In corticospinal hemiparesis, the hip flexes as the trunk flexes and there is an involuntary elevation of the paretic limb off the bed.
- The toes may spread out in a fanlike fashion. The normal limb remains on the bed or rises slightly, but not as high as the paretic one.
- In paraparesis, both legs rise equally. In nonorganic weakness, the normal leg rises and the paretic one does not, or neither leg rises. If the patient tries to sit up with the legs hanging over the edge of the bed, the hip flexes and the knee extends on the involved side.

The Tibialis Sign of Strümpell

- Normally, vigorous flexion of the hip and knee are accompanied by plantarflexion of the foot.
- In lower-extremity weakness due to a corticospinal tract lesion, voluntary flexion of the hip and knee is accompanied by involuntary

dorsiflexion and inversion of the paretic foot; there may also be dorsiflexion of the great toe or of all the toes. The patient is unable to flex the hip and knee without dorsiflexing the foot.

- The response is accentuated if the movement is carried out against resistance. The sign may also be elicited by flexing the knee with the patient lying prone.

Contralateral Coordinated Associated Movements

Coordinated AMs in which the response is contralateral are similar to the symmetric AMs, but the response is not always imitative and may involve muscles other than those used in the primary movement.

Associated Contralateral Contraction of the Triceps

Normally, biceps muscle contraction in one arm is associated with contraction of the contralateral triceps and extension of the opposite elbow. In organic hemiparesis, this contralateral extension is present in the normal arm on forceful flexion of the paretic arm, but absent in the paretic arm on flexion of the normal arm.

Raimiste Leg Sign

- When the sound leg is forcefully abducted or adducted against the therapist resistance, the paretic leg will carry out a movement identical with that attempted on the normal side.
- With the patient supine and the lower extremities abducted, an attempt to adduct the sound leg against resistance causes the paretic leg to also adduct, drawing the legs together.
- With attempted abduction of the sound leg, the paretic leg also abducts. Hoover's sign exploits an automatic walking AM of the legs to detect nonorganic weakness.

Loss of Coordinated Associated Movements

Certain coordinated AMs normally present are abolished in pyramidal lesions. Normal associated and automatic movements, such as swinging of the arms in walking and synergistic movements used in rising and sitting down, are also lost in disorders of the extrapyramidal system, especially parkinsonian syndromes.

The Phenomenon of Grasset and Gaussel

The normal supine patient can raise either leg separately or raise both together. In pyramidal lesions, she may still be able to raise either one separately but cannot raise them together. If she first raises the paretic one, it falls back heavily as soon as she attempts to raise the normal one or if the normal leg is passively raised. If she first raises the normal one and then the paretic leg is passively raised, the sound one remains elevated.

Coordination

Coordinate movements requires that both motor and sensory system should be intact, because any satisfactory voluntary effort requires:
- Efficient, smooth, adequate but not excessive movement of group of muscle.
- Appropriate and smooth relaxation of the correct antagonist, together perhaps with contraction of other muscles, such as joint fixators to ensure efficiency of movement.
- Knowledge of position of moving part before, during and at the end of each movement.
- Knowledge of position of point to which the part is to be moved and the relationship between the two at any moment during the movement.

Coordinate action of muscle is under cerebellar control, and influence by extrapyramidal system, but intact proprioceptive sense combined with an accurate image of one's own body and its relationship with the environment are equally essential for movement to be completed satisfactorily. Lesions in many sites may therefore produce in coordination.

Characteristics of coordinated movements:
- Appropriate speed
- Distance
- Direction
- Timing
- Muscular tension.

Coordinated movement involve:
- Appropriate synergistic influence
- Easy reversal between opposite group of muscles
- Proximal fixation to allow distal motion.

Impairment of coordination is characterized by:
- Awkward
- Extraneous
- Uneven
- Inaccurate movement.

Purpose of coordination assessment:
- Determine the muscle activity during voluntary movement
- Ability of muscle or group of muscle to work together for functional task
- Determine level of skill and efficiency of movement
- Ability to initiate, control and terminate movement
- Timing, sequencing and accuracy of movement
- For diagnosis of underlying impairment
- Determine effect of therapeutic and pharmacological intervention on motor function.

Signs of Cerebellar Disease

- *Scanning speech*:
  - Causes enunciation of individual syllables.
- *Nystagmus*:
  - Fast phase toward side of cerebellar lesion
- *Finger to nose and finger to finger test*:
  - Ask patient to fully extend arm then touch nose or ask them to touch their nose then fully extend to touch your finger
    - You increase the difficulty of this test by adding resistance to the patient's movements or move your finger to different locations
    - Abnormality of this is called *dysmetria*
- *Rapid alternating movements*:
  - Ask patient to place one hand over the next and have them flip one hand back and forth as fast as possible (alternatively you can ask the patient to quickly tap their foot on the floor as fast as possible)
  - If abnormal, this is called *dysdiadochokinesia*
- *Rebound phenomenon (of Stewart and Holmes)*:
  - Have the patient pull on your hand and when they do, slip your hand out of their grasp. Normally the antagonists muscles will contract and stop their arm from moving in the desired direction. A positive sign is seen in a spastic limb where the exaggerated

"rebound" occurs with movement in the opposite direction. However, in cerebellar disease this response is completely absent causing to limb to continue moving in the desired direction (Be careful that you protect the patient from the unarrested movement causing them to strike themselves).

- *Heel to shin test*:
  - Have patient run their heel down the contralateral shin (this is equivalent the finger to nose test)
  - Abnormal exam occurs when they are unable to keep their foot on the shin
- *Hypotonia*:
  - "Pendular" knee jerk, leg keeps swinging after knee jerk more than 4 times (4 or less is normal)
- *Gait*:
  - Commonly wide based and staggering (See "Gaits" section)
    - They may fall to the side of the lesion
  - *Note*: Patients with disease of the vermis and flocculonodular lobe will be unable to stand at all as they will have truncal ataxia—they may not be able to sit.

Clinical features of basal ganglia lesion:

- Bradykinesia
  - Decrease arm swing, slow shuffling gait, difficulty in initiating or changing direction of movement lack of facial expression.
- Rigidity
  - Increase muscle tone
  - *Lead pipe*: Uniform, constant resistance.
  - *Cogwheel*: Lead pipe with tremors characterized by series of brief
  - Relaxations or catches when extremity is passively moved.
- *Tremor*: Involuntary, rhythmic, oscillatory movement. Tremors are of three types—resting, pill rolling and postural.
- *Akinesia*: Inability to initiate movement.
- *Chorea*: Rapid, irregular, jerky movements
- *Athetosis*: Writing, twisting, warm like movement.
- *Choreoathetosis*: Features of both chorea and athetosis.
- *Hemiballismus*:
  - Sudden jerky forceful wild, flailing motion of arm and leg of one side of body.

  - *Hyperkinesia*: Increase muscle activity.
  - *Hypokinesia*: Decrease motor response.
- *Dystonia*
  - Twisting movement caused by involuntary contraction of axial and proximal muscles of extremity.

Clinical features of dorsal column lesion:
- Equilibrium and motor control disturbance
- Slowing of voluntary movement
- *Gait disturbances*: Wide base, swaying, uneven step length, excessive lateral displacement.
- Watching feet during ambulation.

Changes with age:
- Decrease strength
  - Loss of alpha motor neurons. Atrophy of type I and II fibers
  - Reduce size of muscle fibers.
- Slow reaction time
  - Time between application of stimulus and initiation of movement
- Loss of flexibility
  - Increase tightness of joint
- Faulty posture
- Impaired balance
  - Decrease balance
  - Increase postural sway.

Purposes of the Tests

To give patient simple movement to perform which the examiner can from past experiences compare with the normal. A certain stereotyping of the test is required, because the possible number is of course uncountable.

The aim of each test is to decide whether any defect demonstrated is due to:
- Cerebellar dysfunction
- Proprioceptive deficiency
- Some other factor such as muscular weakness, simple lack of comprehension as to what the patient is supposed to do, or and very important perfect comprehension but a determination to do it wrongly for a variety of reasons none representing organic disease.

Testing Procedure

Ask patient to hold both arms outstretched in front of him. Watch the movement and how well the posture is maintained. Then ask him to close his eyes and continue to watch the posture.

Next telling the patient to keep his arms up tap each briskly and observe displacement and return to the previous position when eyes are open and closed. Next press down on each in turn and suddenly release the pressure. Normally very little displacement occurs.

With both elbows flexed ask patient to tap briskly with the middle finger on his thumb. Note the speed and rhythm which are usually swifter and smoother in the dominant hand. Next ask him to tap thumb with each finger tip in sequence, back and forward from index to little finger.

Abnormalities

- On first raising the arms if cerebellar disease the arm on the affected side usually overshoot and have to be brought back to be parallel with the other. Frequent correction of its position has to be made so that arm appears to be bounce and often deviates towards the other. The hand may show hyperextension of the metacarpophalangeal joint with partial flexion of wrist.
- When the eyes are shut these feature may increase in cerebellar disease but if the arm now begins to drift upwards and sideways this indicates postural deficiency.
- If the arm falls slowly this may also indicate postural deficiency but more commonly due to simple muscle weakness.
- External rotation of hand bizarre posturing of fingers and little writing movement of thumb and fingers may also be seen in severe postural deficiency, as well as in dystonic states.

Arm is easily displaced on tapping due to:

- Motor weakness when it remains in displace position each tap displacing it further
- Cerebellar hypotonia, when it tends to return after several bounces to previous position
- Postural deficiency, when with the eyes closed the arm grossly displace without the patient realizing it, and if told to replace it he assumes an entirely incorrect position.

In cerebellar disease with eyes open or closed after releasing pressure the arm will fly upwards, sometimes so vigorously as to hit the patient in the face. In postural deficiency when the eyes are closed the arm tends to remain in new position without much rebound.

Finger tapping is slowed by spasticity and extrapyramidal rigidity and by weakness, whether organic or functional the rhythm is disturbed by cerebellar disease, functional disturbance or genuine involuntary movement such as chorea. It is a most useful screening test in examination of motor system.

Finger Nose Test

Hold your finger about arm's length in front of patient. Ask patient to touch your finger with his index finger and then touch his nose. When he has done it correctly ask him to repeat movement faster. Watch for accuracy and smoothness of movement **(Fig. 7.36)**.

Repeated Movements

Ask patient to pet one hand on the back of other quickly and regularly.

Ask patient to twist his hand as if opening a door or unscrewing a light bulb.

Ask patient to tap his right hand alternately with palm and then the back of his left hand. Repeat with the right hand.

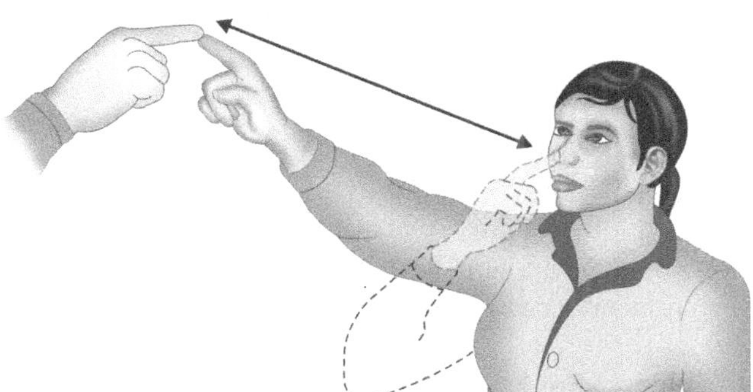

Fig. 7.36 Finger nose test

Abnormality

- In cerebellar disease the arm on the side of lesion may first be flung wildly outward striking nearby objects. The finger moves to the nose in a wavering side to side or up and down but not a jerky fashion at the last moment being brought on to its object fairly accurately. This is increase slightly by eye closure, and emphasized by harder test. In milder lesion all that is seen is wavering to either side of a straight line during the course of the movement, with a tendency to overshoot the object at first, towards the side of the lesion.
- This wavering must not be confused with intention tremor which is a side to side oscillation that develops as the finger approaches the nose, or occurs shortly after finger touches the nose. It may be so wild as to make it impossible for the movement to be completed, so slight as to consist merely of two or three oscillation while the finger is being held on the nose for a few seconds after touching it.
- In postural ataxia the movement from start to finish can be smooth one though it is usually hesitant and the finger hesitates before finally touching the nose. When the eyes are closed however the finger is unable to find the nose and after first touching somewhere else is then dragged along the skin of the face towards its object. If finger is briefly, constantly and confidently placed on the cheek a little to one side of nose, in the same place each time, this almost without exception reflect nonorganic state, and completely without exception if it is still constantly done with the eyes open.

Lower Limb

Preliminary Observation

Exactly the same principles are used as in the arms, but such fine movements cannot be expected.

The patient is told first to raise one leg to touch therapist outstretched hand with his big toe. A patient with normal muscle strength will be able to do this with only with little bounces before it reaches its object, and the knee may be unnecessarily flexed.

The Heel Knee Test

The heel must be placed on the opposite knee. It is wise to touch appropriate heel and knee otherwise some patient whose comprehension is slow flounder helplessly at a simple verbal instruction others always

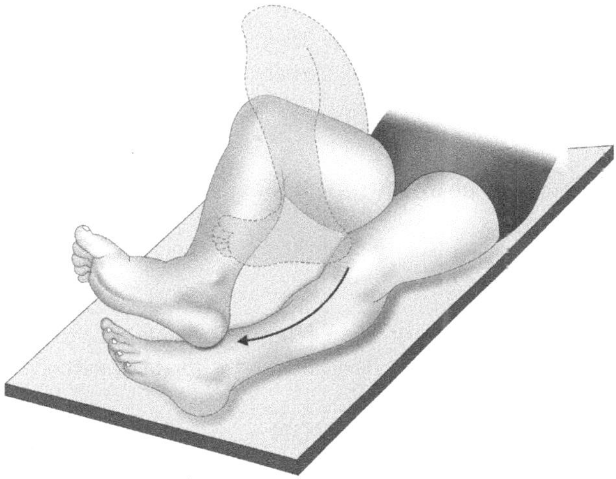

Fig. 7.37 The heel knee test

perform the movement with the opposite limb and some even attempt the discouraging maneuver of trying to place the heel on the knee of the same leg **(Fig. 7.37)**.

When the movement is completed the patient should be told to run the heel down the front of shin to the top of feet. The whole test is repeated on the other side, and finally it is carried out against eyes closed.

Abnormalities

In marked cerebellar disease the heel overshoot the knee sideways, and develop a rotatory oscillation as it approaches it, which is equivalent to intention tremor in the upper limb. As the heel moves down the shin it oscillates from side to side and finally shoots off the opposite foot in uncontrolled manner.

In mild degree of cerebellar ataxia the side to side oscillation may be only obvious defect.

In sensory ataxia the heel is lifted too high in the first place and the patient raises his head to see what the relationship is of two limbs. Deficiencies in the rest of the movement are not rhythmical, though the leg may fall off the other several times during its course. When the eyes are then closed, the patient is only able to find the knee by allowing the heel to land on some part of the thigh and then sliding it downwards.

In combined ataxia, elements of two types of abnormality are present and the movement may be equally diagnosed whether eyes are open or closed, in exactly the same place, usually about 15 cm below knee.

Trunk

Ask the patient to sit up from lying without using his hands. Does he falls on one side?

Abnormality

The patient is unable to sit from lying without falling to one side is present in truncal ataxia. This is associated with ataxic gait.

COORDINATION EXAMINATION

Part I: Nonequilibrium Coordination Tests

Key to Grading

- Normal performance
- *Minimal impairment able to accomplish*: Slightly less than normal speed; requires supervision/minimal contact guarding
- *Moderate impairment*: Able to accomplish activity; movements are slow, awkward. and unsteady: requires moderate contact guarding
- *Severe impairment*: Able only to initiate activity without completion: requires maximal contact guarding
- Activity impossible

Notations should be made under comments section if:
- Lack of visual input renders activity impossible or alters quality of performance
- Verbal cueing is required to accomplish activity
- Alterations in speed affect quality of performance
- Excessive amount of tune required to complete activity
- Changes in arm position alters sitting balance
- Extraneous movements, unsteadiness or oscillations noted on head, neck or trunk.
- Fatigue alters consistency of response.
- Performance impacts patient safety.

Left	Coordination test	Right	Comment
	Finger-to-nose		
	Finger-to-therapist finger		
	Finger-to-finger		
	Alternate nose-to-finger		
	Finger opposition		
	Mass grasp		
	Pronation/supination		
	Rebound phenomenon		
	Tapping (hand)		
	Tapping (foot)		
	Pointing and past-pointing		
	Alternate heel-to-knee: heel-to-toe		
	Toe-to-therapist finger		
	Heel-on-shin		
	Drawing a circle (hand)		
	Drawing a circle (foot)		
	Fixation/position holding (UE)		
	Fixation/position holding (LE)		

Part II: Equilibrium Coordination Tests

Grade	Coordination test	Comment
	Standing in a normal comfortable posture	
	Standing feet together (narrow base of support)	
	Standing on one foot	
	Standing with one foot directly in front of the other in tandem position (toe of one foot touching heel of opposite foot)	
	Standing forward trunk flexion and return to neutral	
	Standing, laterally flex trunk to each side	
	Standing: Eyes open (EO) to eyes closed (EC) (Romberg test)	
	Standing in tandem position: EO to EC (Sharpened Romberg test)	

Contd...

Contd...

Grade	*Coordination test*	*Comment*
	Walk at normal speed	
	Walk as fast as possible	
	Walk as slow as possible	
	Walk: Stop and start abruptly	
	Walk and pivot (turn 90°, 180° or 360°)	
	Walking: Placing the heel of one foot directly in front of the toe of the opposite foot (tandem walking)	
	Walking along a straight line drawn or taped to the floor	
	Walking: Placing feet on floor markers	
	Walk: Sideways	
	Walk: Backwards	
	Walk: Cross-stepping	
	Walk: In a circle, alternate direction	
	Walk: On heels	
	Walk: On toes	
	March in place	
	Walk with horizontal and vertical head turns	
	Step over or around obstacles	
	Stair climbing with handrail	
	Stair climbing without handrail	
	Stair climbing: One step at-a-time	
	Stair climbing: Step-over-step	

Tests Use for Selected Coordination Impairments

Dysdiadokokinesia	Finger-to-nose Alternate nose-to-finger Pronation/supination Knee flexion/extension Walking, alter speed or direction
Dysmetria	Pointing and past pointing Drawing a circle or figure eight Heel to shin Placing feet on floor markers; sitting, standing

Contd...

Contd...

Dyssynergia	Finger-to-nose Finger-to-therapist's finger Alternate heel-to-knee Toe-to-therapist finger
Hypotonia	Passive movement Deep tendon reflexes
Tremor (Intention)	Observation during functional activities (tremor will typically increase as target is approached or movement speed increased) Alternate nose-to-finger Finger-to-finger Finger-to-therapist's finger Toe-to-therapist finger
Tremor (Resting)	Observation of patient at rest; limb or jaw movements Observation during functional activities (tremor will diminish significantly or disappear with movement
Tremor (Postural)	Observation of steadiness of normal posture; sitting, Standing
Asthenia	• Fixation or position holding (upper and lower extremity) • Application of manual resistance to determine ability to hold
Rigidity	• Passive movement • Observation during functional activities • Observation of resting posture(s)
Bradykinesia	• Walking, observation of arm swing and trunk motions • Walking, alter speed and direction • Request that a movement or gait activity be stopped abruptly • Observation of functional activities: timed tests
Disturbances of posture	• Fixation or position holding (upper and lower extremity) • Displace balance unexpectedly in sitting or standing (perturbation) • Standing, alter base of support (e.g. one foot directly in front of the other)
Disturbances of gait	• Walk along a straight line • Walk sideways, backward • March in place • Alter speed and direction of ambulatory activities • Walk in a circle

8 Posture and Balance Control

POSTURE

Functions of Posture

- *Static postural reflexes*:
  - Maintenance of the body in an upright, balanced position
- *Phasic postural reflexes*:
  - Provision of a stable background for voluntary activity

Equilibrium: Maintenance of a normal posture with good alignment.

Posture serves three main behavioral functions:
1. *Antigravity (Static)*: Support head and body against gravity
2. *Alignment with center of gravity (Static)*: Maintain center of body's mass over center of support
3. *Stable background for movement (Dynamic)*: Stabilize supporting parts of body while other parts move.

Mechanisms to Maintain Posture (Flow chart 8.1 and Fig. 8.1)

- *Feed forward*:
  - Modified by experience
  - Stabilizing body prior to movement
- *Feedback*:
  - Evoked by sensory mechanism following loss of balance
  - Automatic

Flow chart 8.1 Postural adjustment

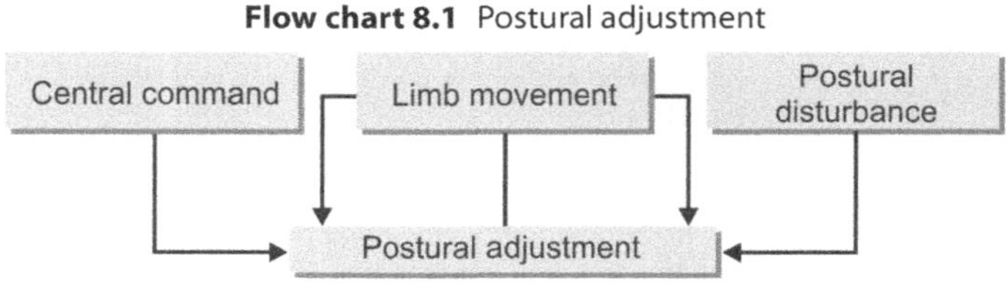

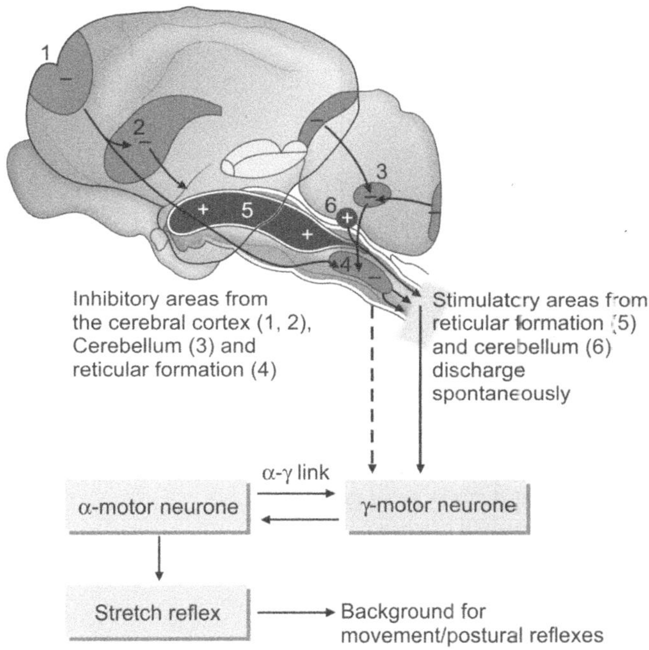

Fig. 8.1 Mechanism for postural reflexes

- Stereotyped
- Appropriately scaled.

Postural Control

- *Higher centers*:
  - *Cerebral cortex*:
    - Optical righting reflex
    - Placing reaction
    - Hopping reaction
  - Cerebellum
  - Basal ganglia
- *Brainstem*:
  - Pons
  - Midbrain

- *The righting reflex*:
  - Labyrinthe
  - Neck
  - Body on head
  - Body on body
- *Medulla*:
  - Tonic labyrinthine reflex
  - Tonic neck reflex

• *Spinal cord*:
  - Positive and negative supporting reaction
  - Stretch reflex.

Static Postural Reflexes

• *The axial muscles functions continuously and unconsciously*:
  - Making tiny adjustments
  - To enable body to keep seated/upright
    - Despite pull of gravity
  - When the center of gravity falls within the area bounded by the feet, the posture is stable.
    - If not, we fall!

• *Antigravity muscles (to maintain natural posture)*:
  - Upright animals - extensor
  - Extensor dominance
    - Masked by higher controls
    - If connection with higher control is loss, this becomes unmasked
    - Seen as extensor rigidity
  - Extensor response—Babinski sign UMN lesion
  - Animals that hang upside down-flexor
  - Flexor dominance
  - Loss of higher control
  - Flexor rigidity

• *Maintenance of position according to center of gravity*:
  - Women in heels
    - Center-of-gravity (COG) shifts forward
    - So pull back shoulders to maintain balance

- Pregnant woman
  - COG shift forward
  - So place hands on hips to lean backwards
- Incorrect posture (like bending forward in gardening)
  - Puts strain on antigravity muscles
- Newborn child can walk
  - But ability suppressed few days later
    - Start lying on belly
    - Head extended, front limbs extended, back limbs flexed (like going up slope)
- Walking patterns redeveloped a year later
- Baby cannot hold up neck until few months later
- Turning the head to one side (integrated in medulla)
  - Extension of ipsilateral limb
  - Flexion of contralateral limb

- *Postural changes—triggered by information from sensory receptors*:
  - Proprioceptors
    - Change in position of joints
  - Visual
    - Detection of movement/orientation
  - Vestibular
    - Motion— speed and direction
  - Cutaneous
    - Shearing forces.

Postural reflexes masked by higher controls. Unmasked when:

- Spinal cord transection in cervical region
- *Decerebration (removal of brain influence)*:
  - Transection at superior border of pons
  - Decerebrate rigidity
- *Decortication (removal of cortical influence)*:
  - Transection at superior border of midbrain
  - Decorticate rigidity
  - *Cardinal Rule of Neurology*:
    - If suprasegmental influences are removed
    - The effect of loss of inhibition are more pronounced than loss of stimulation
    - More inhibitory fibers than facilitatory fibers
  - Activities are then released from control of higher centers.

Spinal Cord Reflex

Stretch Reflex

A muscle contraction in response to stretching within the muscle:

- When muscle lengthens, the spindle is stretched and the activity increases.
- This increases alpha motor neuron activity.
- Therefore the muscle contracts and the length decreases as a result.
- The gamma co-activation is important in this reflex because this allows spindles in the muscles to remain taut therefore sensitive even during contraction.
- *Consider this scenario*: Flexing your arm to touch your nose and while doing that you encounter perturbation which reverses the movement.
  - With Gamma co-activation, monosynaptic stretch reflex return the movement to its previous course and the arm reaches the nose, but without it, spindles are slack and reflex will not be able to correct for the perturbation and the arm will fail to reach the nose.
  - Function of this reflex is to maintain a constant length and has the shortest latency of all spinal reflexes including 'Reflex mediated by the GTO (Golgi Tendon Organ)' and 'Reflexes mediated by pain and cutaneous receptors'.

Medulla Reflexes

- *Tonic neck reflex (primitive reflex found in newborn)* **(Figs 8.2A to D)**:
  - *Head up causes*:
    - Hind limbs to flex
    - Fore limbs to extend
  - *Head down*:
    - Fore limbs flex
    - Hind limbs extend
  - *Head turn to one side*:
    - Limbs on the side where head is turned to extend/straighten
    - Opposite side is bent/flexed
  - Decorticate posturing response (flexor)
  - *Signs*:
    - Arms flexed and bent inwards towards chest
    - Hands clenched into fists
    - Legs extended
    - Feed turned inward

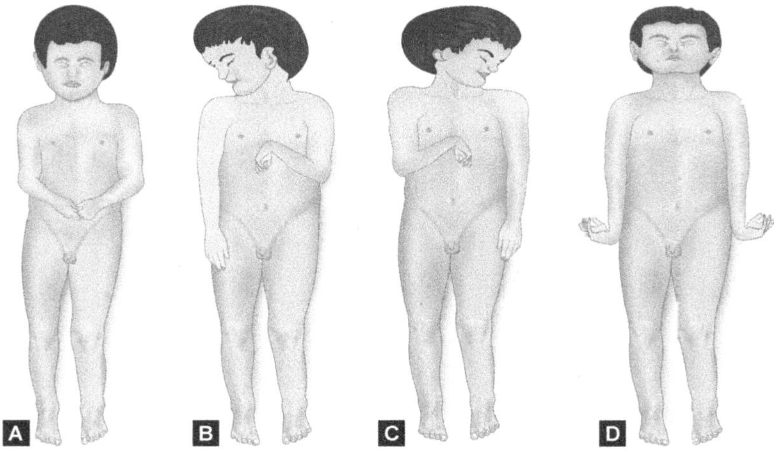

Figs 8.2A to D Tonic neck reflex may be unmasked when suprasegmental control is lost. Decerebrate (hindbrain animal) (medulla oblongata intact): (A) Head position normal, and limbs not extended; (B and C) Extension of limbs on side to which head is urned; (D) Head extended, and limbs rigid

- Seen in corticospinal tract lesion
  - Damage to (level above red nucleus)
    - Cerebral hemispheres
    - Internal capsule
    - Thalamus
    - Midbrain
  - Basal ganglia and reticulo—inhibitory fibers intact

  Glasgow coma scale-3
- *Decerebrate posturing response (extensor)*:
  - *Signs*:
    - Head-arched back
    - Arms extended by the sides and rotated internally (outward)
    - Extended elbows
    - Legs extended and rotated internally
    - Rigid with clenched teeth
- *Damage to (level below red nucleus)*:
  - Brainstem
    - Midbrain
  - Cerebellum

  Glasgow coma scale-2.

Tonic labyrinthine reflex (primitive reflex in newborn):

Gravity
↓
stimulation of otolith organs in labyrinth
↓
medulla
↓
contraction of limb extensor muscles

- Head tilt back while lying on back
  - Back stiffen and arch backwards
- Legs straighten
  - Stiffen and push together
- Toes to point
- Arms to bend at the elbows and wrists
- Hands to become fingers to curl.

Midbrain Righting Reflexes

Dynamic Reflexes

- Restore a normal standing position and keep head upright
- Reflexes seen in midbrain decorticate
- The ability to assume an optimal position when there has been a departure from it
  - *Labyrinthine-righting reflex*:
    - Gravity
      - Otolith organs
      - Head kept level against gravity
  - *Neck-righting reflex*:
    - Stretching of neck muscles
    - Righting of thorax, shoulders and pelvis
    - Body remains tilted, the neck muscles are stretched and initiate a wave of stretch reflexes to right the thorax, abdomen and hindquarters
  - Body on head-righting reflex
    - Head kept level against gravity when body is laid on its side
      - Lift head sideways
  - *Body on body-righting reflex*:
    - Righting of body even when head is held down.

Cerebral Cortex: Reflexes

Optical Righting Reflex

- Visual clues -> righting of the head
- *Placing reaction*:
  - Visual, enteroceptive and proprioceptive clues
  - Foot placed on supporting surface
- *Hopping reaction*:
  - Lateral displacement while standing
  - Cause animal to hop to maintain balance.

BALANCE AND POSTURAL CONTROL

Postural orientation: It involves control of relative position of body parts by skeletal muscle with respect to each other and gravity.

Balance: It is condition in which all forces acting on body are balance such that the COG is within stability limits, the boundaries of BOS.

Balance to be checked:
- *Static*: During static postural control
- *Dynamic*: During dynamic postural balance control
- *Functional*: During functional activities (e.g. walking, stair climbing, transfer).

Static balance can be assessed by following postures:
- Single limb stance
- Double limb stance
- Tandem stance
- Romberg's test

Balance grades for static balance:
- *Normal*: Patient able to maintain steady balance without handhold support.
- *Good*: Patient able to maintain balance without handheld support, limited postural sway.
- *Fair*: Patient able to maintain balance without handheld support, may require minimal assistance.
- *Poor*: Patient require handheld support and moderate to minimal assistance to maintain position.
- No balance.

Dynamic balance: Maintenance of balance during weight shifting or voluntary movement.

- Weight shifting in all direction
- Sit to stand and sit down
- Reaching movements
- Turning
- Step ups

Balance grades for dynamic balance:

- *Normal*: Accept maximal challenge and can shift weight easily within full range in all direction
- *Good*: Accept moderate challenges, able to maintain balance while picking object from floor
- *Fair*: Accept minimal challenges, able to maintain balance while turning head or trunk.
- *Poor*: Unable to accept challenge or move without loss of balance.
- No balance.

Check equilibrium and protective reaction during dynamic balance.

- *Postural control strategy assessment*:
  - Motor strategy
    - Alignment in sitting and standing
  - Voluntary sway
  - Nudge test
- Sensory strategy

Modified clinical test of sensory interaction on balance: This test allows for preliminary assessment of how well a patient can integrate various senses with respect to balance and compensate when one or more of those senses are compromised.

No.	*Condition tested*	*Deficit*
1.	Eyes open standing on normal surface 3 sensory system available (vision, vestibular, somatosensory)	
2.	Eyes close on normal surface (vestibular, somatosensory available)	Visual
3.	Eyes open and standing on foam (vestibular and vision available)	Somatosensory compromised
4.	Eyes close and standing on foam (vestibular available)	Visual and inaccurate somatosensory

Observation of sway in each condition is graded as:

- Minimal sway
- Mild sway
- Moderate sway
- Fall.

Support Strategies

There are three fixed support strategies for maintaining balance **(Fig. 8.3)**:

1. Ankle.
2. Hip.
3. Stepping strategies.

The ankle strategy is usually the first line of defense in maintaining balance. When a patient uses an ankle strategy, the head and hips move in same direction and stay within the patient's limits of stability (LOS). Contractions in the lower extremity occur from distal to proximal musculature.

A hip strategy, most common in the elderly population, results in the head and hips moving in the opposite direction and lower extremity muscle contractions activating proximal to distal.

A stepping strategy has been historically viewed as occurring when a person's center of gravity (COG) exceeds that person's limits of stability

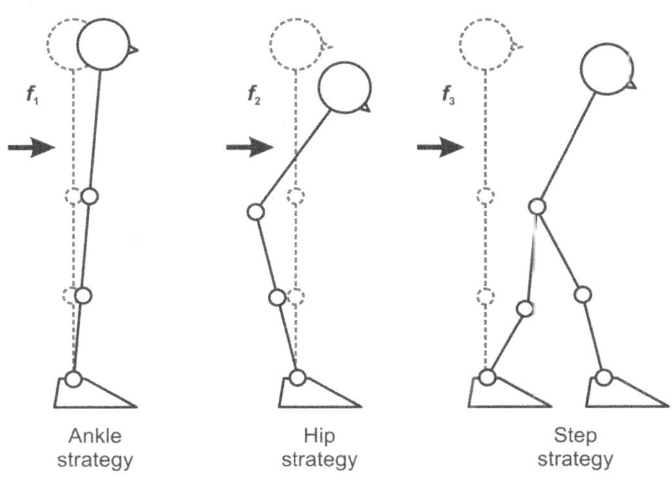

Fig. 8.3 Support strategy

(LOS). A step is taken to prevent a fall to establish a new base of support under a shifting COG.

Stepping strategy and grasping strategy may actually be initiated prior to the COG exceeding the LOS and may also occur prior to a hip strategy. The hip strategy usually occurs when conditions preclude someone from using a stepping or grasping strategy.

Testing

To test for patients' strategy use, first have them do voluntary anterior/posterior and lateral weight shifts on a firm surface that is larger than the patient's feet for evidence of ankle strategy and an unstable surface (e.g. rocker board, foam) or surface that is shorter than the patient's feet (i.e. balance beam or two by four) for a hip strategy **(Fig. 8.4)**.

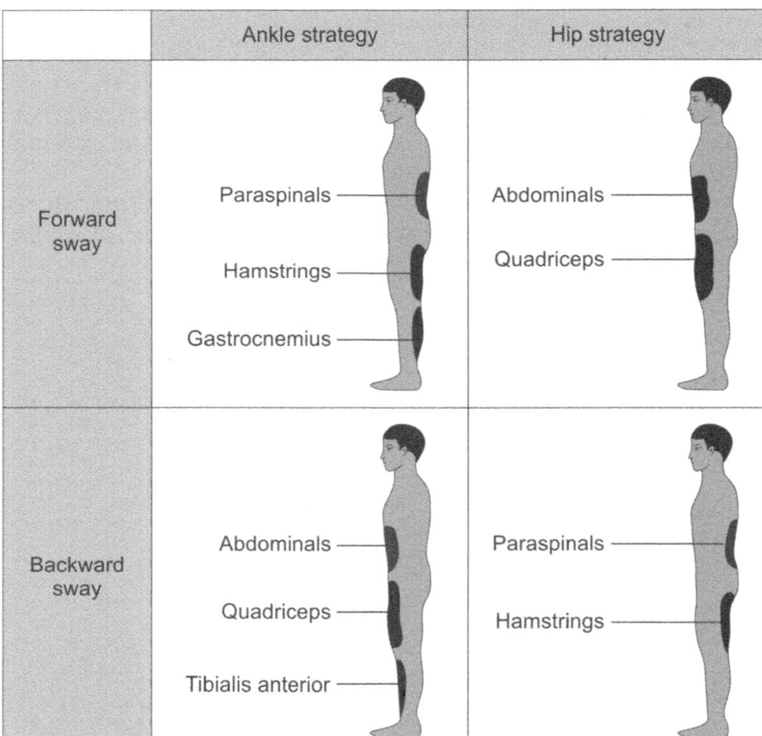

Fig. 8.4 Muscles working in forward and backward sway

Progress to reaching tasks: Reaching 4–6 inches should result in an ankle strategy and 8–10 inches a hip or stepping strategy. Then, progress to perturbations. To test for a patient's ability to use an ankle strategy, use small and slow perturbations. Use large and fast perturbations for a hip strategy. Continue testing by progressing from anticipated perturbations to unpredictable, unexpected perturbations.

9 Abnormal Movements

ABNORMAL INVOLUNTARY MOVEMENTS

Abnormal involuntary movements (AIMs) are also known as "dyskinesias". There are several different varieties of dyskinesia which have different clinical appearances, underlying causes and treatments. Tremor, chorea, dystonia and myoclonus are examples of types of dyskinesia which have different mechanisms and modalities of treatment.

Tics and stereotypes may also be considered to be related, but some experts call these "involuntary" because there is an element of voluntary control.

Classification

Athetosis

- Sinuous writhing movement of the fingers and hands.

Chorea

- Continuous jerky movements in which each movement is sudden and the resulting posture is held for a few seconds. Usually affects head, face or limbs. The focus may move from one part of the body to another at random. Common cause of chorea is adverse effects of drug treatments especially those for *Parkinson's disease, epilepsy* and *schizophrenia*.
  - *Huntington's chorea*: Autosomal dominant inheritance, usually presents in middle age with chorea and *dementia*. Insidious onset with motor, cognitive and psychiatric abnormalities. No treatment.
  - *Sydenham's chorea*: Also known as St Vitus's Dance. Mainly associated with *acute rheumatic fever*. Now rare. Usually presents in children aged 7–12 years, initially with psychological symptoms of behavioral disturbance followed by generalized chorea and

usually recovers in 1–3 months. Penicillin for *rheumatic fever* and diazepam, haloperidol or tetrabenazine for chorea.

Dystonia

Many abnormal involuntary movements occur because of disorders in the basal ganglia.

Dystonia: Muscle spasms contracting the neck, limbs and trunk into typical postures:

- Spasm occurs with intentional movement and may be intermittent and repetitive, so giving a rhythmic appearance to the movement or may be persistent, to give a fixed posture.
- Idiopathic torsion dystonia; condition inherited in autosomal dominant pattern. Usually presents in children, with dystonic spasms of the legs on walking, occasionally of the arms, trunk or neck.
- Normally progressive and spreading to the whole body, causing severe disability within about 10 years. Trial of levodopa as may have dopa-responsive dystonia-Parkinsonism (Segawa's syndrome); otherwise high doses of benzodiazepines and anticholinergics, e.g. benzhexol.

In adults, the condition is not usually inherited and presents with a focal dystonia:

- *Blepherospasm*: Recurrent spasms of eye closure; treated with *botulinum toxin* injection into the orbicularis oculi muscle.
- *Oromandibular dystonia*: Recurrent spasm affecting the mouth and jaw, larynx and pharynx. No effective treatment.
- *Writer's cramp*: Inability to write or use any manual instrument due to abnormal posture of hand and arm. Ask patient to use other hand, injection of botulinum toxin into forearm may help. See *Writer's Cramp article.*

Hemiballismus

Wild flinging/throwing movements of one arm or leg, usually occurring as result of a *cerebrovascular event.* Can vary in intensity from mild to severe and may even cause injury. Usually subsides over 3–6 months but can be treated with a phenothiazine, haloperidol or tetrabenazine. May require neurosurgery.

- *Myoclonus*: Rapid muscle jerks, frequently repetitive and appears as:
  - Benign essential myoclonus; affects much of body, repeated as many as 50 times per minute. Presents in childhood or adolescence with mild disability. Helped by alcohol and beta-blockers.
  - Progressive myoclonic encephalopathies; appear as part of a range of other neurological disorders.
  - Static myoclonic encephalopathies; Lance-Adams syndrome after cerebral anoxia.

  Myoclonic epilepsies, e.g. focal myoclonus—restricted to one part of the body, e.g. spinal-affecting extremities, and *hemifacial spasm* occurring in 1 per 100,000, mainly affecting older women.
- *Spasmodic torticollis*:
  - This usually presents in middle age or elderly with torticollis or sometimes retrocollis or anticollis. Can be repetitive causing tremulous torticollis. Often has a compensatory Lordosis.
  - In one fifth of patients, may remit for a year or more but mostly life-long condition. Condition worsened by stress but patient often finds some manual activity to control the torticollis, e.g. touching jaw with forefinger.
  - Identification of overactive muscle and injection of botulinum toxin often helps. May need local denervation in intractable conditions.
- *Tardive dyskinesia*:
  - Usually occurs following at least six months' treatment with *neuroleptics*; more frequent in older patients; occurs in 20% of those on chronic therapy and persists in 40% of cases after discontinuation of therapy.
  - Characterized by orofacial mouthing with lip-smacking and tongue protrusion, body rocking and distal chorea. In younger patients may cause axial and cranial dystonia.

Tics

Repetitive stereotyped movements. Patient can initiate voluntarily and can also intentionally suppress for a short time.

- *Simple tic*: Sudden rapid twitch always occurring at the same site. Occurs in a quarter of all children and resolves within a year. May persist into adulthood; rarely treated.
- *Complex multiple tics*: More extensive and severe. When occurring with patient speaking, particularly swearing, maybe represent *Gilles*

de la Tourette syndrome. May also appear as symptom of *encephalitis lethargica*, neuroacanthocytosis and be drug induced.

Tremor

Rhythmic movement of part of the body. There are three types of pathological tremor:

- *Static tremor*: Occurs in a relaxed limb when fully supported at rest. Causes include Parkinson's disease, Parkinsonism, other extrapyramidal diseases, *multiple sclerosis*.
- *Postural tremor*: Occurs if a limb is static (can also remain during movement). Types include physiological tremor, exaggerated physiological tremor, e.g. in *thyrotoxicosis*, anxiety states, alcohol abuse, drugs (e.g. sympathomimetics, antidepressants, valproate, lithium), *heavy metal poisoning* ('hatter's shakes' from mercury). Neurological disease, e.g. severe cerebellar lesions, *Wilson's disease, neurosyphilis*, peripheral neuropathies, benign essential (familial) tremor, task-specific tremors, e.g. primary writing tremor.
- *Kinetic or action tremor*: Occurs during voluntary active movement of upper body part. Intention tremor is one that occurs when a tremor worsens as a goal-directed hand movement nears its intended target. Brain stem or *cerebellar disease* including MS, spinocerebellar degenerations, vascular disease, tumors.

Tremors and dystonias that are not secondary to Parkinson's disease may be effectively treated with deep brain electrical stimulation. There are also psychogenic tremors. Benign essential tremor is treated with alcohol in moderation. Beta-blockers or primidone are also used.

Assessment of Abnormal Involuntary Movements

The abnormal involuntary movement (AIM) scale is used to assess tardive dyskinesias and other AIMs. This can be useful to monitor progress and response to treatment.

In evaluating movement disorder, there are three aspects to the examination:

1. *Positive phenomena*:
   - Abnormal position maintained
   - Additional movement seen.
2. *Latent phenomena*: The abnormal phenomena that can be revealed using various maneuvers. Rigidity on testing tone and abnormal postures brought on by writing in writer's clamp.

3. *Negative phenomena*: The inability to do the things, e.g. slowness in imitating action (bradykinesia).

Look at patient's face.
- Are there any additional movements?
- Is the face expressionless?

Look at Patient's Head Position

Look at arms and legs:
- Note position
- Are there any abnormal movements?

Ask the patient to:
- Smile
- Close his eyes
- Hold his hands out in front of him with his wrist cocked back
- Lift his elbows sideways and point his index finger at one another in front of his nose.
- Perform the finger nose test.

If there is tremor note the frequency, the degree of excursion and body parts affected. Look for a tongue tremor.

Test Eye Movements

Test Tone

Test fast repeating movement:
- Bring thumb and index finger rapidly together.
- Touch the thumb with each finger rapidly in turn.
- Tap his toe as if listening to fast music.

Observe speed of movement and weather they break up, compare right with left.
- Test the gait
- Test writing
- Ask patient to:
  - Write his name and address
- Findings.

FACE

Positive Phenomena

Commonly:

- *Lip smacking and twisting of mouth*: Orofacial dyskinesia
- *Flickering of muscle, particularly around eye*: Facial myokymia.

Rarely:

- *Intermittent spasm of muscles around the eye*: Blepherospasm.
- *Intermittent spasm of muscles of one side of face*: Hemifacial spasm.

Negative Phenomena

Facial immobility.

HEAD

Positive Phenomena

- Position
- *Head twisted to one side*: Torticollis
- *Head bent forward*: Anterocollis
- *Head bent backwards*: Retrocollis
- Movement
- Rhythmical
- *Movement of head*: Titubation described as yes-yes or no-no.

ARMS AND LEGS

Positive Phenomena

Tremor

- *Present when limb is at rest*: Rest tremors.
- *Present when limb is maintained in a position*: Postural tremor.
- *Present during an action*: Action tremor.
- *Present and increasing as finger reaches its target*: Intension tremor.

Asterixis

Irregular jerky movements of hands seen during finger to nose or when arms held at 90° flexion.

Latent Phenomena

- On walking the following may occur or increase
- Rest tremor
- Dystonic posturing
- Chorea
- Finger nose testing may reveal
- Action tremor
- Intention tremor
- Myoclonus
- Fast repatriating movements
- *Slowed or break up easily*: Bradykinesia
- *Tone*: Cogwheel rigidity may be found only when the other arm is lifted up and down.
- Writing
- *Writing become progressively slower the hand may go into spasm and the patient often holds the pain in an unusual way*: Writer's clamp.

Negative Phenomena

- *Rigidity*: Lead pipe or cogwheel.
- *Bradykinesia*: Slowness in initiating movement.
- Reduced arm swing on walking.

10 Gait and Station

- Abnormalities of gait are a common clinical problem with numerous causes, both neurologic and non-neurologic. A careful general evaluation is always necessary to exclude a non-neurologic cause.
- Station is the way a patient stands, gait the way she walks. Standing and walking are active processes that depend upon a number of factors and reflex responses. The mechanisms are complex, especially in the human, whose biped gait and erect position over a narrow base require more efficient maintenance and control of equilibrium than is necessary in quadrupeds.
- Normal resting tone, especially in the antigravity muscles, is essential.
- Standing may be considered a postural reflex that is dependent on reflexes mediated through the brainstem and influenced to a major degree by tonic neck and labyrinthine reflexes.
- If the mechanisms mediating static and postural reflexes are impaired, normal standing and walking will be impaired. In addition, proprioceptive sensation must be received, the skeletal system must be intact, the muscles must be functioning normally, and coordination must be adequate.
- Gait and station may be affected by abnormalities of proprioception, abnormalities of muscle power or tone, abnormalities of vestibular function, and by dysfunction of the basal ganglia, the cerebellum, or their connections.

Neurologic causes of an abnormal gait include conditions as varied as:
- Foot drop due to peroneal nerve palsy
- Myopathy
- Hydrocephalus
- Cerebellar degeneration

The various gait abnormalities have different findings on physical examination in regard to the gait itself, such as a steppage pattern as opposed to a pelvic waddle. The differential diagnosis of the gait abnormality is also very dependent on the history and the other clinical signs present.

EXAMINATION OF STATION

- Station is the patient's attitude, posture, or manner of standing.
- The healthy individual stands erect with her head up, chest out, and abdomen in. Abnormality of station may be an important indicator of neurologic disease.
- Station is tested by having the patient stand, feet closely together, noting any unsteadiness or swaying.
- Testing includes having the patient stand eyes open and eyes closed, on one foot at a time, on toes and heels, and tandem with one heel in front of the toes of the other foot. She may be given a gentle push to see whether she falls to one side, forward, or backward.
- Patients with unsteadiness standing often attempt to compensate by placing the feet wide apart in order to stand on a broader and steadier base.
- In cerebellar disease, the patient usually stands on a broad base and there is swaying, to more or less an equal degree, with eyes open and closed. With a lesion of the vermis, the patient may sway backward, forward, or to either side. With a lesion of one hemisphere she sways or falls toward the affected side.
- Unilateral vestibular disease also causes falling toward the affected side. In a unilateral, cerebellar hemispheric lesion, or in a unilateral vestibulopathy, the patient may tilt the head toward the involved side with the chin rotated toward the sound side, with the shoulder on the involved side somewhat higher than the other and slightly in front of it.
- If the patient is given a light push—first toward one side and then toward the other—with a cerebellar hemispheric lesion she will lose balance more easily when pushed toward the involved side.
- If asked to stand on one foot at a time, the patient with a cerebellar hemispheric lesion may be unable to maintain equilibrium standing on the ipsilateral foot, but may stand without difficulty on the contralateral foot.

The Romberg Sign

- When proprioception is disturbed, the patient may be able to stand with eyes open, but sways or falls with eyes closed (Romberg's or Brauch-Romberg sign).
- The essential finding is a difference between standing balance with eyes open and closed.

- In order to test this function, the patient must have a stable stance eyes open and then demonstrate a decrease in balance with eyes closed, when visual input is eliminated and the patient must rely on proprioception to maintain balance.
- The Romberg test can be difficult to interpret. There is some variability, even among expert examiners, in how the Romberg test is performed and interpreted. Many patients sway slightly with eyes closed, and minimal amounts of sway, especially in elderly patients, is seldom significant. Minor, normal swaying may stop if the patient is simply asked to stand perfectly still. Most clinicians discount sway at the hips, and insist on seeing sway at the ankles before calling the test positive; some require the patient take a corrective step to the side; and some that the patient nearly fall. Some require the patient be barefoot.
- The "sharpened" or tandem Romberg is done by having the patient stand in tandem position with eyes open and closed; the limits of normality for this variation are conjectural.

Use of Romberg's Sign

- Test of proprioceptive
- Useful in separating tabes dorsalis from cerebellar disease
- Acute unilateral vestibulopathy

False Romberg's sign: Some histrionic patients will sway with eyes closed in the absence of any organic neurological impairment.

The instability can often be eliminated by diverting the patient's attention. Effective distracters are to ask the patient to detect numbers the examiner writes with her finger on the forehead, wiggle the tongue, or to perform the finger-to-nose testing.

Having the shoes off and watching the toe movements may be very informative. The toes of the patient with histrionic sway are often extended; the patient with organic imbalance flexes the toes strongly and tries to grip the floor.

PHYSIOLOGY OF GAIT

The brainstem and spinal cord in lower forms contain "central pattern generators", which are groups of interneurons that coordinate the activity in pools of motor neurons to produce patterned movements.

The pattern generators control the activity in lower motor neurons that execute the mechanics of walking.

Higher centers in the sub thalamus and midbrain, particularly the pedunculopontine nucleus, modulate the activity in the spinal cord pattern generators through the reticulospinal tracts.

Normal Gait

Gait is the medical term to describe human locomotion, or the way that we walk. Interestingly, every individual has a unique gait pattern.

Definitions

- *Physiological*:
  - It is a mechanism which depends upon closely integrated action of the subjects, bones, muscles and nervous system (including peripheral and central nervous system)
  - The degree of integration determines the different gait patterns. Any defect of any part of them or all of them will lead to pathological gait.
- *Mechanical*:
  - It is a form of bipedal locomotion as there is an alternating action between lower extremities. One leg is in touch with the ground for restraining, supporting and propulsion.
  - The other leg is in swing phase for creating a new step forward. So gait is the result of a series of rhythmic alternating movement of arms, legs, and trunk which create forward movement of the body.

Prerequisites of Gait

There are four major criteria essential to walking:

1. *Equilibrium*: The ability to assume an upright posture and maintain balance.
2. *Locomotion*: The ability to initiate and maintain rhythmic stepping.
3. *Musculoskeletal integrity*: Normal bone, joint, and muscle function.
4. *Neurological control*: Must receive and send messages telling the body how and when to move. (Visual, vestibular, auditory, sensori-motor input.)

Forces for Gait

- Muscular force
- Gravitational force
- Forces of momentum
- Floor reaction force

Gait Cycle

- *The gait cycle* is used to describe the complex activity of walking, or our gait pattern. This cycle describes the motions from initial placement of the supporting heel on the ground to when the same heel contacts the ground for a second time.
- *Phases of gait*: Each gait cycle can be described in the phasic terms.

Stance Phase

- It is defined as the interval in which the foot is on the ground (60% of the gait cycle).
- *Stance phase is divided into*:
  - Heel strike to flat foot
  - Flatfoot to mid stance
  - Mid stance through heel off
  - Heel-off to toe-off
- *The stance period consists of the first four phases*: Initial contact, loading response, mid-stance and terminal stance.

Initial Contact

Initial contact is an instantaneous point in time only and occurs the instant the foot of the leading lower limb touches the ground. Most of the motor function that occurs during initial contact is in preparation for the loading response phase that will follow. Initial contact represents the beginning of the stance phase. Heel strike and heel contact serve as poor descriptors of this period since there are many circumstances when initial contact is not made with the heel alone. The term "foot strike" sometimes is used as an alternative descriptor.

Loading Response

The loading response phase occupies about 10% of the gait cycle and constitutes the period of initial double-limb support. During loading response, the foot comes in full contact with the floor, and body weight is fully transferred onto the stance limb.

The initial double-support stance period occasionally is referred to as initial stance. The term foot flat (FF) is the point in time when the foot becomes plantar grade. The loading response period probably is best described by the typical quantified values of the vertical force curve. The ascending initial peak of the vertical force graph reveals the period of loading response.

Mid-stance

Mid-stance represents the first half of single support, which occurs from 10 to 30% periods of the gait cycle. It begins when the contralateral foot leaves the ground and continues as the body weight travels along the length of the foot, until it is aligned over the forefoot. The descending initial peak of the vertical force graph reveals the period of mid-stance.

Terminal Stance

Terminal stance constitutes the second half of single-limb support. It begins with heel rise and ends when the contralateral foot contacts the ground. Terminal stance occurs from 30% to 50% periods of the gait cycle. During this phase, body weight moves ahead of the forefoot.

- The term heel off (HO) is a descriptor useful in observational analysis and is the point during the stance phase when the heel leaves the ground. The ascending second peak of the vertical force graph demonstrates the period of terminal stance.
- Roll off describes the period of late stance (from 40% to 50% periods of the gait cycle) when there is an ankle plantar-flexor moment and simultaneous power generation of the triceps surae to initiate advancement of the tibia over the fulcrum of the metatarsal heads in preparation for the next phase.

Swing Phase

- It is defined as the interval in which the foot is not in contact with the ground (40% of the gait cycle). Denotes the time when the foot is in the air, constituting the remaining 38% of the gait cycle. The swing phase could be defined as the phase when all portions of the foot are in forward motion. Swing is divided into two phases:
  1. Acceleration to mid swing.
  2. Mid-swing to deceleration.

- *The swing period primarily is divided into* three phases: Initial swing, mid-swing and terminal swing. Preswing, however, prepares the limb for swing advancement and in that sense could be considered a component of swing phase.

Preswing

- *Preswing* is the terminal double-limb support period and occupies the last 12% of stance phase, from 50% to 62%. It begins when the contralateral foot contacts the ground and ends with ipsilateral toe off. During this period, the stance limb is unloaded and body weight is transferred onto the contralateral limb. The descending portion of the second peak of the vertical force graph demonstrates the period of preswing.
- Terminal contact (TC), a term rarely used, describes the instantaneous point in the gait cycle when the foot leaves the ground. It thus represents either the end of the stance phase or the beginning of swing phase. In pathologies where the foot never leaves the ground, the term foot drag is used. In foot drag, the termination of stance and the onset of swing may be somewhat arbitrary.
- The termination of stance and the onset of swing is defined as the point where all portions of the foot have achieved motion relative to the floor. Likewise, the termination of swing and the onset of stance may be defined as the point when the foot ends motion relative to the floor. Toe off occurs when terminal contact is made with the toe.

Initial Swing

The initial one-third of the swing period, from 62% to 75% periods of the gait cycle is spent in initial swing. It begins the moment the foot leaves the ground and continues until maximum knee flexion occurs, when the swinging extremity is directly under the body and directly opposite the stance limb.

Mid-swing

Mid-swing occurs in the second third of the swing period, from 75% to 85% periods of the gait cycle. Critical events include continued limb advancement and foot clearance. This phase begins following maximum knee flexion and ends when the tibia is in a vertical position.

Terminal Swing

In the final phase of terminal swing from 85% to 100% periods of the gait cycle, the tibia passes beyond perpendicular, and the knee fully extends in preparation for heel contact.

GAIT TERMINOLGY

We are calculating the two basic parameters:

1. Time.
2. Distance.

Temporal Variable

- Stance time
- Single limb and double time
- Swing time
- Stride and step time
- Cadence
- Speed

Stance time: It is the amount of time that elapses during the stance phase of one extremity in a gait cycle.

Single support time: Only one extremity is on the supporting surface in a gait cycle.

Double support time: It is the amount of time spent with both feet on the ground during one gait cycle

- Increased in elderly persons and in those with balance disorders
- Decreases as the speed of walking increases

Stride duration: Amount of time it takes to complete one stride

- Stride duration and gait cycle are synonymous
- For normal adult the stride duration lasts for 1 sec.

Distance Variable

- Stride length
- Step length
- Width
- Degree of toe-out

Stride length: It is the linear distance between two successive events that are accomplished by the same lower extremity.

- It is measured from the point of one heel strike of one lower extremity to the point of the next heel strike of the same extremity
- ↓ - elderly patients and ↑ - speed of gait increases

Step length: It is the linear distance between two successive points of contact of opposite extremities

- Measured from the heel of one extremity to the heel strike of the opposite extremity
- If there pain in an extremity, step duration decrease on the affected side and increase on the normal side

Cadence: No of steps/unit of time, it is usually measured steps/min

- Adult men—110 steps/min
- Adult women—116 steps/min

Walking velocity: It is the rate of linear forward motion of the body, which can be measured in meters or cm/sec, m/min, miles/hour

- Meters/sec is preferred
- Walking velocity (m/sec) = distance walked (meters)/time (sec)
- Increases in velocity up to 120 steps/min—increases both cadence and stride length
- Above 120 steps/min, step length levels off, speed increases are achieved only with cadence increases.

Speed:

- Free speed of gait refers to a person's normal walking speed
- Slow and fast speeds of gait refers to speeds slower or faster than the person's normal comfortable walking speed

Step width: Measuring the linear distance between the midpoint of the heel of one foot and the same point on the other foot

- Step width ↑ in elderly persons and children as they demand more stability
- In young children, COG is higher than in adults, as wide base of support is necessary for stability
- Normal width - 3.5 inches and varies between 1 and 5 inches

Degree of toe out: Measuring the angle formed by each foot's line of progression and a line intersecting the center of the heel and the second toe

- Angle of degree for normal men–7
- Degree of toe out ↓ as the speed of walking ↑ in normal men

- Gait terminology
- *Power generation*: Power generated or absorbed across a joint is the product of the net internal moment and the net angular velocity across the joint
- When work is positive in value, the internal moment and joint angular velocity are acting in the same direction, a concentric muscle contraction is indicated, and mechanical energy is being generated
- During periods of energy generation, the muscle is working on the limbs to produce movement.

ABNORMAL GAITS

Five major components those are lost in pathological gait are:
1. Stability and stance.
2. Sufficient foot clearance during swing.
3. Appropriate swing phase repositioning of the foot.
4. Adequate step length.
5. Energy conservation.

Abnormal gait different area like may be caused by diseases in many:
- Vestibular disorders (the inner ear is responsible for maintaining balance, and damage results in *vertigo*)
- *Central nervous system* (disorders of the brain that cause muscular problems resulting in gait disturbance such as *multiple sclerosis* and *cerebral palsy*)
- Spinal cord abnormalities (disease, trauma, degeneration)
- Degenerative muscle diseases (*muscular dystrophy, myositis*)
- Neurodegenerative illnesses (Parkinson's disease)
- Skeletal abnormalities and disease
- *Arthritis*
- Foot conditions (*plantar warts, bunions, ingrown toenails,* pressure ulcers)
- Toxic reactions (alcohol, drugs, allergens)
- Peripheral nerve diseases (nerves from the spinal cord to the muscles may be damaged by disease or trauma and result in gait abnormalities).

Causes of Abnormal Gait

- Trauma
- Foot problems (such as a callus, corn, ingrown toenail, wart, pain, skin ulcer, swelling, spasms)

- *Fracture*
- *Hemophilia*
- Immunization (soreness in the leg or buttocks)
- Legs that are different lengths myositis
- Tight or uncomfortable shoes
- Shin splints
- Infection
- *Tendonitis*
- *Conversion disorder* (a psychological disorder)

Cerebellar Ataxia

The gait of cerebellar disease is caused by involvement of the coordinating mechanisms in the cerebellum and its connecting systems.

Characteristics

- Clumsy
- Staggering
- Unsteady
- Irregular
- Lurching
- Titubating
- Wide-based gait
- The patient may sway to either side, back, or forward
- Leg movements are erratic, and step length varies unpredictably.
- The patient is unable to walk tandem or follow a straight line on the floor.
- There may be tremors and oscillatory movements involving the entire body. With a lesion of the cerebellar vermis, the patient will exhibit a lurching, staggering gait, but without laterality, the ataxia will be as marked toward one side as the other.
- Cerebellar ataxia is present with eyes both open and closed; it may increase slightly with eyes closed, but not so markedly as in sensory ataxia.
- A gait resembling cerebellar ataxia is seen in acute alcohol intoxication. With a hemispheric lesion, the patient will stagger and deviate toward the involved side.

Causes

- Disease localized to one cerebellar hemisphere
- In unilateral vestibular disease
- There is persistent swaying or deviation toward the abnormal side. As the patient attempts to walk a straight line or to walk tandem she deviates toward the side of the lesion.
- Walking a few steps backward and forward with eyes closed may bring out "compass deviation" or a "star-shaped gait". When attempting to walk a fixed circle around a chair, clockwise then counterclockwise, the patient will tend to fall toward the chair if it is on the side of the lesion, or to spiral out away from the chair if on the opposite side.
- Either unilateral cerebellar or vestibular disease may cause turning toward the side of the lesion on the Fukuda stepping test.
- For all the tests that bring out deviation in one direction, other findings must be used to differentiate between vestibulopathy and a cerebellar hemispheric lesion. Unilateral ataxia may be demonstrated by having the patient attempt to jump on one foot, with the eyes either open or closed.
- The patient with bilateral vestibular disease may seek to minimize head movement during walking, holding the head stiff and rigid; having the patient turn the head back and forth during walking may bring out ataxia.

Sensory Ataxia

- The difference in walking ability with and without visual input is the key feature of sensory ataxia. If the condition is mild, locomotion may appear normal when the patient walks eyes open; more commonly it is wide based, and poorly coordinated.
- The term "steppage gait" refers to a manner of walking in which the patient takes unusually high steps. Sensory ataxia is one of the causes of a steppage gait.
- The patient takes a high step, throws out her foot, and slams it down on the floor in order to increase the proprioceptive feedback.
- The heel may land before the toe, creating an audible "double tap". An additional sound effect may be the tapping of a cane, creating a "slam, slam, tap" cadence.
- The patient with sensory ataxia watches her feet and keeps her eyes on the floor while walking.

- With eyes closed, the feet seem to shoot out, the staggering and unsteadiness are increased, and the patient may be unable to walk.
- There is less reeling and lurching in sensory ataxia than with a comparable degree of cerebellar ataxia.
- The difficulty is even worse walking backward, since the patient cannot see where she is going. The patient with bilateral foot drops, however, also has a steppage gait and a double tapping.
- In all of these tests, sensory ataxia can be differentiated from predominantly cerebellar ataxia by accentuation of the difficulty with eyes closed; and unilateral cerebellar or vestibular disease from vermis involvement by laterality of unsteadiness.

The Gait of Spastic Hemiparesis

- The patient stands with a hemiparetic posture, arm flexed, adducted, and internally rotated, and leg extended. There is plantar flexion of the foot and toes, either due to foot dorsiflexion weakness or to heel cord shortening, rendering the lower extremity on the involved side functionally slightly longer than on the normal side, referred to as an equinus deformity.
- When walking, the patient holds the arm tightly to the side, rigid and flexed; she extends it with difficulty and does not swing it in a normal fashion. She holds the leg stiffly in extension and flexes it with difficulty.
- Consequently, the patient drags or shuffles the foot and scrapes the toes. With each step, she may tilt the pelvis upward on the involved side to aid in lifting the toe off the floor (hip hike) and may swing the entire extremity around in a semicircle from the hip (circumduction).
- The stance phase is shortened because of weakness, and the swing phase shortened because of spasticity and slowing of movement.
- The sound produced by the scraping of the toe, as well as the wear of the shoe at the toe, may be quite characteristic.
- The patient is able to turn toward the paralyzed side more easily than toward the normal side. Loss of normal arm swing and slight circumduction of the leg may be the only gait abnormalities in very mild hemiparesis.

Scissoring

- This gait pattern occurs in patients who have severe spasticity of the legs.

- It occurs in patients who have congenital spastic diplegia (Little's disease, cerebral palsy) and related conditions, and in chronic myelopathies due to conditions such as multiple sclerosis and cervical spondylosis.
- There is characteristic tightness of the hip adductors causing adduction of the thighs, so that the knees may cross, one in front of the other, with each step (scissors gait).
- The patient walks on an abnormally narrow base, with a stiff shuffling gait, dragging both legs and scraping the toes.
- The steps are short and slow; the feet seem to stick to the floor. There may be marked compensatory sway of the trunk away from the side of the advancing leg. Swaying and staggering may suggest an element of ataxia, but usually there is no true loss of coordination.
- The shuffling, scraping sound—together with worn areas at the toes of the shoes—are characteristic.
- The equinus position of the feet and heel cord shortening often cause the patient to walk on tiptoe.

The Spastic-Ataxic Gait

- Some neurological disorders cause involvement of both the corticospinal and the proprioceptive pathways (e.g. combined system disease due to vitamin B_{12} deficiency, or multiple sclerosis), resulting in a gait that has features of both spasticity and ataxia.
- The relative proportion of each abnormality depends on the particulars of the case. The ataxic component may be either cerebellar or sensory.
- In vitamin B_{12} deficiency, it is predominantly sensory; in multiple sclerosis, both components may be present.
- In amyotrophic lateral sclerosis, there may be bilateral foot drops, as well as spasticity, resulting in an abnormality in walking that may suggest a spastic ataxic gait.
- The gait has been described as "jiggling" or "bobbing", with tremulous, bouncing, up-and-down body movements.

The Parkinsonian Gait

- The gait in most akinetic-rigid, parkinsonian syndromes is characterized by rigidity, bradykinesia, and loss of associated movements.

- The patient is stooped, with head and neck forward and knees flexed; the upper extremities are flexed at the shoulders, elbows, and wrists, but the fingers are usually extended.
- The gait is slow, stiff, and shuffling; the patient walks with small, mincing steps. Difficulty walking may be one of the earliest symptoms of the disease.
- The same gait disorder can occur with any condition causing parkinsonism, such as drug side effects.

The Myopathic (Waddling) Gait

- Myopathic gaits occur when there is weakness of the hip girdle muscles, most often due to myopathy, and most characteristically due to muscular dystrophy.
- If the hip flexors are weak, then there may be a pronounced lordosis.
- The hip abductor muscles are vital in stabilizing the pelvis while walking. Trendelenburg's sign is an abnormal drop of the pelvis on the side of the swing leg due to hip abductor weakness.
- When the weakness is bilateral, there is an exaggerated pelvic swing that results in a waddling gait. The patient walks with a broad base, with an exaggerated rotation of the pelvis, rolling or throwing the hips from side to side with every step to shift the weight of the body.
- In the extreme forms, this gait pattern has a bizarre appearance. The patient walks with a pronounced waddle, shoulders thrown back and pelvis thrust forward.
- This form of gait is particularly common in facioscapulohumeral muscular dystrophy.
- The myopathy patient has marked difficulty climbing stairs, often needing to pull herself up with the hand rail. Patients also have difficulty going from a lying to standing position without placing the hands on the knees and hips to push themselves up.

Cautious ('Senile') Gait

- A cautious gait is seen in older patients who have no neurological disease but are uncertain of their balance and postural reflexes.
- The gait takes on the characteristics seen when a healthy person walks on an icy surface: velocity slows, steps shorten, and the base widens.

Hyperkinetic Gait

- In conditions such as Sydenham's chorea, Huntington's disease, other forms of transient or persistent chorea, athetosis, and dystonia the abnormal movements may become more marked while the patient is walking, and the manifestations of the disease more evident.
- Walking may accentuate not only the hyperkinesis, but also the abnormalities of power and tone that accompany them.
- In Huntington's disease, the gait may be grotesque, dancing or prancing with abundant extraneous movement. It may look histrionic but is all too real.
- In athetosis, the distal movements, and in dystonia the proximal movements, may be marked during walking, and in both there are accompanying grimaces.

Gaits Associated with Focal Weakness

- In addition to the steppage gait that accompanies foot drop, weakness limited to other muscle groups may cause gait difficulties.
- With paralysis of the *gastrocnemius* and *soleus* muscles, the patient is unable to stand on the toes, and unable to push off to enter the swing phase with the affected leg. This may cause a shuffling gait that is devoid of spring.
- In weakness of *the quadriceps* muscle (e.g. femoral neuropathy), there is weakness of knee extension, and the patient can only accept weight on the affected extremity by bracing the knee. When walking the knee is held stiffly, and there is a tendency to fall if the knee bends. The patient has less difficulty walking backward than forward.
- *Lumbosacral radiculopathy* may cause either foot drop or a unilateral Trendelenburg gait, or both. In addition, the patient with acute radiculopathy may walk with a list or pelvic tilt, accompanied by flattening of the normal lumbar lordosis because of low back muscle spasm. The patient may walk with small steps; if the pain is severe, she may place only the toes on the floor, since dorsiflexion of the foot aggravates the pain. Patients commonly use a cane to avoid bearing weight on the involved leg.

11 Neurological Signs

MISCELLANEOUS NEUROLOGIC SIGNS

Miscellaneous neurologic signs—some of them reflexes, some closely related to the defense and postural reflex mechanisms, and others more varied in nature—are elicited in certain diseases of the nervous system. Some of these are quite important, especially the signs of meningeal irritation; others are arcane and primarily of historical interest.

SIGNS OF MENINGEAL IRRITATION

- Meningeal signs are elicited most frequently when the meanings are inflamed—from infection (e.g. bacterial meningitis) or from the presence of a foreign material (e.g. blood in the subarachnoid space).
- Meningismus is a term that refers to the presence of nuchal rigidity and other clinical signs of meningeal inflammation.
- Meningism is sometimes used synonymously with meningismus, but it is also used to refer to a syndrome characterized by neck stiffness without meningeal inflammation, seen in patients with systemic infections, particularly young children.
- The clinical manifestations of meningeal irritation are varied and depend on the severity of the process. Accompaniments depend on etiology but commonly include headache, pain and stiffness of the neck; irritability; photophobia; nausea and vomiting; and other manifestations of infection, such as fever and chills.
- The various maneuvers used to elicit meningeal signs produce tension on inflamed and hypersensitive spinal nerve roots, and the resulting signs are postures, protective muscle contractions, or other movements that minimize the stretch and distortion of the meninges and roots.

Nuchal (Cervical) Rigidity

- Nuchal rigidity is the most widely recognized and frequently encountered sign of meningeal irritation, and the diagnosis of meningitis is rarely made in its absence.

- It is characterized by stiffness and spasm of the neck muscles, with pain on attempted voluntary movement as well as resistance to passive movement.
- The degree of rigidity varies. There may be only slight resistance to passive flexion, or marked spasm of all the neck muscles.
- Nuchal rigidity primarily affects the extensor muscles, and the most prominent early finding in meningeal irritation is resistance to passive neck flexion.
- The physician is unable to place the patient's chin on his chest, but the neck can be hyperextended without difficulty; rotatory and lateral movements may also be preserved.
- With more severe nuchal rigidity there may be resistance to extension and rotatory movements as well.
- Extreme rigidity causes retraction of the neck into a position of opisthotonos, the body assuming a wrestler's bridge or *arc de cercle* position, with the head thrust back and the trunk arched forward.
- Rigidity may be absent in meningitis when the disease is fulminating or terminal, when the patient is in coma, or in infants.
- Stiffness and rigidity of the neck may occur in other conditions.
- A common problem is to distinguish restricted neck motion due to cervical spondylosis or osteoarthritis from nuchal rigidity.
- Patients with osteoarthritis typically have difficulty with rotation and lateral bending of the neck; these motions are usually preserved in patients who have meningismus, unless the meningeal irritation is extremely severe.
- Restricted neck motion may also occur with retropharyngeal abscess, cervical lymphadenopathy, neck trauma, and as a nonspecific manifestation in severe systemic infections.
- Extrapyramidal disorders, particularly progressive supranuclear palsy, may also cause diffuse rigidity of the neck muscles.
- Meningeal signs may occur with increased spinal fluid pressure, and nuchal rigidity may be a manifestation of cerebellar tonsillar (foramen magnum) herniation. Meningeal irritation may also cause resistance to movement of the legs and back, with the patient lying with his legs drawn up and resisting passive extension.

Kernig's Sign

- There is some variability in the descriptions of how to elicit a Kernig sign.

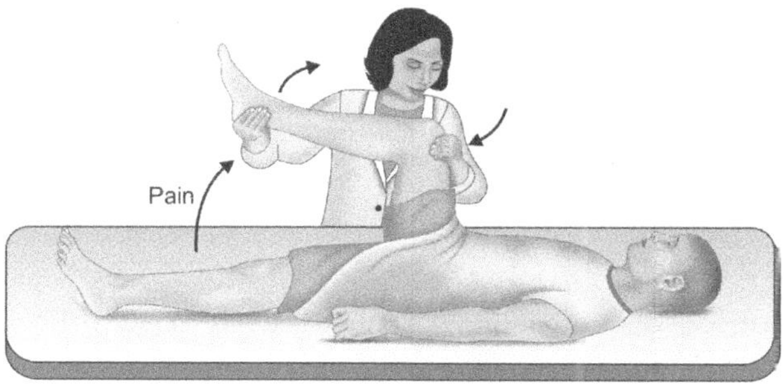

Fig. 11.1 Testing for meningeal irritation—Kernig's sign

- Kernig described an involuntary flexion at the knee when the examiner attempted to flex the hip with the knee extended **(Fig. 11.1)**.
- The more common method is to flex the hip and knee to right angles, and then attempt to passively extend the knee.
- This movement produces pain, resistance, and inability to fully extend the knee; another definition of Kernig's sign is inability to extend the knee to over 135° while the hip is flexed.
- There is some overlap between Kernig's sign and the Lasègue (straight leg raising) sign. The technique is similar, but the Lasègue sign is used to check for root irritation in lumbosacral radiculopathy.
- Both the Kernig sign and straight leg raising are positive in meningitis because of diffuse inflammation of the nerve roots and meninges, and positive with acute lumbosacral radiculopathy because of focal inflammation of the affected root.
- In radiculopathy the signs are usually unilateral, but in meningitis they are bilateral.

Brudzinski's Neck Sign

- Placing one hand under the patient's head and flexing the neck while holding down the chest with the other hand causes flexion of the hips and knees bilaterally **(Fig. 11.2)**.
- With severe meningismus, it may not be possible to hold the chest down, and the patient may be pulled into a sitting position with only the therapist hand behind the head.
- Occasionally there may be extension of the hallux and fanning of the toes, and sometimes arm flexion.

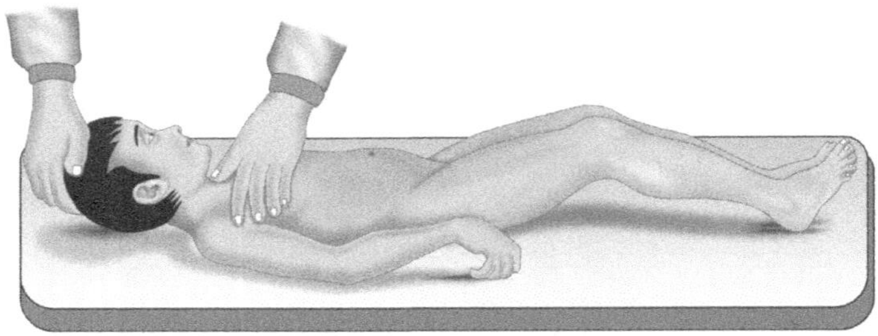

Fig. 11.2 Brudzinski's sign

- The leg may fail to flex on one side when meningeal irritation and hemiplegia coexist.

Other Meningeal Signs

To avoid spinal flexion, the patient with meningitis may sit in bed with the hands placed far behind, the head thrown back, the hips and knees flexed, and the back arched (Amoss's, Hoyne's, or tripod sign). Brudzinski described several signs of meningeal inflammation in patients with tuberculous meningitis that likely reflected involvement of the parenchyma more than the meninges.

Signs of Tetany

- The clinical manifestations of tetany include spasm and tonic contractions of the skeletal muscles, principally the distal muscles of the extremities.
- There may be carpopedal spasm, with tonic contraction of the muscles of the wrists, hands, fingers, feet, and toes.
- There is hyperexcitability of the entire peripheral nervous system, as well as the musculature, to even minimal stimuli. Sensory nerve involvement may cause paresthesias in the hands, feet, and perioral region.
- Tetany is related to a disturbance of calcium metabolism or alkalosis, causing a decrease in the ionized calcium level.
- Certain neurologic signs may be present that aid in making a diagnosis on the basis of the clinical examination alone.
- They are more easily obtained if the patient first hyperventilates for a few minutes (latent tetany). Severe tetany may cause seizures, laryngospasm, stridor, and respiratory arrest.

Chvostek's Sign

- Tapping over the facial nerve causes spasm or a tetanic, cramp like contraction of some or all of the facial muscles.
- *Two points of stimulation have been described*: Just below the zygomatic process of the temporal bone, in front of the ear (Chvostek's sign); and midway between the zygomatic arch and the angle of the mouth (Schultz's sign) **(Fig. 11.3)**.
- Sometimes the response may be elicited merely by stroking the skin in front of the ear.
- The sign is minimal if only a slight twitch of the upper lip or the angle of the mouth results; moderate if there is movement of the ala nasi and the entire corner of the mouth; maximal if the muscles of the forehead, eyelid, and cheek also contract.
- When the response is marked, even muscles supplied by the trigeminal nerve may respond. Chvostek's sign is the result of a hyperexcitability of the motor nerves, in this instance the facial nerve, to mechanical stimulation.
- It is an important sign in tetany, but may occur in other conditions in which there is hyperreflexia, such as in lesions of the corticospinal tract.
- It is present in a majority of neonates and disappears during childhood.

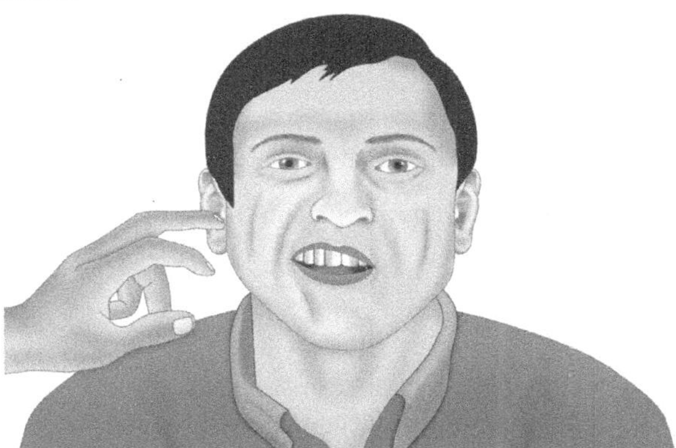

Fig. 11.3 Ask the patient to relax his facial nerves. Next, stand directly in front of him and tap the facial nerve either just anterior to the earlobe or below the zygomatic arch and the corner of the mouth. A positive response varies from twitching of the lip at the corner of the mouth to spasm of all facial muscles, depending on the severity of hypocalcemia

Sign Technique Finding Significance

Bikele sign with elbow flexed, shoulder abducted, elevated, and externally rotated, examiner attempts to passively extend the elbow resistance to elbow extension similar to Kernig's sign in that it stretches irritated nerve roots; positive in meningeal inflammation and in brachial plexitis.

Brudzinski's Contralateral Leg Sign

- Passive flexion of one hip, especially with the knee extended, or passive knee extension after the hip has been flexed to a right angle flexion of the opposite hip and knee.
- Meningeal inflammation.

Brudzinski's Reciprocal Contralateral Leg Sign

- One knee and hip are flexed with the other leg extended; then the flexed limb is lowered contralateral extended leg goes into flexion
- Meningeal inflammation.

Brudzinski's Cheek Sign

- Pressure against the cheeks on or just below the zygoma
- Flexion at the elbows with an upward jerking of the arms
- Meningeal inflammation.

Brudzinski's Symphysis Sign

Pressure on the symphysis pubis flexion of both lower extremities meningeal inflammation.

Guilland's Sign

- Pinching the skin over the quadriceps femoris muscle or squeezing the muscle on one side flexion of contralateral hip and knee
- Meningeal inflammation.

Edelmann Great Toe Phenomenon

- Flexion of the hip with the knee extended extension of the great toe
- Meningeal inflammation.

Tonic Plantar Reflex

- Stroking sole of foot slow flexion and adduction of toes and distal part of the foot that persists for a minute or two
- Prefrontal and extrapyramidal involvement; may be contralateral, ipsilateral, or bilateral with respect to the lesion.

Soderbergh Pressure Reflex

- Firm stroking of certain bony prominences slow muscular contraction (e.g. stroking the ulna causing flexion of the medial three fingers, stroking the radius causing thumb flexion)
- Pyramidal and extrapyramidal disorders.

Schrijver-Bernhard Reflex

- Percussing anterior surface of the leg or tapping over tibia or anterior leg muscles just below the knee
- Plantar flexion of toes pyramidal and extrapyramidal disorders; a distant toe flexor reflex.

Lomadtse Sign

- Pressure over anterior aspect of tibia
- Plantar flexion of toes pyramidal and extrapyramidal disorders; a distant toe flexor reflex.

Trousseau's Sign

Ischemia of the peripheral nerve trunks increases nerve excitability and causes spontaneous discharges.

Compression of the arm by manual pressure, a tourniquet, or a sphygmomanometer cuff is followed first by distal paresthesias that progress centripetally, then twitching of the fingers, and finally by cramping and contraction of the muscles of the fingers and hand with the thumb strongly adducted and the fingers stiffened, slightly flexed at the metacarpophalangeal joints, and forming a cone clustered about the thumb (obstetrician's or accoucheur's hand, *main d'accoucheur*) **(Fig. 11.4)**.

There may be a latent period of 1–4 minutes. Similar pressure around the leg or thigh will cause pedal spasm. A modification is to keep a

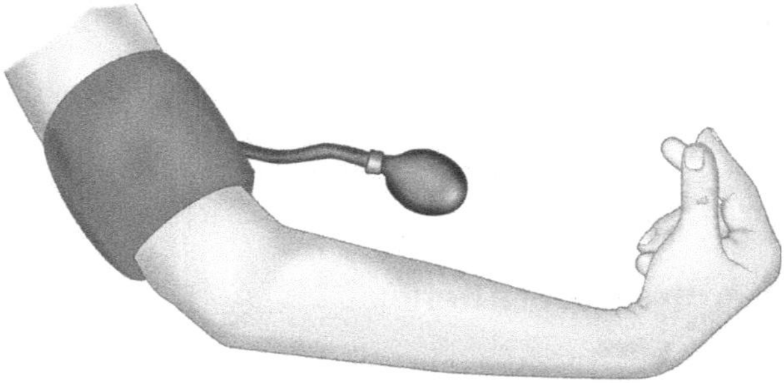

Fig. 11.4 Trousseau's sign

moderately inflated sphygmomanometer cuff on one arm for about 10 minutes, and then remove it and have the patient hyperventilate; typical titanic spasm occurs earlier in the previously ischemic arm.

12 Autonomic Nervous System

INTRODUCTION

The autonomic nervous system (ANS) is the system that controls nonstriated muscles and glands. There are three divisions of the ANS: sympathetic (thoracolumbar), parasympathetic (craniosacral), and enteric.

The sympathetic and parasympathetic divisions are characterized by a two-neuron chain with two anatomic elements:

- A preganglionic (first order) neuron within the central nervous system (CNS) that terminates in a ganglion outside the CNS.
- A postganglionic (second order) neuron that carries impulses to a destination in the viscera.
- The enteric nervous system is located in the walls of the gastro-intestinal tract.

In addition, dorsal root ganglion neurons convey afferent visceral impulses that arise in both sympathetic and parasympathetic fibers. There are also autonomic neurons within the CNS at various levels from the cerebral cortex to the spinal cord. Autonomic functions are beyond voluntary control and for the most part beneath consciousness.

THE PERIPHERAL AUTONOMIC NERVOUS SYSTEM

- The parasympathetic division is composed of the general visceral efferent fibers of cranial nerves III, VII, IX, X, and bulbar portion of XI (the cranial outflow), together with fibers arising in the S2-S4 segments of the spinal cord (the sacral outflow).
- The parasympathetic nerves have long preganglionic fibers that end in peripheral ganglia near or in the viscera they supply, and short postganglionic fibers that arise in proximity to or within the viscus innervated.
- It consists of the Edinger-Westphal nucleus, the superior and inferior salivatory nuclei, the dorsal motor nucleus of the vagus, and neurons in the vicinity of the nucleus ambiguus.

- The sacral parasympathetic fibers arise from cells in the intermediolateral cell column at the S2-S4 levels of the sacral spinal cord, travel through the sacral nerves, and are collected into the pelvic splanchnic nerves (nervi erigentes), which proceed to the pelvic plexuses and their branches.
- Some postganglionic fibers may travel from these plexuses to the pelvic viscera, where postganglionic fibers supply the bladder, descending colon, rectum, anus, and genitalia.
- The sympathetic division is composed of preganglionic fibers that arise from cells in the intermediolateral columns from the T1 to the L3 segments of the spinal cord. Postganglionic fibers go to the viscera.
- The sympathetic ganglia are arranged into two plexuses: paravertebral and prevertebral.
- *Paravertebral*: The prevertebral ganglia lie anterior to the vertebral column.
- The prevertebral ganglia innervate the viscera of the abdomen and pelvis.
- The paravertebral sympathetic chain consists of two elongated plexuses, each composed of a series of ganglia that are segmentally arranged and bound together by ascending and descending nerve fibers.
- The sympathetic trunks have from 22 to 24 ganglia and extend from the level of C2 to the coccyx.
- There are 3 cervical, 10–12 thoracic, 4 lumbar, and 4–5 sacral ganglia.
- The chains usually join at the level of the coccyx in an unpaired coccygeal ganglion (ganglion impar).
- Preganglionic fibers leave the spinal cord through the anterior root and mixed spinal nerve to reach the anterior primary ramus, and then exit as finely myelinated fibers (white rami communicantes) to enter the ganglionic chain. They may synapse immediately or ascend or descend before synapsing.
- The postganglionic fibers return to the anterior primary ramus as unmyelinated fibers (gray rami communicantes). The T1-T3 segments innervate the head and neck, the T3-T11 segments innervate the upper extremities and viscera in the thorax and abdomen, and the T12-L2 segments innervate the lower extremities and pelvic viscera.
- The cervical portion of the sympathetic chain consists of the superior, middle, and inferior cervical ganglia. These innervate structures within the head, upper extremities, and thorax.

- The superior cervical ganglion, the largest, lies opposite the C2-C3 vertebrae and behind the internal carotid artery. It is primarily supplied by the first two thoracic segments.
- The internal carotid nerve, a direct continuation of the superior cervical ganglion, gives rise to postganglionic filaments that supply the internal carotid and terminate as the internal carotid and cavernous plexuses.
- Anterior branches from the ganglion form plexuses around the middle meningeal and external carotid and maxillary arteries.
- The sympathetic innervations of the ciliary ganglia travel through the long ciliary nerves from the cavernous plexus. The sphenopalatine ganglion is supplied by the internal carotid plexus through the deep petrosal and vidian nerves.
- The optic ganglion receives its sympathetic innervations from the plexus around the middle meningeal artery, and the sub-maxillary ganglion from that around the external maxillary artery.
- The inferior cervical ganglion communicates with the seventh and eighth cervical nerves to form the inferior cardiac nerve and nerves to the blood vessels.
- The superior cervical ganglion (T1-T2) provides pupil dilator and sudomotor fibers to the face.
- The stellate ganglion (T2-T6) innervates the upper limb through branches of the brachial plexus, and the lumbar sympathetic ganglia (T9-L1) innervate the lower limb through branches of the lumbosacral plexus.
- The postganglionic sympathetic fibers join the peripheral somatic nerves via the gray rami communicantes, and thus their distribution is similar to that of the corresponding somatic nerve.
- The upper five ganglia provide branches to the cardiac and pulmonary plexuses. The abdominal portion of the sympathetic trunk is situated in front of the vertebral column along the medial margin of the psoas major muscle, and the pelvic portion is in front of the sacrum.
- All of these ganglia send gray rami communicantes to the corresponding spinal nerves and many branches to the various plexuses and collateral ganglia. The postganglionic fibers terminate on blood vessels, sweat glands, and other smooth muscle and glandular structures.
- Branches of the lower seven thoracic ganglia unite to form the three splanchnic nerves that penetrate the diaphragm and supply the abdomen and the pelvic viscera.

- The celiac plexus is the largest of the three sympathetic plexuses, and innervates all the abdominal viscera except for the descending colon.
- The renal and inferior mesenteric plexuses and their branches are also supplied by the lowest splanchnic nerve.
- The hypogastric plexus is located in front of the last lumbar vertebra and the promontory of the sacrum, between the two common iliac arteries, and is formed by the union of many elements from the aortic plexus and the lumbar sympathetic chain, together with some fibers from the inferior mesenteric plexus.
- It is divided into the two pelvic plexuses formed by fibers from the hypo gastric plexus; preganglionic sympathetic fibers from the second, third, and fourth sacral nerves; and a few filaments from the sacral sympathetic ganglia.
- Branches are distributed to the pelvic viscera and the internal and external genitalia through the middle hemorrhoidal, vesical, prostatic, vaginal, and uterine plexuses.

Autonomic Afferents

- General visceral afferent fibers convey both conscious and unconscious sensations from the viscera, and are involved in autonomic reflexes.
- Small myelinated and unmyelinated fibers carry impulses from visceral receptors to cell bodies in the dorsal root and cranial nerve ganglia.
- The visceral afferents that enter the spinal cord synapse on neurons in the dorsal horn and intermediolateral gray column.
- Centrally, sensation from the viscera travels mainly in the spinothalamic and spinoreticular tracts, but some visceral afferents—especially those related to bowel and bladder control—are carried in the posterior columns.
- After a synapse in the thalamus, visceral sensory fibers project to areas of the cortex involved in autonomic function.
- The vagal afferents transmit impulses from the heart, great vessels, lungs, and gastrointestinal (GI) tract; the glossopharyngeal afferents convey information from the carotid sinus.
- These afferents synapse in the nucleus of the solitary tract and are involved in autonomic reflexes as well as such functions as coughing and swallowing.

Neurotransmitters

- Acetylcholine is the neurotransmitter at sympathetic and parasympathetic preganglionic neurons, and at postganglionic parasympathetic neurons **(Fig. 12.1)**.
- Norepinephrine is the primary postganglionic sympathetic neurotransmitter, except at sweat glands, which are cholinergic.
- There are two subtypes of acetylcholine receptor:
  1. Nicotinic.
  2. Muscarinic.
- Most of the postganglionic acetylcholine receptors are muscarinic.
- They mediate the cardiac effects and cause pupillary constriction, lacrimal and salivary secretion, bronchoconstriction and erection.
- They also stimulate GI tract motility and cause evacuation of the bladder and rectum.
- There are two main subtypes of adrenergic receptors:
  1. Alpha.
  2. Beta.
- The alpha-adrenergic receptors mediate pupillary dilatation, vasoconstriction, and ejaculation, and they also control the internal sphincters of the bladder and rectum.
- Beta-adrenergic receptors control the heart, and cause vasodilatation, bronchial dilatation, and mediate metabolic effects.

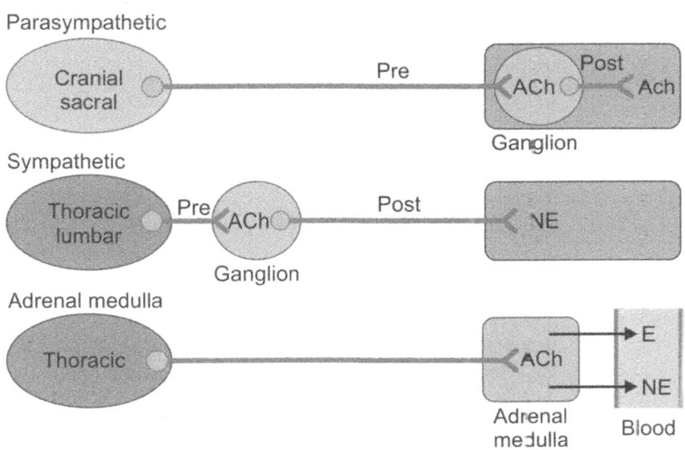

Fig. 12.1 Neurotransmitters for autonomic nervous system

The Physiology of the Peripheral Autonomic Nervous System

- The ANS governs the activities of cardiac and smooth muscle, including the smooth muscle of the blood vessels and the functions of most glandular structures.
- It regulates such important functions as respiration, circulation, digestion, temperature adjustment, and metabolism—all vital to normal existence—and combats forces acting from within or without that would tend to cause undesirable changes in the normal function of the body.
- By homeostasis the constancy of the internal environment of the body and the uniformity and stability of the organism are maintained.
- The sympathetic division supplies all parts of the body. Its functions are catabolic and directed toward the utilization of energy.
- It prepares the organism for combat or escape (fight-or-flight response). It acts whenever rapid adjustment to the environment is required.
- It accelerates the heart, dilates the coronary vessels, increases the arterial blood pressure, empties the blood reservoirs, dilates the bronchi, liberates glucose, and inhibits GI activity **(Table 12.1)**.

Table 12.1: Effects of sympathetic and parasympathetic systems on various effector organs

Organ	*Effect of sympathetic stimulation*	*Effect of parasympathetic stimulation*
Heart	Increased rate, increased force of contraction (of whole heart)	Decreased rate, decreased force of contraction (of atria only)
Blood vessels	Constriction	Dilation of vessels supplying the penis and clitoris only
Lungs	• Dilation of bronchioles (airways) • Inhibition (?) of mucus secretion	• Constriction of bronchioles • Stimulation of mucus secretion
Digestive tract	• Decreased motility (movement) • Contraction of sphincters (to prevent forward movement of contents) • Inhibition (?) of digestive secretions	• Increased motility • Relaxation of sphincters (to permit forward movement of contents) • Stimulation of digestive secretions

Contd...

Contd...

Organ	*Effect of sympathetic stimulation*	*Effect of parasympathetic stimulation*
Urinary bladder	Relaxation	Contraction (emptying)
Eye	• Dilation of pupil • Adjustment of eye for far vision	• Constriction of pupil • Adjustment of eye for near vision
Liver (glycogen stores)	Glycogenolysis (glucose released)	None
Adipose cells (fat stores)	Lipolysis (fatty acids released)	None

- It is an emergency protective mechanism that is called into action under emotional stress and causes the individual to react strongly to stimuli of rage and fear. The parasympathetic division supplies special structures, such as the pupils, salivary glands, heart, lungs. GI tract, bladder, and portions of the genital system.
- In certain parasympathetic functions, as in bladder, rectal, and genital activity, contraction of striated muscles are closely integrated with those of smooth muscle. The parasympathetic division conserves energy **(Fig. 12.2)**.
- It controls anabolic, excretory, and reproductive functions, and conserves and restores bodily resources and energy.
- The viscera receive a dual autonomic supply, both sympathetic and parasympathetic. In general these two divisions are antagonistic and reciprocal in their functions, but there are exceptions.

THE CENTRAL REGULATION OF AUTONOMIC FUNCTION

- The peripheral ANS is under the control of higher centers in the cerebral cortex, especially the amygdale, hypothalamus, basal forebrain, ventral striatum, brainstem, and spinal cord that regulate and influence the function of its peripheral components.
- The centers in the CNS that are involved in autonomic function are referred to as the central autonomic network.
- The neurons of the central autonomic network are interconnected and make up a functional unit. The most important of these centers is the hypothalamus.

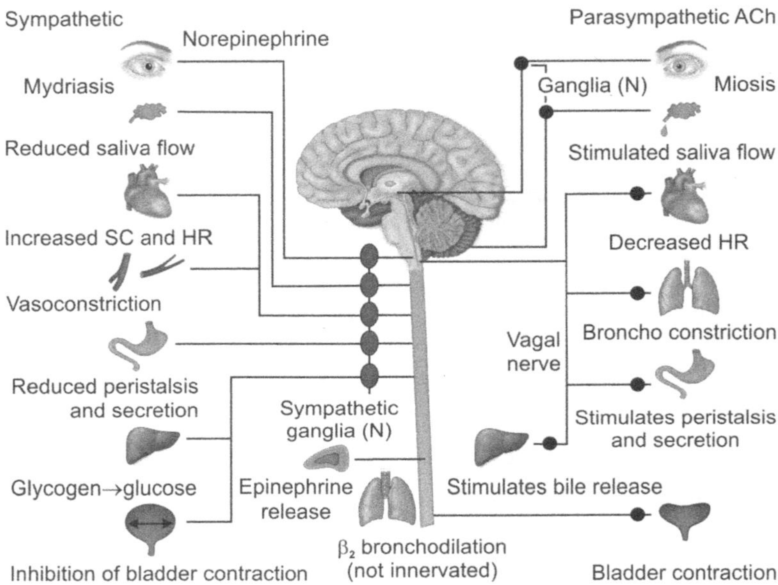

Fig. 12.2 The autonomic nervous system

EXAMINATION

The history in patients with autonomic insufficiency may reveal symptoms related to orthostatic hypotension, abnormalities of sweating, or dysfunction of the GI or genitourinary tracts.

The Vasovagal Reflex

Stimulation of Vagus Nerve

Some of the more common triggers are the sight of blood, standing quickly or for too long, emotional upset and traumatic experiences. When the vagus nerve is suddenly stimulated, it sets off a chain of events within the body, most notably a rapid reduction of blood pressure and heart rate. This action can then cause a variety of physical symptoms, such as:

- Dizziness
- Sweating

- Light-headedness
- Nausea
- Person turns pale
- Fainting, a condition known as *vasovagal syncope*
- Neurocardiogenic mechanism.

On Changing Posture

- Shift of venous blood from central to periphery
- Decrease in cardiac filling pressure
- Stroke volume decreased by 40%
- Decreased afferent sensitivity of baroreceptor and HR rises due to withdrawal of parasympathetic activity and later due to increase in sympathetic activity.

Normal Response

- Stimulate baroreceptor
  - Reduced sympathetic outflow
- Release vasoconstrictor tone
- Decrease total peripheral resistance

Drop of BP up to 20 mm Hg

↓

It remains for few seconds then comes to normal

↓

Due to squeezing of capacitance vessels

↓

Venous return increases

↓

So, BP comes to normal

- Tests of cardiac and vascular autonomic regulation
- Afferent impulses originate from the cardio-mechanoreceptor, pulmonary stretch receptors and arterial baroreceptors.
- Sympathetic stimulation increase the HR, myocardial contractibility, dilate coronary vessels and constricts resistance vessels.
- Parasympathetic opposite effect
- Regulation of CVAF negative feedback mechanism.

Test of Cardiac and Vascular Autonomic Regulation

- Cardiovascular response to standing and 30:15 R-R ratio
- Head up tilt table testing
- Heart rate variation with respiration
- Valsalva maneuver and Valsalva ratio
- Miscellaneous tests.

Heart rate and blood pressure recording:

- Beat-to-beat heart rate analysis is useful
- Heart rate documented on electrocardiogram or on EMG equipment
- Active recording electrode is placed over midline posteriorly between the inferior angle of scapulae and the reference on mid axillary line
- Heart rate is inversely related to R-R interval
- HR = sweep speed (mm/s)/ R-R interval in mm × 60
- It assumes that patient is in a sinus rhythm.
- Blood pressure is recorded from standard sphygmomanometer.
- The level of measurement should be maintained at the level of heart.
- Beat-to-beat BP measurement formerly required invasive intra-arterial measurement.

Cardiovascular response to standing and 30:15 R-R ratio:

- It will assess the integrity of the sympathetic system and HR changes of parasympathetic cholinergic function.
- Normally on standing mechanical effect on venous capacitance and arterial resistance vessels becomes operative due to gravitational changes.
- Squeezing of capacitance vessels by postural muscles result in displacement of blood towards heart it with which in turn leads to increase venous return, cardiac output and BP.
- It lasts for 6–8 secs then HR increasing immediately upon standing and continues to rise for next several seconds and then slows to a max 20 secs.

Technical and normal value:

- HR and BP measured after 20 minutes of resting position.
- First it measured at baseline then serially for 1–3 minutes after standing.
- *ECG 30:15 R–R ratio*: Longest R–R interval/shortest R–R interval
- Orthostatic hypotension is determined by fall of 20 mm Hg systolic and 10 mm Hg diastolic after assuming erect posture.

- Orthostatic tachycardia = sustain increase of HR > 25 beats/min.
- 30:15 R–R ratio normally > 1.04 abnormal < 1.0
- This test is simple, direct easily accessible and quantitative.
- *Limitations*:
  - Complex underlying physiology
  - Lack of reproducibility
  - Poor sensitivity.
- The hallmark of orthostatic hypotension due to absence of compensatory tachycardia indicating autonomic failure is the absence of both cardiac and vascular reflexes.
- Disruption of baroreflex occurs due to transaction of glossopharyngeal nerve, bilateral resection if carotid body.
- Baroreflex failure is uncommon condition
  - Labial hypertension
  - Tachycardia
  - Palpitation
  - Headache
  - Sweating
  - Pallor
  - Flushing

Head up tilt table testing:
- Testing the integrity of autonomic cardiovascular and neuro-cardiogenic reflexes.
- Early response will be obtained within 30–60 secs → (autonomic cardiovascular)
- Late response will be obtained within after 30–60 minutes → (neurocardiogenic reflex).
- *Method*: Conducted after standard period of supine. Baseline ECG and BP are recorded. Patient is positioned at 80° of inclination from horizontal on a tilt table with foot rest and monitored for a period of 3–5 minutes.
- ECG measured continuously and BP at 1 minutes and every 3 minutes.
- In laboratories inclination is 60° and monitored for 45–60 minutes.
- Orthostatic hypotension is defined as reduction of systolic BP of at least 20 mm Hg or diastolic BP of 10 mm Hg within 3 minutes following change of posture (Neurocardiogenic mechanism).
- Sympathetic activity increases vascular tone and total peripheral vascular resistance due to that cardiac output drops by 20%.

- Neurocardiogenic syncope (paradoxical bradycardia) occurs by reflex it with may be precipitated by stress, fear, micturation, defecation, coughing, sneezing.
- Increased wall tension leads to increase afferent activity which in turn leads to activate parasym reflex and withdraws sympathetic reflex to produce bradycardia, hypotension, vasodilatation.
- Tests are useful for multisystem atrophy and recurrent syncope.
- *Disadvantage:* Special equipment is needed.
- *Normal response*: It differs from active testing → exercise reflex and mechanical squeeze on capacitance and resistance vessels are less.

Valsalva Maneuver and Valsalva Ratio

- To assess parasympathetic cholinergic (cardiovagal) functions.
- Consists of respiratory strain which leads to increase intrathoracic and intra-abdominal pressure and alters hemodynamic and cardiac function.
- *Four phases*:

Phase 1: Onset of strain, transient increase in BP lasting for few second.

Due to increase intrathoracic pressure:
Mechanical squeeze of great vessels HR does not change

Phase 2: During straining

Early part	**Later part**
Venous return decreases baseline	BP returns towards
↓	↓
Reduction in - Stroke volume - Cardiac output - Blood pressure - Lasts about 4 secs	Increased peripheral Vascular resistance ↓ Sympathetic vasoconstriction

- Throughout phase 2 HR increases steadily due to vagal withdrawal early and increased sympathetic in the later part of stage 2.

Phase 3: Following releasing of strain there will be transient decrease in BP for few secs caused by mechanical displacement of blood to pulmonary vascular bed which was under increase intrathoracic pressure.

No change in HR.

Phase 4: Further cessation of strain, BP slowly increase, HR decreases.

- Since the BP rise to above and HR falls below baseline level leads to overshoot phenomenon
  - Occurs following 15–20 secs after release of strain, lasts for 10 min/longer
- *Overshoot phenomena*: Cause due to—increase in venous return
  - Stroke volume
  - Cardiac output

Valsalva ratio: Max HR in phase 2/min HR in phase 4.

Calculated as: Longest R–R interval in 4/shorted R–R interval in 2

- *Variables*:
  - Age
  - Position of patient
  - Expiratory pressure
  - Duration of strain and medication
- *Method*: Supine with head slightly elevated to about 30°. Patient strains for 15 secs against 40 mm Hg by blowing into mouthpiece attached to a sphygmomanometer. The system should have a slow leak to ensure that the patient strains continuously and not falsely maintain pressure by glottic closure of the airway or tongue closure of mouthpiece.
- After cessation of strain, patient relaxes and breathes at a normal comfortable rate. ECG is monitored during the strain and 30–45s after release.
- Maximum HR of phase 2 occurs about 1 sec following cessation of strain HR.
- Minimum HR occurs about 15–20 sec after releasing the strain.
- Repeat 3 times after a brief rest.
- Valsalva ratio
  - Less than 1.2 → abnormal
  - 1.2–1.45 → borderline
  - Greater than 1.45 → normal
- Ratio decreases with age
- Valsalva ratio
- *Advantages:* Simple sensitive and fast
- *Disadvantages:* It may be difficult to carry out in debilitated persons.
- MSA → abnormality in ratio 90%.

TESTS OF THERMOREGULATORY FUNCTIONS

Skin Response

Erythema

Scratching the skin will produce a line surrounded by a spreading flare and followed by a wheal with central pallor. This is often exaggerated below level of transverse cord lesion and according to the lesion may be unilateral or bilateral, often becoming apparent after testing cutaneous sensation to pin prick. At the level of lesion even normal response may be absent. Exaggerated response unfortunately can occur in normal psychoneurotic individual—this dermatographia is however not simply limited to skin below segmental level.

Temperature

The measurement of temperature show:
- Increase temperature below recently denervated level
- Decrease temperature following chronic neurological lesions which have caused prolonged immobility
- Increase response to warming of the part or of distant parts over the denervated area in sympathetic lesions but
- Decrease response to warming in areas where deficit is circulatory rather than neurogenic.

Pilomotor Responses

These are similar in significance to erythematous responses. They are produced by sharp scratching or by touching the warmed body with cold metal.

Scrotal Response

Touching the scrotum with a cold object normally results in vermicular contraction of the dartos, without elevation of testicles, thus differing from the cremasteric reflex. This is absent in sympathetic paralysis.

Tests of thermoregulatory functions:
- Sympathetic skin responses (SSR)
- Thermoregulatory sweat test

- Sweat imprint test
- Miscellaneous tests

Sympathetic Skin Responses

- Useful in studying the integrity of peripheral sympathetic cholinergic (sudomotor) function by evaluating the changes in resistance of skin to electric conduction (Low et al.)
- Changes are regulated by the sweat gland of dermis and may be generated by pre-secretory rather than secretory activity.

Method: Recorded on EMG equipment. Low frequency filters should be set at 0.1–0.5 Hz.

- Gain → set to record a potential of 0.5–3 mV.
- Sweep → set to record 5 secs after the stimulus.

Recordings are obtained simultaneously from hands and feet:

- Active electrodes → on the palm or sole
- Reference → over the dorsum after cleaning the part
- Temperature of skin → maintained above 30°C
- Disc electrodes with electrodes gel are used
- Give adequate stimulation
- Best potentials are chosen
- SSR → mono, bi or triphasic and varies from stimulus to stimulus. symmetric in homologous body region that have higher amplitude and shorter latency in hands.
- *Age dependent*: Present in both hands and feet till 60 years.
- SSR parameters are affected by composition of surface electrode, frequency and mental state.
- Cooling → prolongation of latency and reduction of amplitude
- So measurement of temperature is mandatory.
- In MSA and progressive autonomic failure, SSR abnormalities → 88%
- In diabetics → 66–83%

Thermoregulatory Sweat Test

For evaluating sympathetic cholinergic function. Evaluate overall autonomic regulation of body temperature, especially cooling by providing physiological stimulus, heat and then recording the body's ability to dissipate it.

Method:

Patient
↓
Placed in controlled heat environment
↓
45–50°C
Relative humidity
↓
45–50%

Core body temperature is warmed to 38°C

Patient has an indicator powder (alizarin red mixed with cornstarch and sodium carbonate applied to body

- Other indicators that can be used → iodinated cornstarch or iodine solution which is painted on the body.
- This indicators change color when wet to indicate area of sweating. Alizarin red is slight orange when dry and changes to purple when wet.
- Sweating reaches to max after 35–45 minutes warming
- Sweating area of the body are recorded. Normally, it is generalized, symmetrical and variable involvement of proximal limbs and legs.
- The abnormal pattern includes distal anhydrosis, segmental or regional anhydrosis and focal or global anhydrosis
- *Advantage:* Sensitive assess overall fun
- *Disadvantage:* Time consuming, messy, require special equipment.

Tests of Pupillary and Exocrine Function

To study parasympathetic cholinergic and sympathetic adrenergic functions:

- *Denervation hypersensitivity*: Cannon's law
- *For parasympathetic*: Use parasympathetic mimetics
- *For sympathetic*: Use parasymlytic or sympathomimetics
- Schirmer's test.

Tests of Genitourinary Autonomic Regulation

- Patient with dysphagia, constipation, gastroparesis, fecal incontinence → autonomic dysfunction
- Barium swallow is useful
- Barium enema

- Manometer and solid state pressure transducers placed in different location of GI tract help to localize the site of stasis.
- System denervation → diagnosed by prompt rise of epinephrine and norepinephrine following IV edrophonium.

Tests of Genitourinary Autonomic Regulation

- Cystometrogram measures intravesical pressure as function of Saline infusion permitted to flow into bladder.
- Rise of intravesical pressure as 500 mL of saline solution is allowed to flow gradually, the volume at which the patient reports a sensation of bladder fullness are recorded.
- *Method*: To assess bladder atony is to measure the residual urine by catheterization immediately after voluntary voiding.

DISORDERS OF THE AUTONOMIC NERVOUS SYSTEM

Autonomic disorders can be divided into:

- Those that affect the central autonomic elements and are typically associated with other evidence of CNS disease, and
- Those that affect the peripheral autonomic nervous system. Multiple system atrophy (MSA) is a degenerative neurologic disorder, which is usually accompanied by prominent dysautonomia.

Autonomic Failure Produces

- Orthostatic hypotension
- Impotence
- Constipation
- Urinary incontinence
- It may be associated with respiratory symptoms such as laryngeal stridor and sleep apnea.

Autonomic dysfunction may also occur in patients with Parkinson's disease, but usually late in the illness and not to the degree typical of MSA.

Autonomic disturbances may accompany:

- Seizures
- Flushing
- Pallor
- Sweating

- Shivering
- Piloerection
- Vomiting
- Respiratory abnormalities

Seizure-induced cardiovascular abnormalities include:
- Sinus tachycardia
- Bradyarrhythmia
- Sinus arrest
- Ventricular tachyarrhythmias, including
- Ventricular fibrillation

Hypothalamic disorders may cause many abnormalities of autonomic function, including:
- Deficiencies in osmoregulation and thermoregulation
- Abnormalities of appetite, body weight; sleep disturbances
- Changes in carbohydrate, fat and water metabolism and respiratory abnormalities; together with, in many instances
- Behavioral abnormalities
- Personality changes
- Hyperthermia or hypothermia
- Disturbances of the sleep cycle

Brainstem disorders commonly cause autonomic dysfunction, including:
- Paroxysmal hypertension
- Profound bradycardia
- Intractable vomiting
- Central hypoventilation
- Neurogenic pulmonary edema
- Horner's syndrome

Peripheral autonomic failure results in dysautonomia occurs commonly in some peripheral nerve disorders.

It may develop acutely in:
- Guillain-Barré syndrome
- Porphyria
- Paraneoplastic neuropathies

The most common cause of autonomic neuropathy is diabetes mellitus. Patients typically develop orthostatic hypotension, impotence, gastroparesis, constipation alternating with diarrhea, nocturnal diarrhea, and difficulty voiding.

Dysautonomia may accompany disorders of neuromuscular transmission, particularly Lambert-Eaton syndrome and botulism, in which the defect is presynaptic and acetylcholine release is impaired at autonomic synapses as well as at neuromuscular junctions.

Dysautonomia primarily involving the vascular system may cause Raynaud's phenomenon, acrocyanosis, erythromelalgia (Weir Mitchell syndrome), and livedo reticularis.

Autonomic dysfunction of the genitalia causing erectile dysfunction and other abnormalities is common, especially in diabetes mellitus.

Abnormalities of sweating occur frequently and are sometimes the only manifestation of the autonomic disturbance. Autonomic dysregulation is a common component of complex regional pain syndromes (reflex sympathetic dystrophy) and occurs in the same distribution as the pain.

ANATOMY OF BLADDER

- Urinary bladder is the temporary storage house of urine which gets emptied through urethra.
- The bladder varies in its shape, size and position according to the amount of urine it contains.
- When empty it is entirely within the pelvis but as its fills it expands up to the umbilicus or even higher.
- An empty bladder is tetrahedral in shape and it has apex, base, neck, 3 surfaces and 4 borders.
- A full bladder is ovoid in shape and it has an apex, neck, 2 surfaces.
- *Blood supply*: Superior and inferior vesicle artery.
- *Nerve supply*: Supplied by the vesicle plexus of nerves.
- It contains both sympathetic and parasympathetic component **(Fig. 12.3)**.
- *Sympathetic efferent fibers*: T11 to L2. It is inhibiting contraction of the detrusor and stimulate closer of the sphincter **(Fig. 12.4)**.
- *Parasympathetic efferent fibers*: S2 to S4. It is stimulate contraction of the detrusor and inhibit closer of the sphincter.
- *Sensory nerves*: Pain sensation caused by distension or spasm of the bladder wall are carried mainly parasympathetic and partly sympathetic nerves.
- In SC pain arising in the bladder passes through lateral spinothalamic tract and awareness of bladder distension is mediated through the posterior columns.

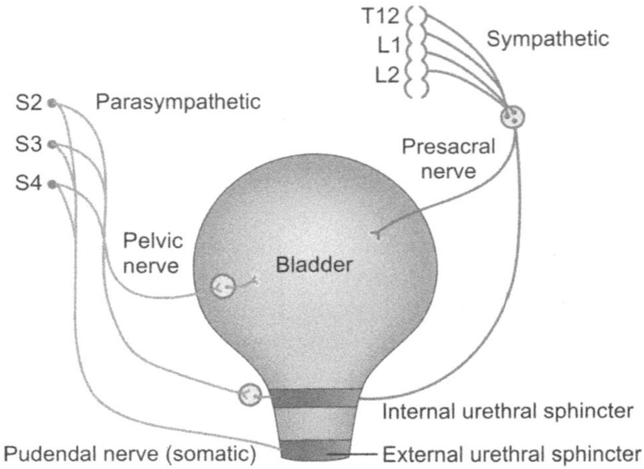

Fig. 12.3 Nerve supply of bladder

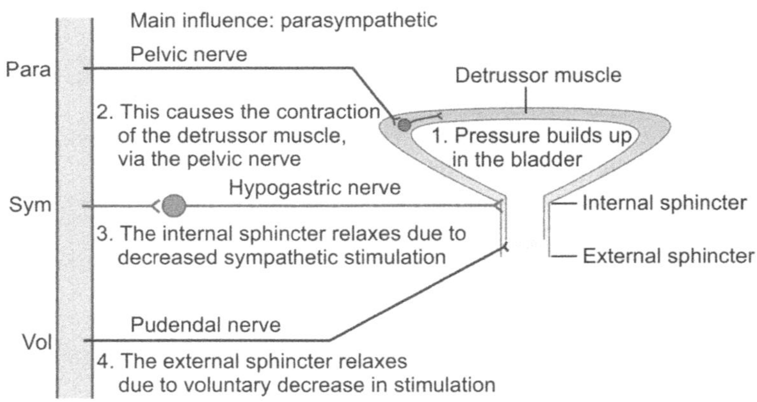

Fig. 12.4 Regulation of the bladder

- *Two main function of bladder is*:
  1. Storage
  2. Voiding
- *Normal bladder requires intact spinal connection between*:
  - Pontine micturition center
  - The sacral spinal cord.
- Disruption of spinobulbospinal micturition reflex pathway results in impaired storage and/or voiding.

PROCESS OF MICTURITION

- *Cortical center*: Removal of conscious inhibition of micturition.
- *Voiding*: Wave like detrusor muscle contraction with relaxation of internal and external sphincters.
- *Voiding completed*: Detrusor muscle relaxation
- Contraction of internal sphincter
- Contraction of external sphincter
- Relaxation of detrusor muscle
- Voiding may be voluntarily interrupted before complete bladder emptying by forced voluntary contraction of the external sphincter.

NEUROGENIC BLADDER

- A urinary tract dysfunction
- Condition may be congenital or acquired
- No cure but can be managed
- Most cases managed with medication and intermittent catheterization.

CAUSES

- Spinal cord injury
- Diabetes mellitus
- Heavy metal poisoning
- Acute infections
- Spinal cord tumors
- Syphilis
- Benign prostatic hyperplasia

OTHER CAUSES

- Bladder dysfunction
- Neurological
- Other causes

Types of Neurogenic Bladder

Following spinal shock, one of two types of bladder conditions will develop, depending on location of lesions, i.e.

- UMN bladder (Failure to store)
- LMN bladder (Failure to void)
- Uninhibited bladder

UMN Bladder

- Injury above the sacral micturition center
- Sign and symptoms of UMN bladder
- Frequent involuntary urination
- Small capacity <300 mL
- Scanty amount
- Associated with spasticity of lower extremities
- Lack of bladder sensation
- Upper tract dilation—reflux/obstruction
- Voiding may be triggered by stimulation of skin of perineum/genitalia
- Urinary infection.

LMN Bladder

- Injury at/below the sacral micturition center
- Sign and symptoms of LMN bladder
- Overflow incontinence (dribbling of urine)
- Reduced sphincter tone
- Sensation loss—perianal area
- LMN signs in lower limbs

UNINHIBITED BLADDER

Hyperactive Neurogenic Bladder

- The lesion in the midbrain causes continuous excitation of spinal micturition centers resulting in frequent and uncontrollable micturition
- Barrington's nucleus in brainstem is a center of micturition
- It is the urinary bladder with frequent and uncontrollable micturition
- Continuous dribbling of urine.

INCONTINENCE (TABLE 12.2)

Urge incontinence:

It is the involuntary loss of urine associated with a strong desire to void two types:

1. Sensory urgency is related to the infection, urinary calculi or bladder tumor.

Table 12.2: Structural causes of persistent urinary incontinence

	Cause	*Symptoms*	*Signs*	*Post-void residual*
Urge	Detrusor instability	• Urge • Enuresis • Large volume	Often none	Low
Stress	Sphincter insufficiency	• Triggers • No enuresis • Small volume	• Atrophy • Prolapse • Cystocele	Low
Overflow	• Outlet obstruction • Detrusor underactive	• Small volume • Enuresis • Frequency	• Benign prostatic hyperplasia • +/- palpable bladder • Neurodeficits	High
Functional	• Environment • Musculoskeletal disease congnitive • Impairment	• Varied volume • Restraints		Low

2. Motor urgency is due to the detrusor muscle instability and mostly seen in elderly patient.

Genuine stress incontinence:

- It is the voluntary small leak of urine occurring when intra-abdominal pressure raised
- If high intra-abdominal pressure exceeds the urethral pressure and the outlet mechanism are incompetent, urine is voided.

Bladder and Bowel Assessment

Bladder

- Frequency of urination
- Urgency
- Incontinence
- Hesitancy
- Distention
- Retention
- *Neurogenic bladder*: Present or absent.

Bowel

- Urgency of defecation
- Precipitancy
- Constipation
- Incontinence.

Sexual Function

Disturbed sexual function is common in dysautonomia. In the genital (sex, ejaculatory, coital) reflex, arousal causes penile erection and sometimes ejaculation. Erection is a parasympathetic function mediated through S2-S4; ejaculation is a largely sympathetic function mediated by the lumbar nerves. Autonomic insufficiency usually causes impotence, but pathologic exaggeration of the sexual reflex may occur as part of the mass reflex, a spinal defense reflex seen in severe myelopathy, and may produce priapism and occasionally ejaculation after minimal stimulation. In autonomic neuropathy, especially from diabetes, retrograde ejaculation may precede the development of impotence. Because the internal vesical sphincter does not close, semen goes into the bladder rather than externally through the urethra. The patient with retrograde ejaculation may notice milky-appearing urine.

13 Assessment of Unconscious Patient

COMA

Coma is a state of unconsciousness caused by temporary or permanent impairment of the ascending reticular system in the brainstem, or both cerebral hemispheres.

The key components of the neurological examination of the comatose patient are:

- Level of consciousness (Glasgow Coma Score — list the components; e.g. E4V5M6 = GCS 15)
- The pattern of breathing
- Size and reactivity of the pupils
- Eye movements and oculovestibular responses
- Motor responses (tone, reflexes and posturing)
- Meningism and signs of the underlying cause.

In particular, assessment of asymmetry for the presence of focal neurological deficits is vital.

CAUSES OF COMA

Causes with Focal Signs

- *No meningism*: Stroke, space occupying lesions (e.g. tumor, hemorrhage, abscess), injury, inflammation.
- *Meningism*: Meningoencephalitis, subarachnoid hemorrhage (SAH).

Systemic Causes without Focal Signs

- Toxins
- Organ failures
- *Metabolic*: Check COATPEGS (CO_2, O_2, ammonia, temperature, pH, electrolytes, glucose, serum osmolality)
- Endocrine
- Seizures

Remember that systemic causes can sometimes have focal signs! (e.g. Todd's paresis, hemiparesis due to hypoglycemia).

GENERAL EXAMINATION

General examination is also important:

- Consider the neurological findings in light of the vital signs, evidence of trauma, acute or chronic illness, and/or drug ingestion
- Cranial scars, drains, ICP monitors and VP shunts
- Neck stiffness
- Track marks and drug paraphernalia
- Infusions (e.g. sedatives, nimodipine, vasopressors)
- Ventilator (evidence of spontaneous breaths?)

LEVEL OF CONSCIOUSNESS

- GCS is most commonly used
- Other scores such as the Richmond Agitation-Sedation Score (RASS) are used to titrate sedation.

PATTERN OF BREATHING

Breathing pattern is often forgotten in intubated patients, but is important as the pattern of breathing correlates with the level of the lesion, and may suggest other causes

- Cheyne-Stokes respiration is not specific but is seen in lesions above the brainstem
- Central hyperventilation, or prolonged inspiratory pauses or irregular ataxic breathing indicates various brainstem lesions as does apnea
- Also look for deep rapid Kussmaul breathing, secondary to a metabolic acidosis, as in diabetes ketoacidosis
- Look for spontaneous breaths in the ventilated patient (may be supressed if hyperventilated).

PUPILLARY RESPONSES

- We need to assess the pupils for size, asymmetry and reactivity to light
- Different sized pupils correspond to different types of lesions
- Pinpoint pupils occur in pontine lesions and certain overdoses (e.g. opioid, clonidine)
- Fixed mid-sized pupils occur in midbrain lesions
- One dilated pupil suggests CN3 compression—e.g. ICH, PCOM aneurysm or raised ICP (parasympathetic nerves are in the superficial

parts of the nerve, so tend to be more vulnerable to compressive lesions—ptosis and 'down and out' eye positioning tends not to occur due to sparing of the more central motor fibers)

OCULAR DEVIATION AND DYSCONJUGATE GAZE

Dysconjugate Gaze

- Most individuals have a degree of exophoria when drowsy for any reason and any underlying strabismus tends to worsen
- Thus dysconjugate gaze is difficult to interpret in the stupor or comatose patient.

Tonic Deviation

- A frontal lobe lesion on the same side as the eye deviation, commonly a stroke. This can also be a result of a Todd's paralysis following a seizure (whereas during the seizure the eyes deviate in the *opposite* direction—*away* from the origin of the 'irritative' focus).
- A pontine lesion on the opposite side to the eye deviation. 'Wrong way eyes' may also be seen in thalamic hemorrhage.
- Lateral gaze deviation from a pontine lesion *cannot* be overcome by stimulating oculocephalic or ocular vestibular reflexes (see below), whereas supranuclear (e.g. frontal lesions) *can*. Hence, they can be distinguished clinically.

Skew Deviation

- Vertical separation of the ocular axes is called skew deviation
- This is suggestive of a pontine or vestibulocerebellar lesion on the side of the inferior eye, or a medial longitudinal fasciculus lesion on the side of the superior eye.

Abnormal eye position can also result from cranial nerve palsies (CN 6 is particularly at risk due to its long course) and orbital entrapment in trauma.

OCULOVESTIBULAR REFLEXES

Oculocephalic Reflex ('Doll's Eye' Reflex)

- Ensure the C-spine is cleared
- The patient's eyes are held open

- The head is briskly turned from side to side with the head held briefly at the end of each turn.
- A positive response occurs when the eyes rotate to the opposite side to the direction of head rotation, thus indicating that the brainstem (CN 3,6,8) is intact.
- A similar result is seen when the head is flexed and extended—a positive result is downward deviation of the eyes during extension, and upward deviation during flexion (the eyelids, if closed, may also open as part of the 'doll's head phenomenon'). These vertical responses indicates that the brainstem (CN 3,4,8) is intact.
- The eyes should gradually return to the mid-position in a smooth, conjugate movement if the brainstem is intact.
- Patients with metabolic coma (e.g. hepatic failure) may have exaggerated, brisk oculocephalic reflexes.

Oculovestibular Reflex (Caloric Stimulation)

- The head is elevated to 30° above horizontal so that the lateral semicircular canal is vertical, and so that stimulation with generate a maximal response.
- Check that the tympanum is intact and that the external ear canal is clear—C-spine clearance is not necessary.
- Introduce iced water into the external ear canal through a small cather until one of the following occurs:
  - Nystagmus (in the intact brainstem the slow phase is towards the irrigated ear)
  - Ocular deviation
  - 200 mL of iced water has been instilled
- Allow 5 minutes between testing ears to allow re-equilibration of the oculovestibular system
- As consciousness is lost, the fast component (towards the non-irrigated ear) is lost and the slow component tonically deviates the eye in the direction of the irrigated ear.

Vertical oculovestibular eye responses can be assessed by irrigated both ears simultaneously.

If the brainstem is intact, cold water causes the eyes to deviate downwards and warm water causes the eyes to deviate upwards.

Causes

- Brainstem encephalitis, deep metabolic coma and certain drugs may mimic brainstem death.

- Drugs include recently administered antiepileptics such as phenytoin and barbiturates. Like phenytoin, tricyclic overdose may cause bilateral vestibular failure, as might aminoglycoside vestibulotoxicity. Baclofen overdose can also mimic brain death.
- Another cause pertains to the trauma patient—ocular movements may be impaired if a blowout fracture has trapped the extraocular muscles.

Typical findings for various lesions are shown in **Figures 13.1A to E** from Posner et al. (2008):

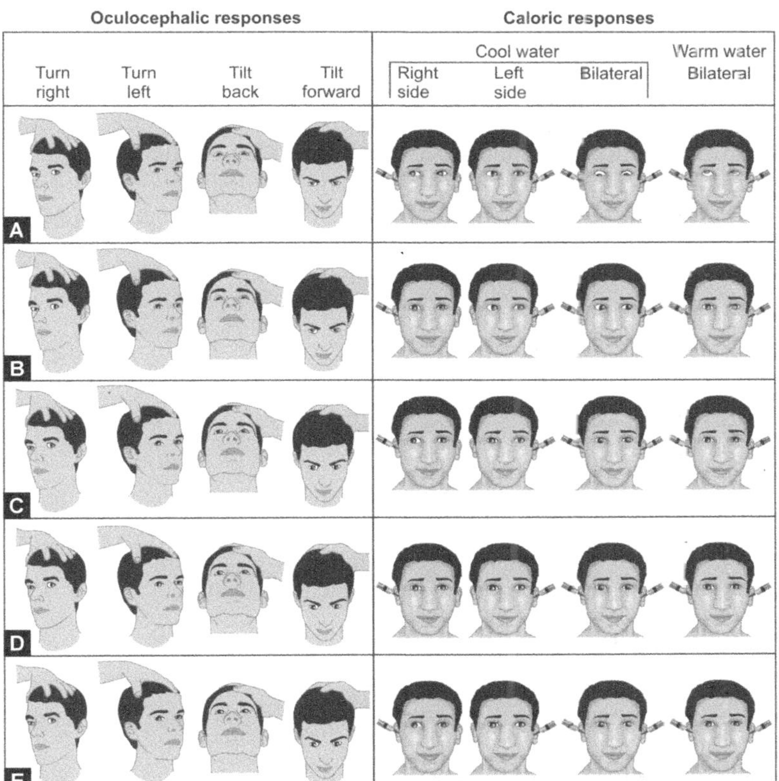

Figs 13.1A to E (A) Brainstem intact (metabolic encephalopathy); (B) Right lateral pontine lesion (gaze paralysis); (C) MLF lesion (bilateral internuclear ophthalmoplegia); (D) Right paramedian pontine lesion (1-1/2 syndrome); (E) Midbrain lesion (bilateral)

CORNEAL REFLEX

Corneal reflex is of limited use:

- Patients that chronically wear contact lenses may have diminished corneal reflexes.
- Loss of the corneal reflex is usually a late sign in coma.

Assessment

- Traditional method is to stroke the cornea with cotton wool
- Corneal stimulation can also be performed by dropping a few drops of sterile saline onto the cornea from a height of 10 cm (less traumatic)
- Reflex is present and intact if the patient blinks and eyes roll upwards
- *Afferent*: Cranial nerve 5
- *Efferent*: Cranial nerve 7 (blink) and cranial nerve 3 (eye movement)
- Indicates that the pons and midbrain are intact (the reflex pathway involves the trigeminal nerve, the spinal CN5 nucleus, the lateral brainstem tegmentum, and the CN3 and CN7 nuclei)
- If the eye turns upwards but the eyelid does not close there is a CN7 lesion (Bell's phenomenon)
- If the eye does not turn upwards and the eyelid does not close there is a CN5 lesion.

GAG AND COUGH REFLEXES

Gag Reflex

- Sensory = CN9, motor = CN10
- May be absent in normal people and those accustomed to an endotracheal tube.
- Best assessed using a laryngoscope and a tongue depressor in intubated patients, look for bilateral palatal elevation.

Cough Reflex

- Mediated by cranial nerve 10
- Can be stimulated by a suction catheter down and endotracheal tube.

MOTOR RESPONSES

Posturing can occur spontaneously or in response to a stimulus:

- Abnormal flexion is decorticate posturing—adduction of arm, internal rotation of shoulder, pronation of forearm, flexion of wrist (lower limbs are extended); indicates a lesion above the brainstem

- Extension is decerebrate posturing—abduction of arm, external rotation of shoulder, supination of forearm, extension of wrist (lower limbs are extended); indicates a lesion extending to the midbrain or below.

Assess for:
- Tone
- Clonus
- Deep tendon reflexes
- Plantar reflex
- Involuntary movements (such as subtle signs of seizures and myoclonus).
  Look for asymmetry.

SIGNS OF THE UNDERLYING CAUSE

- Consider the neurological findings in light of the vital signs, evidence of trauma or shock, acute or chronic illness, and/or drug ingestion
- Cranial scars, drains, ICP monitors and VP shunts
- Neck stiffness
- Track marks, drug paraphernalia and toxidromes
- Infusions (e.g. sedatives, nimodipine, vasopressors)
- Ventilator (evidence of spontaneous breaths?)
- Look in the fundi for papilloedema, diabetic or hypertensive retinopathy, or subhyaloid hemorrhage

FUNDOSCOPY

Important findings include:
- *Papilloedema*: Optic disc swelling due to raised intracranial pressure. However, the absence of papilloedema does not rule out intracranial hypertension.
- *Evidence of Terson syndrome*: Vitreous, subhyaloid, or retinal bleeding in association with subarachnoid hemorrhage.

14 Functional Assessment

The main aim of any rehabilitation program is to return the individual to a life style that is close to pre-morbid status of function as possible or alternatively to maximize the current potential for function and maintain it.

Purpose of functional assessment:

- It measures how a person does certain task or fulfills certain roles in various dimension of living. Data collected in functional assessment is used for provide base line information for setting functional oriented goals and outcomes of intervention.
- Indicator of patients initial abilities and progress towards more complex functional levels.
- Criteria for placement decisions.
- Evidence of the effectiveness of a specific intervention.

Terminologies for functional assessment:

- *Independent*: Patient is able to perform skill safely with no one present.
- *Supervision*: Patient requires someone within arm's reach as a precaution, low probability of patient having problem requiring assistance.
- *Close guarding*: Person assisting is positioned as if to assist with hand raised but not touching patient. Full attention on patient but not giving any assistance, fair probability of patient requiring assistance.
- *Contact guarding*: It is positioned as close guarding with hands on patient but not giving any assistance, high probability of patient requiring assistance.
- *Minimum assistance*: Patient is able to complete majority of activities without assistance.
- *Moderate assistance*: Patient is able to complete part of activity without assistance.
- *Maximum assistance*: Patient is unable to complete any part of activity.

Descriptive terminologies:

- *Bed mobility*:
  - *Independent*: No cuing is given
  - Supervision
  - Minimum assistance
  - Moderate assistance
  - Maximum assistance
- *Transfer*: Ambulation
  - *Independent*: No cuing is given
  - Supervision
  - Close guarding
  - Contact guarding
  - Minimum assistance
  - Moderate assistance
  - Maximum assistance

} —May require cues (Minimum, Moderate and Maximum assistance under Bed mobility)

} —May require cues (Close guarding through Maximum assistance under Transfer)

Functional balance grades:

- *Normal*: Patient is able to maintain steady balance without support. Accept maximum challenges and can shift weight in all directions.
- *Good*: Patient is able to maintain balance without support. Accept moderate challenges able to maintain balance while picking object off floor.
- *Fair*: Patient is able to maintain balance with hand hold accept minimal challenge. Able to maintain balance while turning head or trunk.
- *Poor*: Patient requires handhold and assistance. Unable to accept challenge or move without loss of balance.
- No balance.

Functional Skill Level

- *Codes*: I = Independent D = Dependent A = Assisted sitting: Floor Bench transfers: ______________________________
  - Describe: ______________________________
  - Self care: ______________________________
  - Feeding: ______________________________
  - Dressing: ______________________________
  - Hygiene: ______________________________
  - Toileting: ______________________________

15 Neurological Diagnostic Test

Diagnostic tests and procedures are vital tools that help physicians confirm or rule out the presence of a neurological disorder or other medical condition.

LABORATORY SCREENING TESTS

- Blood, urine, or other substances are used to help diagnose disease, better understand the disease process, and monitor levels of therapeutic drugs.
- Certain tests, ordered by the physician as part of a regular check-up, provide general information, while others are used to identify specific health concerns.
- Blood and blood product tests can detect brain and/or spinal cord infection, bone marrow disease, hemorrhage, blood vessel damage, toxins that affect the nervous system, and the presence of antibodies that signal the presence of an autoimmune disease.
- Blood tests are also used to monitor levels of therapeutic drugs used to treat epilepsy and other neurological disorders.
- Genetic testing of DNA extracted from white cells in the blood can help diagnose Huntington's disease and other congenital diseases.
- Analysis of the fluid that surrounds the brain and spinal cord can detect meningitis, acute and chronic inflammation, rare infections, and some cases of multiple sclerosis.
- Chemical and metabolic testing of the blood can indicate protein disorders, some forms of muscular dystrophy and other muscle disorders, and diabetes.
- Urinalysis can reveal abnormal substances in the urine or the presence or absence of certain proteins that cause diseases including the mucopolysaccharidoses.

GENETIC TESTING

It help parents who have a family history of a neurological disease determine if they are carrying one of the known genes that cause the disorder or find out if their child is affected. Genetic testing can identify many neurological disorders, including spina bifida, *in utero* (while the child is inside the mother's womb).

Genetic tests include the following:

- *Amniocentesis*, usually done at 14–16 weeks of pregnancy, tests a sample of the amniotic fluid in the womb for genetic defects (the fluid and the fetus have the same DNA). Under local anesthesia, a thin needle is inserted through the woman's abdomen and into the womb. About 20 milliliters of fluid (roughly 4 teaspoons) is withdrawn and sent to a lab for evaluation. Test results often take 1–2 weeks.
- *Chorionic villus sampling*, or CVS, is performed by removing and testing a very small sample of the placenta during early pregnancy. The sample, which contains the same DNA as the fetus, is removed by catheter or fine needle inserted through the cervix or by a fine needle inserted through the abdomen. It is tested for genetic abnormalities and results are usually available within 2 weeks. CVS should not be performed after the tenth week of pregnancy.
- *Uterine ultrasound* is performed using a surface probe with gel. This noninvasive test can suggest the diagnosis of conditions such as chromosomal disorders.

NEUROLOGICAL EXAMINATION

It assesses motor and sensory skills, the functioning of one or more cranial nerves, hearing and speech, vision, coordination and balance, mental status, and changes in mood or behavior, among other abilities. Items including a tuning fork, flashlight, reflex hammer, ophthalmoscope, and needles are used to help diagnose brain tumors, infections such as encephalitis and meningitis, and diseases such as Parkinson's disease, Huntington's disease, amyotrophic lateral sclerosis (ALS), and epilepsy. Some tests require the services of a specialist to perform and analyze results.

X-rays

- X-ray of the patient's chest and skull are often taken as part of a neurological work-up.
- X-rays can be used to view any part of the body, such as a joint or major organ system. In a conventional X-ray, also called a radiograph, a technician passes a concentrated burst of low-dose ionized radiation through the body and onto a photographic plate.
- Since calcium in bones absorbs X-rays more easily than soft tissue or muscle, the bony structure appears white on the film.
- Any vertebral misalignment or fractures can be seen within minutes.
- Tissue masses such as injured ligaments or a bulging disc are not visible on conventional X-rays.
- This fast, noninvasive, painless procedure is usually performed in a doctor's office or at a clinic.

Fluoroscopy

- It is a type of X-ray that uses a continuous or pulsed beam of low-dose radiation to produce continuous images of a body part in motion.
- The fluoroscope (X-ray tube) is focused on the area of interest and pictures are either videotaped or sent to a monitor for viewing.
- A contrast medium may be used to highlight the images.
- Fluoroscopy can be used to evaluate the flow of blood through arteries.

Diagnostic Tests

Based on the result of a neurological exam, physical exam, patient history, X-rays of the patient's chest and skull, and any previous screening or testing, physicians may order one or more of the following diagnostic tests to determine the specific nature of a suspected neurological disorder or injury.

These diagnostics generally involve either *nuclear medicine imaging,* in which very small amounts of radioactive materials are used to study organ function and structure, or *diagnostic imaging,* which uses magnets and electrical charges to study human anatomy.

The following list of available procedures—in alphabetical rather than sequential order—includes some of the more common tests used to help diagnose a neurological condition.

Angiography

- It is a test used to detect blockages of the arteries or veins.
- A *cerebral angiogram* can detect the degree of narrowing or obstruction of an artery or blood vessel in the brain, head, or neck.
- It is used to diagnose stroke and to determine the location and size of a brain tumor, aneurysm, or vascular malformation.
- This test is usually performed in a hospital outpatient setting and takes up to 3 hours, followed by a 6 to 8 hours resting period.

Procedure

- The patient, wearing a hospital or imaging gown, lies on a table that is wheeled into the imaging area.
- While the patient is awake, a physician anesthetizes a small area of the leg near the groin and then inserts a catheter into a major artery located there.
- The catheter is threaded through the body and into an artery in the neck.
- Once the catheter is in place, the needle is removed and a guide wire is inserted. A small capsule containing a radiopaque dye (one that is highlighted on X-rays) is passed over the guide wire to the site of release.
- The dye is released and travels through the bloodstream into the head and neck. A series of X-rays is taken and any obstruction is noted.
- Patients may feel a warm to hot sensation or slight discomfort as the dye is released.

Biopsy

- It involves the removal and examination of a small piece of tissue from the body.
- *Muscle* or *nerve biopsies* are used to diagnose neuromuscular disorders and may also reveal if a person is a carrier of a defective gene that could be passed on to children.

Procedure

- A small sample of muscle or nerve is removed under local anesthetic and studied under a microscope.

- The sample may be removed either surgically, through a slit made in the skin, or by needle biopsy, in which a thin hollow needle is inserted through the skin and into the muscle.
- A small piece of muscle or nerve remains in the hollow needle when it is removed from the body.
- The biopsy is usually performed at an outpatient testing facility. A *brain biopsy,* used to determine tumor type, requires surgery to remove a small piece of the brain or tumor.
- Performed in a hospital, this operation is riskier than a muscle biopsy and involves a longer recovery period.

Brain Scans

- They are imaging techniques used to diagnose tumors, blood vessel malformations, or hemorrhage in the brain.
- These scans are used to study organ function or injury or disease to tissue or muscle.
- Types of brain scans include computed tomography, magnetic resonance imaging, and positron emission tomography.

Cerebrospinal Fluid Analysis

- It involves the removal of a small amount of the fluid that protects the brain and spinal cord.
- The fluid is tested to detect any bleeding or brain hemorrhage, diagnose infection to the brain and/or spinal cord, identify some cases of multiple sclerosis and other neurological conditions, and measure intracranial pressure.

Procedure

- The procedure is usually done in a hospital.
- The sample of fluid is commonly removed by a procedure known as *lumbar puncture,* or *spinal tap.*
- The patient is asked to either lie on one side, in a ball position with knees close to the chest, or lean forward while sitting on a table or bed.
- The doctor will locate a puncture site in the lower back, between two vertebrate, then clean the area and inject a local anesthetic.

- The patient may feel a slight stinging sensation from this injection. Once the anesthetic has taken effect, the doctor will insert a special needle into the spinal sac and remove a small amount of fluid (usually about three teaspoons) for testing.
- Most patients will feel a sensation of pressure only as the needle is inserted.
- A common after-effect of a lumbar puncture is headache, which can be lessened by having the patient lie flat.
- Risk of nerve root injury or infection from the puncture can occur but it is rare. The entire procedure takes about 45 minutes.

Computed Tomography

- It is also known as a CT scan, is a noninvasive, painless process used to produce rapid, clear two-dimensional images of organs, bones, and tissues.
- Neurological CT scans are used to view the brain and spine. They can detect bone and vascular irregularities, certain brain tumors and cysts, herniated discs, epilepsy, encephalitis, spinal stenosis (narrowing of the spinal canal), a blood clot or intracranial bleeding in patients with stroke, brain damage from head injury, and other disorders.
- Many neurological disorders share certain characteristics and a CT scan can aid in proper diagnosis by differentiating the area of the brain affected by the disorder.

Procedure

- Scanning takes about 20 minutes (a CT of the brain or head may take slightly longer) and is usually done at an imaging center or hospital on an outpatient basis. The patient lies on a special table that slides into a narrow chamber.
- A sound system built into the chamber allows the patient to communicate with the physician or technician.
- As the patient lies still, X-rays are passed through the body at various angles and are detected by a computerized scanner.
- The data is processed and displayed as cross-sectional images, or "slices", of the internal structure of the body or organ.
- A light sedative may be given to patients who are unable to lie still and pillows may be used to support and stabilize the head and body.

- Persons who are claustrophobic may have difficulty taking this imaging test.
- Occasionally a contrast dye is injected into the bloodstream to highlight the different tissues in the brain. Patients may feel a warm or cool sensation as the dye circulates through the bloodstream or they may experience a slight metallic taste.
- Although very little radiation is used in CT, pregnant women should avoid the test because of potential harm to the fetus from ionizing radiation.

Discography

- It is often suggested for patients who are considering lumbar surgery or who's lower back pain has not responded to conventional treatments.
- This outpatient procedure is usually performed at a testing facility or a hospital. The patient is asked to put on a metal-free hospital gown and lie on an imaging table.
- The physician numbs the skin with anesthetic and inserts a thin needle, using X-ray guidance, into the spinal disc. Once the needle is in place, a small amount of contrast dye is injected and CT scans are taken.
- The contrast dye outlines any damaged areas. More than one disc may be imaged at the same time. Patient recovery usually takes about an hour.
- Pain medicine may be prescribed for any resulting discomfort.

Intrathecal Contrast-enhanced CT Scan

- It is used to detect problems with the spine and spinal nerve roots.
- This test is most often performed at an imaging center.

Procedure

- The patient is asked to put on a hospital or imaging gown. Following application of a topical anesthetic, the physician removes a small sample of the spinal fluid via lumbar puncture.
- The sample is mixed with a contrast dye and injected into the spinal sac located at the base of the lower back.

- The patient is then asked to move to a position that will allow the contrast fluid to travel to the area to be studied.
- The dye allows the spinal canal and nerve roots to be seen more clearly on a CT scan.
- The scan may take up to an hour to complete. Following the test, patients may experience some discomfort and/or headache that may be caused by the removal of spinal fluid.

Electroencephalography, or EEG

- It monitors brain activity through the skull.
- EEG is used to help diagnose certain seizure disorders, brain tumors, brain damage from head injuries, inflammation of the brain and/or spinal cord, alcoholism, certain psychiatric disorders, and metabolic and degenerative disorders that affect the brain.
- EEGs are also used to evaluate sleep disorders, monitor brain activity when a patient has been fully anesthetized or loses consciousness, and confirm brain death.
- This painless, risk-free test can be performed in a doctor's office or at a hospital or testing facility.

Procedure

- Prior to taking an EEG, the person must avoid caffeine intake and prescription drugs that affect the nervous system.
- A series of cup-like electrodes are attached to the patient's scalp, either with a special conducting paste or with extremely fine needles.
- The electrodes (also called leads) are small devices that are attached to wires and carry the electrical energy of the brain to a machine for reading.
- A very low electrical current is sent through the electrodes and the baseline brain energy is recorded. Patients are then exposed to a variety of external stimuli—including bright or flashing light, noise or certain drugs—or are asked to open and close the eyes, or to change breathing patterns.
- The electrodes transmit the resulting changes in brain wave patterns. Since movement and nervousness can change brain wave patterns, patients usually recline in a chair or on a bed during the test, which takes up to an hour. Testing for certain disorders requires performing an EEG during sleep, which takes at least 3 hours.

- In order to learn more about brain wave activity, electrodes may be inserted through a surgical opening in the skull and into the brain to reduce signal interference from the skull.

Electromyography or EMG

- It is used to diagnose nerve and muscle dysfunction and spinal cord disease.
- It records the electrical activity from the brain and/or spinal cord to a peripheral nerve root (found in the arms and legs) that controls muscles during contraction and at rest.
- During an EMG, very fine wire electrodes are inserted into a muscle to assess changes in electrical voltage that occur during movement and when the muscle is at rest.
- The electrodes are attached through a series of wires to a recording instrument. Testing usually takes place at a testing facility and lasts about an hour but may take longer, depending on the number of muscles and nerves to be tested.
- Most patients find this test to be somewhat uncomfortable.

Procedure

- An EMG is usually done in conjunction with a *nerve conduction velocity (NCV)* test, which measures electrical energy by assessing the nerve's ability to send a signal.
- This two-part test is conducted most often in a hospital.
- A technician tapes two sets of flat electrodes on the skin over the muscles. The first set of electrodes is used to send small pulses of electricity (similar to the sensation of static electricity) to stimulate the nerve that directs a particular muscle.
- The second set of electrodes transmits the responding electrical signal to a recording machine.
- The physician then reviews the response to verify any nerve damage or muscle disease.
- Patients who are preparing to take an EMG or NCV test may be asked to avoid caffeine and not smoke for 2–3 hours prior to the test, as well as to avoid aspirin and non-steroidal anti-inflammatory drugs for 24 hours before the EMG.
- There is no discomfort or risk associated with this test.

Electronystagmography (ENG)

It describes a group of tests used to diagnose involuntary eye movement, dizziness, and balance disorders, and to evaluate some brain functions.

Procedure

- The test is performed at an imaging center.
- Small electrodes are taped around the eyes to record eye movements.
- If infrared photography is used in place of electrodes, the patient wears special goggles that help record the information.
- Both versions of the test are painless and risk-free.

Evoked Potentials

- It measures the electrical signals to the brain generated by hearing, touch, or sight. These tests are used to assess sensory nerve problems and confirm neurological conditions including multiple sclerosis, brain tumor, acoustic neuroma (small tumors of the inner ear), and spinal cord injury.
- Evoked potentials are also used to test sight and hearing (especially in infants and young children), monitor brain activity among coma patients, and confirm brain death.

Procedure

- Testing may take place in a doctor's office or hospital setting. It is painless and risk-free. Two sets of needle electrodes are used to test for nerve damage.
- One set of electrodes, which will be used to measure the electrophysiological response to stimuli, is attached to the patient's scalp using conducting paste. The second set of electrodes is attached to the part of the body to be tested.
- The physician then records the amount of time it takes for the impulse generated by stimuli to reach the brain. Under normal circumstances, the process of signal transmission is instantaneous.
  - *Auditory evoked potentials* (also called brain stem auditory evoked response) are used to assess high-frequency hearing loss, diagnose any damage to the acoustic nerve and auditory pathways in the brainstem, and detect acoustic neuroma. The patient sits in a soundproof room and wears headphones. Clicking sounds are

delivered one at a time to one ear while a masking sound is sent to the other ear. Each ear is usually tested twice, and the entire procedure takes about 45 minutes.

- *Visual evoked potentials* detect loss of vision from optic nerve damage (in particular, damage caused by multiple sclerosis). The patient sits close to a screen and is asked to focus on the center of a shifting checkerboard pattern. Only one eye is tested at a time; the other eye is either kept closed or covered with a patch. Each eye is usually tested twice. Testing takes 30–45 minutes.
- *Somatosensory evoked potentials* measure response from stimuli to the peripheral nerves and can detect nerve or spinal cord damage or nerve degeneration from multiple sclerosis and other degenerating diseases. Tiny electrical shocks are delivered by electrode to a nerve in an arm or leg. Responses to the shocks, which may be delivered for more than a minute at a time, are recorded. This test usually lasts less than an hour.

Magnetic Resonance Imaging

- It uses computer-generated radio waves and a powerful magnetic field to produce detailed images of body structures including tissues, organs, bones, and nerves.
- Neurological uses include the diagnosis of brain and spinal cord tumors, eye disease, inflammation, infection, and vascular irregularities that may lead to stroke.
- MRI can also detect and monitor degenerative disorders such as multiple sclerosis and can document brain injury from trauma.
- The equipment houses a hollow tube that is surrounded by a very large cylindrical magnet.
- The patient, who must remain still during the test, lies on a special table that is slid into the tube.
- The patient will be asked to remove jewelry, eyeglasses, removable dental work, or other items that might interfere with the magnetic imaging.
- The patient should wear a sweat shirt and sweat pants or other clothing free of metal eyelets or buckles.
- MRI scanning equipment creates a magnetic field around the body strong enough to temporarily realign water molecules in the tissues.

- Radio waves are then passed through the body to detect the "relaxation" of the molecules back to a random alignment and trigger a resonance signal at different angles within the body.
- A computer processes this resonance into either a three-dimensional picture or a two-dimensional "slice" of the tissue being scanned, and differentiates between bone, soft tissues and fluid-filled spaces by their water content and structural properties.
- A contrast dye may be used to enhance visibility of certain areas or tissues. The patient may hear grating or knocking noises when the magnetic field is turned on and off. (Patients may wear special earphones to block out the sounds).
- Unlike CT scanning, MRI does not use ionizing radiation to produce images. Depending on the part(s) of the body to be scanned, MRI can take up to an hour to complete.
- The test is painless and risk-free, although persons who are obese or claustrophobic may find it somewhat uncomfortable. (Some centers also use open MRI machines that do not completely surround the person being tested and are less confining).
- However, open MRI does not currently provide the same picture quality as standard MRI and some tests may not be available using this equipment). Due to the incredibly strong magnetic field generated by an MRI, patients with implanted medical devices such as a pacemaker should avoid the test.
  - *Functional MRI (fMRI)* uses the blood's magnetic properties to produce real-time images of blood flow to particular areas of the brain. An fMRI can pinpoint areas of the brain that become active and note how long they stay active. It can also tell if brain activity within a region occurs simultaneously or sequentially. This imaging process is used to assess brain damage from head injury or degenerative disorders such as Alzheimer's disease and to identify and monitor other neurological disorders, including multiple sclerosis, stroke, and brain tumors.

Myelography

- It involves the injection of a water- or oil-based contrast dye into the spinal canal to enhance X-ray imaging of the spine.
- *Myelograms* are used to diagnose spinal nerve injury, herniated discs, fractures, back or leg pain, and spinal tumors.

Procedure

- The procedure takes about 30 minutes and is usually performed in a hospital. Following an injection of anesthesia to a site between two vertebrae in the lower back, a small amount of the cerebrospinal fluid is removed by spinal tap (see *cerebrospinal fluid analysis*, above) and the contrast dye is injected into the spinal canal.
- After a series of X-rays is taken, most or all of the contrast dye is removed by aspiration. Patients may experience some pain during the spinal tap and when the dye is injected and removed. Patients may also experience headache following the spinal tap. The risk of fluid leakage or allergic reaction to the dye is slight.

Positron Emission Tomography

- The scans provide two- and three-dimensional pictures of brain activity by measuring radioactive isotopes that are injected into the bloodstream.
- PET scans of the brain are used to detect or highlight tumors and diseased tissue, measure cellular and/or tissue metabolism, show blood flow, evaluate patients who have seizure disorders that do not respond to medical therapy and patients with certain memory disorders, and determine brain changes following injury or drug abuse, among other uses.
- PET may be ordered as a follow-up to a CT or MRI scan to give the physician a greater understanding of specific areas of the brain that may be involved with certain problems.

Procedure

- Scans are conducted in a hospital or at a testing facility, on an outpatient basis. A low-level radioactive isotope, which binds to chemicals that flow to the brain, is injected into the bloodstream and can be traced as the brain performs different functions.
- The patient lies still while overhead sensors detect gamma rays in the body's tissues.
- A computer processes the information and displays it on a video monitor or on film.
- Using different compounds, more than one brain function can be traced simultaneously.

- PET is painless and relatively risk-free. Length of test time depends on the part of the body to be scanned.
- PET scans are performed by skilled technicians at highly sophisticated medical facilities.

Polysomnogram

- It measures brain and body activity during sleep.
- It is performed over one or more nights at a sleep center.

Procedure

- Electrodes are pasted or taped to the patient's scalp, eyelids, and/or chin. Throughout the night and during the various wake/sleep cycles, the electrodes record brain waves, eye movement, breathing, leg and skeletal muscle activity, blood pressure, and heart rate.
- The patient may be videotaped to note any movement during sleep.
- Results are then used to identify any characteristic patterns of sleep disorders, including restless legs syndrome, periodic limb movement disorder, insomnia, and breathing disorders such as obstructive sleep apnea.
- Polysomnograms are noninvasive, painless, and risk-free.

Single Photon Emission Computed Tomography (SPECT)

- A nuclear imaging test involving blood flow to tissue, is used to evaluate certain brain functions.
- The test may be ordered as a follow-up to an MRI to diagnose tumors, infections, degenerative spinal disease, and stress fractures.
- As with a PET scan, a radioactive isotope, which binds to chemicals that flow to the brain, is injected intravenously into the body.
- Areas of increased blood flow will collect more of the isotope.

Procedure

- As the patient lies on a table, a gamma camera rotates around the head and records where the radioisotope has traveled.

- That information is converted by computer into cross-sectional slices that are stacked to produce a detailed three-dimensional image of blood flow and activity within the brain.
- The test is performed at either an imaging center or a hospital.

Thermography

- It uses infrared sensing devices to measure small temperature changes between the two sides of the body or within a specific organ.
- Also known as digital infrared thermal imaging, thermography may be used to detect vascular disease of the head and neck, soft tissue injury, various neuromusculoskeletal disorders, and the presence or absence of nerve root compression.

Procedure

- It is performed at an imaging center, using infrared light recorders to take thousands of pictures of the body from a distance of 5–8 feet.
- The information is converted into electrical signals which results in a computer-generated two-dimensional picture of abnormally cold or hot areas indicated by color or shades of black and white.
- Thermography does not use radiation and is safe, risk-free, and noninvasive.

Ultrasound Imaging

- It is also called ultrasound scanning or sonography, uses high-frequency sound waves to obtain images inside the body.
  - *Neurosonography* (ultrasound of the brain and spinal column) analyzes blood flow in the brain and can diagnose stroke, brain tumors, hydrocephalus (build-up of cerebrospinal fluid in the brain), and vascular problems.
- It can also identify or rule out inflammatory processes causing pain. It is more effective than an X-ray in displaying soft tissue masses and can show tears in ligaments, muscles, tendons, and other soft tissue masses in the back.
  - *Transcranial Doppler ultrasound* is used to view arteries and blood vessels in the neck and determine blood flow and risk of stroke.

Procedure

- During ultrasound, the patient lies on an imaging table and removes clothing around the area of the body to be scanned.
- A jelly-like lubricant is applied and a transducer, which both sends and receives high-frequency sound waves, is passed over the body.
- The sound wave echoes are recorded and displayed as a computer-generated real-time visual image of the structure or tissue being examined.
- Ultrasound is painless, noninvasive, and risk-free.
- The test is performed on an outpatient basis and takes between 15 and 30 minutes to complete.

16 Normal Development

GROSS MOTOR DEVELOPMENT (FIG. 16.1)

0–1 Months

- Predominant head lag
- Head falls on chest
- May extend momentarily.

0–2 Months

- Lifts head momentarily from prone
- Turns head to both sides in supine.

3 Months

- Supports himself on forearms and raises thorax and head off bed when prone
- Rolls supine to side lying.

4 Months

- Holds head steady
- Pulls to sit with head in midline
- Sits if propped
- Bears part of weight when held upright
- Reaches for and grasps toy
- Has symmetrical postures.

5–6 Months

- Lifts head while supine
- Bears large amount of weight on legs
- Rolls from prone to supine
- Sits by leaning on hands, head erect

- Displays protective reactions forward
- Rolls from supine to prone.

7–8 Months

- Transfers object from hand to hand
- Sets in hand-knee position (4-point kneel)
- Helps hold bottle when being fed
- Pivots on abdomen, using hands and feet
- Sits indefinitely unsupported
- Has equilibrium reactions.

9–10 Months

- Creeps with true alternating creeping
- Gets into sitting position without help and recovers lost balance
- Pulls to standing
- Drinks from cup if assisted
- Moves about independently and explores
- Can side sit.

11–12 Months

- Balances momentarily while standing alone
- Cruises holding onto furniture
- Walks when one hand is held.

13–15 Months

- Walks alone—unequal steps on broad base
- Rises to standing and lowers independently
- Stops and starts walking without falling
- Climbs stairs when hand is held.

16–18 Months

- Runs stiffly with only occasional falls
- Climbs onto chair and bed
- Creeps up and down stairs
- Stands on one foot with help.

19–21 Months

- Runs well with little falling
- Climbs stairs holding onto rail, both feet on same step (marking time)
- Walks backwards.

22–24 Months

- Runs without falling but headlong
- Picks up object from floor
- Squats to roll and catch a ball.

2–2½ Years

- Can walk on tip toes
- Jumps with both feet in place
- Stands up from the floor without support
- Kicks ball with one hand 5–7 feet

3 Years

- Goes up stairs alternating feet, both feet on same step (marking time) going down
- Jumps from bottom step
- Rides tricycle
- Shows reciprocal arm and leg gait pattern
- Runs on toes
- Stands on one foot for two seconds.

4 Years

- Goes up and down stairs alternating feet without rail
- Balances on one foot for four to eight seconds
- Throws ball overhand.

5 Years

- Gallops
- Skips with alternating feet
- Stands on one foot for more than eight seconds
- Tandem walks forward

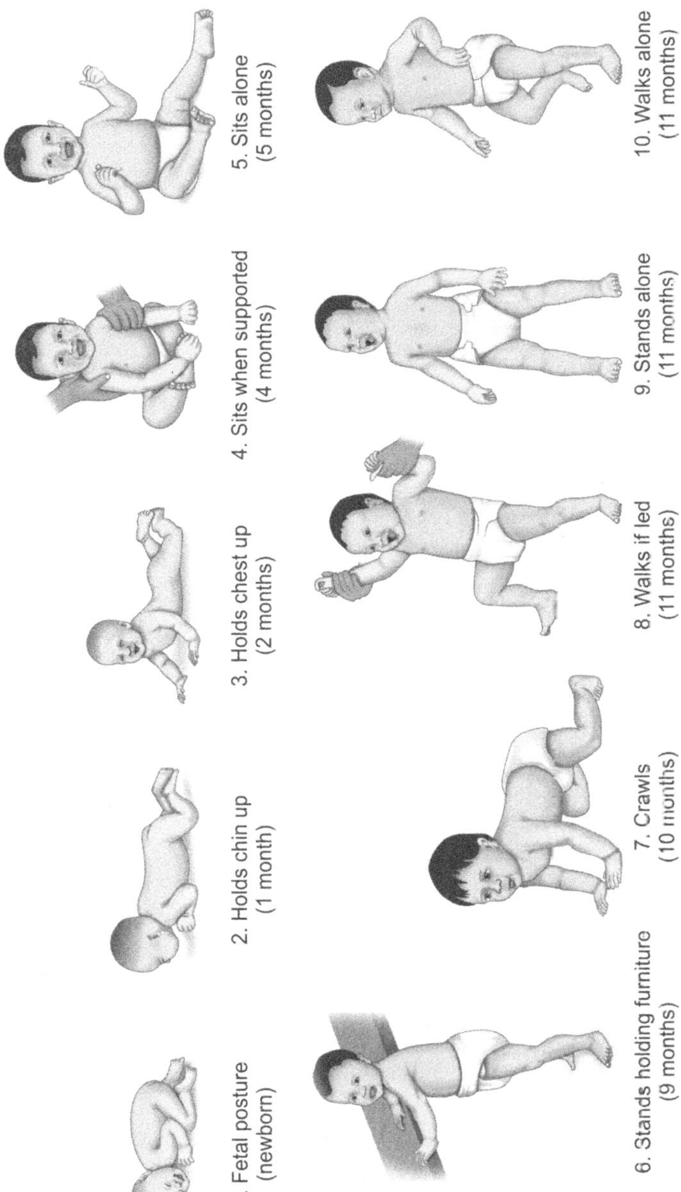

Fig. 16.1 Gross motor development

- Catches thrown playground ball with both hands
- Uses a swing.

6 Years

- Jumps from 12-inch height, landing on toes
- Stands on alternating feet with eyes closed
- Shows advanced throwing (mature pattern)
- With accurate placement
- Walks forward, backwards, sideways on balance beam
- Hops on one foot
- Tandem walks backwards.

FINE MOTOR/VISUAL MOTOR DEVELOPMENT (FIG. 16.2)

0–2 Months

- Moves arms symmetrically
- Shows grasp reflex
- Responds to different light intensities.

1–3½ Months

- Shows asymmetrical reach
- Brings hands to midline in supine
- Attempts to reach towards object
- Recognizes hands
- Begins vertical tracking downward, often loses object.

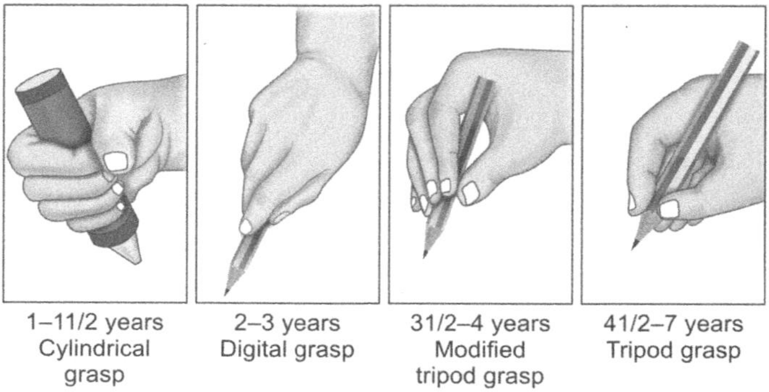

Fig. 16.2 Fine motor development

2–4 Months

Grasps toy actively.

3–5 Months

- Has ulnar palmar grasp—wrist flexed with no thumb involvement
- Exhibits inhibited grasp reflex
- Shows bilateral symmetrical reach
- Moves head to track a moving object
- Shows prolonged looking at objects at midline
- Looks for lost object outside visual field.

4–5 Months

- Demonstrates palmar grasp—using all fingers, thumb not opposed
- Begins to move hand under visual control
- Controls wrist and fingers with arm extended
- Demonstrates object permanence.

5–7 Months

- Has raking grasp
- Transfers object from one hand to the other
- Has radial palmar grasp
- Under reaches, adjusts, and obtains
- Exhibits accidental release
- Tracks vertically and diagonally with jerky eye movements.

7–10 Months

- Exhibits inferior pincer grasp
- Exhibits radial digital grasp
- Exhibits three-jaw chuck grasp
- Exhibits lateral pinch
- Drops object into large container opening.

10–12 Months

- Exhibits neat pincher grasp
- Bangs two objects together

- Shows development of supinated grasp
- Reaches overhead in sitting position
- Manipulates an object with one hand while the other stabilizes.

15 Months

- Places objects in and out of container with small opening
- Points with index finger.

18 Months

- Builds three-block tower
- Puts peg in 1" hole
- Turns pages two to three at a time
- Scribbles spontaneously.

3 Years

- Builds nine-block tower
- Assists with one hand
- Screws lid on jar
- Places ten pellets in bottle (30 seconds)
- Grasps with extended wrist and thumb opposition
- Turns doorknob with forearm rotation
- Imitates building cube bridge
- Snips with scissors.

3–4 Years

- Exhibits definite hand preference
- Begins to color
- Copies circle, imitates a cross
- Traces diamond, angles rounded
- Draws designs without detail
- Begins to cut with scissors on wide lines
- Throws ball overhead
- Catches large ball with arms
- Scribbles with intense spots of color
- Completes shape form boards and simple puzzles.

4–5 Years

- Exhibits dominant hand is established
- Shows finger isolation
- Traces simple designs and mazes
- Copies cross and square
- Colors within lines
- Draws simple picture of person
- Cuts straight or simple curved lines
- Cuts circle and square
- Catches ball using hands and arms.

5–6 Years

- Copies diagonal lines and triangle
- Prints name
- Begins to form letters
- Colors small area of detail
- Draws detailed pictures of person
- Draws designs with detail
- Cuts convex and concave shapes
- Shows controlled tracking skills in vertical, horizontal, circular, and diagonally (no head movement).

6–7 Years

- Uses a mature pattern when manipulating a writing instrument (movements generated from fingers)
- Copies letters (still some inverted or reversed)
- Writes upper and lower case letters with differences in sizes and limited spacing
- Shows mature figure-ground skills
- Shows body awareness has been established.

7–9 Years

- Writes more neatly and legibly spaced
- Begins cursive writing
- Exhibits position in space development complete
- Shows directional concept.

RELEASE

The following is the developmental sequence of release:

0–9 Months

Drops objects.

9 Months

Releases against another surface.

10 Months

Exhibits crude release, systematic dropping (voluntary).

11 Months

- Releases large objects with ease, clumsy
- Releases small objects.

12 Months

- Exhibits smooth voluntary release of large objects
- Exhibits crude but voluntary release of small objects.

15 Months

Exhibits voluntary smooth controlled release of all objects.

GRASP

The following is the developmental sequence of grasp:

- 12 weeks Reflexive, ulnar side strongest
- 16 weeks Ulnar side weakening
- 20 weeks Primitive squeeze; no thumb or palm involved; raking
- 24 weeks Palmar; no thumb participation
- 28 weeks Radial palmar; whole hand grasp, thumb adducted
- 32 weeks Scissors, thumb abducted to side curled index finger
- 36 weeks Radial digital, thumb opposed to end of fingers
- 40 weeks Inferior finger, thumb moves toward dip joint of index finger; other fingers inhibited

- 44 weeks Neat pincer, with slight wrist extension
- 52 weeks Opposed grasp
- 3–4 years Static tripod posture; pencil grasped proximally; crude approximation of thumb, index, and middle fingers; continual adjustments by other hand; ring and little fingers only slightly flexed, no fine, localized movements of components
- 4–6 years Dynamic tripod posture; pencil grasped distally; precise opposition of distal phalanges of thumb, index, and middle fingers; ring and little fingers flexed to form stable arch; metacarpal joints stabilized during fine localized movements of interphalangeal joints
  Lateral prehension; key or card held between pad of thumb and lateral surface of index near dip joint
  Spherical grasp; ball or door knob grasped with flexion at all finger joints, hand cupped over object
  Cylindrical grasp; small jar or large peg

These ages are approximations and may vary when other resources are used. This is not designed to be a complete description at each age level. Use as a quick reference.

FEEDING DEVELOPMENT

0–3 Months

- Gag reflex (diminished by 7 months)
- Rooting reflex
- Suck-swallow reflex
- Drools
- Anticipates feeding
- Brings fingers to mouth.

3–6 Months

- Phasic bite-and-release pattern used for most things placed in mouth (biting is not controlled or sustained)
- Uses tongue to move pureed food in mouth
- Swallows pureed food
- Gumming action on solid food like cracker (jaw movements are up and down).

6–9 Months

- Holds bottle without assistance, may remove and replace
- Feeds self-cracker, munching pattern
- Tongue retraction in sucking
- Absence of tongue protrusion during spoon feeding
- Can protrude tongue
- Can lateralize tongue.

9–12 Months

- Finger feed dry cereal, soft foods, mashed table foods
- Voluntary biting on food and objects
- Helps guide spoon and cup to mouth
- Controls drooling.

12–18 Months

- Distinguishes edible versus no edible
- Uses fork
- Unwraps edible item
- Gives up bottle
- Drinks from cup

18–24 Months

- Finger feeds part of meal
- Bites and chews food well (rotary chewing)
- Holds own spoon, pronated grasp
- Scoops food
- Directs spoon to mouth without spillage, palm down
- Turns spoon over in mouth
- Drinks well independently, few spills (good coordination of suck, swallow, and breathing).

2–3 Years

- Sucks through a straw
- Tongue-tip elevation used for swallowing
- Holds small cup in one hand
- Brings spoon to mouth, palm up

- Eats meats and raw vegetables
- Feeds self independently with set up with little spillage
- Uses a rotary chew pattern
- Lips are closed during chewing
- Opens jars
- Pours from a small container.

3–4 Years

- Get drink from faucet
- Attempts to cut with knife.

4–5 Years

- Holds spoon with fingers for solid foods
- Holds fork with fingers
- Uses straw without mashing the end
- Fixes dry cereal
- Pours from large container
- Uses napkin.

5–6 Years

- Cuts with knife soft foods
- Carries drink without spillage.

6–7 Years

- Cuts independently with knife
- Makes simple sandwich.

PERSONAL CARE DEVELOPMENT

9–12 months

Removes socks in sitting position.

1–2 Years

- Assists with dressing, holds arms out, putting foot up for shoe
- Pushes leg through pants

- Takes off hat
- Pulls off shoes
- Pulls of sock
- Indicates when wet or soiled.

2–3 Years

- Removes unfastened garments and elastic waist pants
- Removes coat, with help with fasteners
- Puts on front-button shirt and jacket with help with fasteners
- Puts on socks with difficulty with heel placement
- Helps push down pants (standing)
- Unzips front or side zipper
- Unsnaps
- Indicates need for using the bathroom but may need reminders
- Needs supervision for brushing or combing hair.

3–4 Years

- Needs assistance to remove and put on pullover shirt
- Independent with pull-down garments (pants and underpants)
- Puts on socks with heel placement
- Puts on shoes, may be on wrong feet
- Puts on jacket
- Unlaces shoes
- Unbuttons and buttons large buttons
- Unsnaps and snaps
- Unzips and zips jacket.

4–5 Years

- Laces with supervision for sequencing
- Buttons large buttons
- Zips, locking tab
- Zips, aligning separating zipper
- Washes and dries face
- Brushes teeth
- Puts belt in loops
- Manages shoes with Velcro
- Unbuckles and buckles shoes or belt

- Covers mouth when coughing upon request
- Washes and dries hands
- Blows and wipes nose
- Goes to bathroom independently, able to on and off commode without assistance.

5–6 Years

- Puts on pullover garment correctly
- Buttons medium buttons
- Dresses self with assistance for back fasteners, small buttons, bows
- Puts shoes on correct feet
- Laces
- Ties a knot
- Cleans and wipes nose independently
- Completely cares for toileting needs.

6–7 Years

- Ties a bow
- Buttons small buttons
- Closes back zipper
- Brushes or combs hair independently.

17 General Neurological Assessment

Name : ______________________

Age : ______________________

Sex : ______________________

Address : ______________________

Occupation : ______________________

Chief complaints : ______________________

CASE HISTORY

History indicates probable pathology:

- *History of presenting condition*: Chronological occurrence of manifestation with the character, exact date, duration and other treatment.
  - Information about mode of onset:

Mode of onset	*Probable cause*
Abrupt/instantaneous	Vascular/trauma
Deterioration over period of time	Inflammatory/demyelinating disease
Deterioration over months	Chronic inflammation/malignancy
Relapsing and remitting symptoms	Multiple sclerosis
Recurrent headaches	Migraine

  - Information about negative symptoms:
    - Hemiparesis
    - Memory loss
    - Muscle weakness
    - Micturition control
    - Numbness, loss of feeling, perception, anesthesia.
  - Information about positive symptoms:
    - Pill rolling tremor of finger and thumb
    - Flashing lights preceding headache

    - Repetitive twitching of fingers
    - A hallucination of an odd smell
    - Paresthesia, tingling, dysesthesia
  - *Information about vertigo*: Subjective/objective
  - *Information about mental symptom*: Delirium, confusion, personality changes, tension, drug abuse
  - *Information about disturbance in sleep rhythm*: Drowsiness, hypersomnia, insomnia.
  - Information about trauma.
- Past medical and surgical history
- Treatment history
- Socio-economic history
- Family history
  - Screen carefully before declaring a negative family history
- Personal history
- Functional history
  - Past and current functional status in self-care
  - Growth and developmental history
  - Dominance of hand and foot
  - Occupational and employment history and other activities
- History of toxin exposure
- Environmental history

Associated Problem

- Diabetes
- Blood pressure
- Cardiac disease
- Other orthopedic dysfunction

Vital Signs

- *Four vital signs*:
  1. Body temperature
  2. Pulse rate
  3. Blood pressure
  4. Respiratory rate

Pain is considered as fifth vital sign, as perceived by the patient on a pain scale 0–10.

PAIN ASSESSMENT

- Onset : ____________________
- Nature : ____________________
- Duration : ____________________
- Intensity : ____________________
- Type of pain : ____________________
- Radiating or nonaddicting : ____________________
- Aggravating factors : ____________________
- Relieving factors : ____________________
- Intensity of pain : ____________________
- Visual analogue scale : ____________________

On Observation

- *General appearance*:
  - Agitation
  - Vomitus
  - Urinary or fecal incontinence
- *Body built*:
  - Ectomorphic (thin, prominence of structures from ectoderm)
  - Mesomorphic (muscular, prominence of structure from mesoderm)
  - Endomorphic (heavy, fat body built, prominence of structure from endoderm).
- *Posture evaluation (mention the position of patient)*:
  - *Anterior view*: Both eyes, acromion process, iliac crests, ASIS, greater trochanter of femur, patella and melleoli should be horizontally level, waist angles are symmetrical. Patella and feet face anteriorly.
  - *Posterior view*: Ear lobes, shoulders, inferior angle of scapula, iliac crests, PSIS, greater trochanter, buttocks and knee creases and melleoli should be in level. Spine should be straight with medial border of scapula equidistance from spine bilaterally. Varus and valgus deformity of knee and calcareous should be noted.
  - *Lateral view*: The line of gravity should be bisect the external auditory meatus, acromion process, greater trochanter, posterior to patella and approximately two inches anterior to lateral malleolus. The cervical and lumbar spine should exhibit moderate lordosis and thoracic spine exhibit kyphotic curve.

- *Attitude of the limbs/body part:*
  - To know stage and severity of disease
  - Observe for synergy
  - Observe ipsilateral pushing
- *Alignment of trunk and extremity*:
  - Lateral flexion to convexity on affected side
  - Upper quadrant is in excessive forward flexion
  - Excessive spinal flexion throughout the spine the convexity on the weak side and spinal rotation towards the affected side
  - Lateral translation of thoracic spine from hyper mobile point of T10.
- *Presence of any inflammatory sign*
- *Presence of joint effusion/edema/swelling*
  - Indicates disease originating from lymphatic, neurological, vascular or cardiac problems
  - Proximal edema due to renal dysfunction
  - Distal edema suggest cardiac involvement
  - Focal due to loss of muscle tone.
- *Bony deformities*:
  - Indicate stage of presenting condition
  - Observe for deformity from head to toe.
- *Trophic changes*:

  Wound/scar/skin
  - *Skin*: Color and texture indicate state of circulation.
    - *Cyanosis*: Blue discoloration of skin and nail bed indicates lack of O_2 and excessive CO_2 in superficial blood vessel.
    - *Pallor*: Noted with decrease in blood flow/blood hemoglobin.
    - *Erythema*: Localize redness indicate increase blood flow and inflammation.
    - *Generalize redness*: Fever, sunburn, CO poisoning.
    - *Yellow skin*: Increase carotene intake or liver disease.
    - Brown highly pigmented hairy areas sometime overlay bony defects like spina bifida.
    - Skin tissue thickening, e.g. Callus can indicate chronic over loading and stress.
    - Thin glossy skin with decrease elasticity and hair loss indicates peripheral nerve lesion or neurovascular disorder.
    - Observe areas most vulnerable to pressure injury in prolong recumbence:

Supine	*Prone*	*Side lying*
Occiput	Ears	Ears
Spine of scapula	Anterior shoulders	Lateral shoulder
Spinous process	Iliac crests	Greater trochanter
Olecranon process	Patella	Head of fibula
Sacrum	Dorsum of feet	Medial aspect of knee
Coccyx		Lateral and medial malleolus
Back of heels		

- *External aids*:

  To know patient's functional status and extent of injury functional aids, walking aids and catheter
  - *Protective aids*: Orthotics and prosthetics
  - *Catheter*: Suggest site of injury
  - *Calipers*: Paralysis of concerned muscles
  - *Wheelchair*: Patient with severe disability.
- *Wasting of muscles*:
  - It suggests less chances of developing spasticity
  - Seen in neuromuscular disorder
  - Seen in UMN type of lesion.
- *Attitude of the patient*:
  - Alert and mobile/attentive and pleasant
  - Placid and cheerful/sulky/perplexed
  - Distressed/fearful/mask like face.
- *Gait*:
  - Observe stride length, step length, frequency, time of swing, speed of walking and duration of the complete walking cycle.
  - Circumductory gait indicates hemiplegia, festinating gait indicates parkinsonism, ataxic gait indicates incomplete spinal cord injury or cerebellar problem, scissoring gait indicates spastic cerebral palsy, cautious gait, dystonic gait, antalgic gait, waddling gait, foot drop gait, gluteus maximus gait.
- *Breathing pattern*:
  - Observe shape of chest
  - Use of accessory muscles
  - *Pattern of breathing*
    - *Normal breathing pattern*:
      1. Thoracoabdominal seen in females
      2. Abdominothoracic seen in males

- If patient is using accessory muscles of respiration commonly because of weakness of diaphragm, it may indicate problem with C_4 root level.
- Cheyne-Stokes indicates bilateral cerebral dysfunction.
- Hyperventilation indicates low midbrain or upper pons dysfunction
- Apneusis indicates middle and caudal pons dysfunction.

- *Facial expression*:
  - It can indicate about what the presenting condition is, e.g. parkinson patient has mask like face
  - Patient with lack of frowning or dropping of angle of mouth suggest Bell's palsy.
  - Frontal baldness, ptosis, jaw hanging, wasting of muscle of mastication are the typical features of the myotonic dystrophy.
- *Eye movements and pupils*:
  - Fix uncreative pupils
  - Anisocoria indicates transtentorial herniation, pharmacological, Horner's syndrome
  - Absent eye movement indicates muscle paralysis, pontine dysfunction
  - Gaze preference indicates hemispheric infract, seizures, pontine dysfunction.
- *Involuntary movements*:
  - *Tremor*: Simple, resting, intentional, postural, physiological, psychogenic
  - Shivering/rigor
  - Fasciculation
  - Myoclonus
  - Chorea
  - Hemiballismus
  - Athetosis
  - Dystonia
  - Spasms
  - Tics
  - Cramp
- *Cranial nerve observation*:
  - Ptosis (III)
  - Facial drop/Asymmetry (VII)
  - Hoarse voice (X)
  - Articulation of words (V, VII, X, XII)

- Abnormal eye position (III, IV, VI)
- Abnormal or asymmetrical pupils (II, III)
- *Shoulder observation*:
  - Drooping of shoulder/contour of shoulder
  - Abnormal prominence of acromion
  - Sulcus sign, abnormal swelling, atrophy
  - Ecchymosis, venous distension, winging of scapula

On Palpation

- *Warmth/variation in temperature*:
  - Warmth is one of the cardinal signs of inflammation. The dorsum of hand which is more sensitive to heat changes is use for comparing skin temperature above, over and below an inflamed area.
- *Texture of skin*: Dryness or excessive moisture
- *Tenderness*:
  - *Grade I:* Patient complains of pain
  - *Grade II:* Patient complains of pain and winces
  - *Grade III:* Patient winces and withdraws joint
  - *Grade IV:* Patient will not allow palpation of the joint
- Tissue tension
- *Edema*: It is an abnormal accumulation of fluid in the intracellular spaces.
  - It is pitting/non-pitting
  - *Mild:* < ¼" depth of depression
  - *Moderate:* ¼" to ½" depth of depression
  - *Severe:* ½" to 1" depression
- *Swelling*:
  - *Acute*: Soft, fluctuating thickening
  - *Chronic*: Leathery thickening
  - *Blood*: Harder, tense or thick gel like feeling with warmth and develops immediately or in 2–4 hours after injury.
  - Pus (Thick and less fluctuant with warmth and elevated temperature)
  - Synovial swelling of joints (boggy, spongy feeling and develops evident after 8–24 hours)
  - Inflammation (swelling evident after 8–42 hours)
  - Bony/hard swelling (due to osteophytes/new bone formation)
  - Soft tissue swelling
  - Skin callus.
- Bony irregularities

- Pulses
- Synovial membrane thickening
- Crepitus

ON EXAMINATION

Higher Mental Functions (For further detail, Refer Chapter 2)

- *Level of consciousness*
  - *Awake and alert*: Attentive to normal stimulation
  - *Obtunded*: Reduce alertness, slow response
  - *Lethargic*: Drowsy may fall asleep if not stimulated
  - *Stupor*: Responsive only with vigorous and repeated stimuli
    - arousable with voice, gentle stimulation, painful/vigorous stimulation
  - *Comatose*: Cannot be aroused
- *Language* (For further detail, Refer Chapter 3)
  - Fluency
  - Naming
  - Repetition
  - Reading
  - Writing
  - Comprehension
  - Aphasia versus dysarthria
- *Memory*
  - Immediate-recall a measure of attention rather than memory
  - Remote
  - 3 objects at 0/3/5 minutes
  - Historical events
  - Personal events
- *Orientation*
  - Person–not who they are but who you are
  - Place
  - Time
- *Other cognitive functions*
  - Calculation
  - Abstraction
  - Similarities/differences
  - Judgment

- Personality/behavior
- *Attention*: Divided, alternating, sustained.

- *Perception* (For further detail, Refer Chapter-2)
  - Body scheme/Body image
  - Spatial relation
  - Agnosias
  - Aprexia.
- Cranial nerve exam (For further detail, Refer Chapter 4)

  I (olfactory)
  - Do not use a noxious stimulus
  - Coffee, lemon extract

  II (optic)
  - Visual acuity
  - Visual fields
  - Fundoscopic exam

  III/IV/VI (oculomotor, trochlear, abducens)
  - Pupillary response
  - Eye movements
  - 9 cardinal positions
  - Observe lids for ptosis

  V (trigeminal)
  - Motor-jaw strength
  - Sens-all 3 divisions

  VII (facial)
  - Observe for facial asymmetry
  - Forehead wrinkling, eyelid closure, whistle/pucker

  VIII (vestibular)
  - Acuity
  - Rinne, weber

  IX/X (glossopharyngeal, vagus)
  - Gag

  XI (spinal accessory)
  - Sternocleidomastoid m
  - Trapezius muscle

  XII (hypoglossal)
  - Tongue strength
  - Right thrusts tongue to left.

- *Motor examination* (For further detail, Refer Chapter 5)
  - *Range of motion*: Active and passive
  - *Muscle tone*
  - *Voluntary control assessment*
  - *Strength*
  - Graded 0–5
  - 0-no movement
  - 1-flicker
  - 2-movement with gravity removed
  - 3-movement against gravity
  - 4-movement against resistance
  - 5-normal strength

  Strength examination:
  - Upper and lower extremities
  - Distal and proximal muscles
  - Grip strength is a poor screening tool for strength
  - Subtle weakness
  - Toe walk, heel walk
  - Out of chair
  - Deep knee bend
  - Subtle signs of weakness on a cortical/subcortical basis
  - Pronator drift
  - Orbiting

  Muscle observation:
  - Atrophy
  - Fasciculations
  - Abnormal movements
  - Muscle tightness and contracture assessment

  Upper extremity:
  - Pectoralis
  - Biceps
  - Triceps
  - Flexor digitorum profundus and superficialis
  - Extensor digitorum
  - Lumbrical

  Lower extremity:
  - Hip flexors
  - Rectus femoris

  - Hamstrings
  - Tensor fascia lata
  - Gastrocnemius

  Tremor
  - Rest
  - With arms outstretched
  - Intention
  - Chorea
  - Athetosis
- *Abnormal posture reflexes* (For further detail, Refer Chapter 7)
- *Muscle stretch reflexes* (deep tendon reflexes)
  - Graded 0–5
  - 0-absent
  - 1-present with reinforcement
  - 2-normal
  - 3-enhanced
  - 4-unsustained clonus
  - 5-sustained clonus

  Deep tendon reflexes
  - Biceps
  - Brachioradialis
  - Triceps
  - Knee
  - Ankle

  Other reflexes
  - Upper motor neuron dysfunction
  - Babinski
  - Present or absent
  - Toes downgoing/flexor plantar response
  - Hofman's
  - Jaw jerk.
- *Sensory exam* (For further detail, Refer Chapter 6)
  Superficial sensation:
  - Touch
  - Pain
  - Temperature
  - Vibration

- *Deep sensation*
  - 128 hz tuning fork
  - Joint position sense
  - Pin prick

  Higher cortical sensations
  - Graphesthesia
  - Stereognosis
  - Double simultaneous stimulation
  - Textures
- *Gait evaluation*
  - Include walking and turning
  - Examples of abnormal gait
  - High steppage
  - Waddling
  - Hemiparetic
  - Shuffling
  - Turns en bloc
- Cerebellar function (For further detail, Refer Chapter 7)
  - Rapid alternating movements
  - Finger to finger to nose testing
  - Heel to shin
  - Gait
  - Tandem
  - Romberg sign
  - Stand with feet together—assure patient stable—have them close eyes
  - Romberg is positive if they do worse with eyes closed

  Measures
  - Frequently poor balance with eyes open and closed
  - Proprioception
  - Frequently do worse with eyes closed
  - Vestibular system

  Frontal release signs
  - Grasp
  - Snout
  - Suck
  - Palmomental.

18 Case-wise Physiotherapy Assessment

CEREBRAL PALSY ASSESSMENT

Assessment of the child gives a baseline to appropriate treatment and management aims and techniques. Re-assessment should be continuing part of treatment, which allows for improvement or deterioration to be noted, thus enabling treatment to be more effective.

Subjective Examination

- Subjective information should be obtained from the parents especially mother or from relatives and through case-sheet.
- *General details includes*:
  1. Name : ______________________
  2. Age : ______________________
  3. Gender : ______________________
  4. Address : ______________________
  5. Telephone number : ______________________
  6. Informant : ______________________
  7. Religion : ______________________
  8. Mother tongue : ______________________
  9. Diagnosis : ______________________
  10. Type of cerebral palsy : ______________________
  11. Mother's name : ______________________
  12. Father's name : ______________________
  13. Age of mother : ______________________
  14. Age of father : ______________________
  15. Mother's education : ______________________
  16. Father's education : ______________________
  17. Mother's occupation : ______________________
  18. Father's occupation : ______________________
  19. Primary care giver : ______________________
  20. Family income : ______________________
  21. Family history (Family tree) : ______________________

DIAGNOSIS

History

Prenatal or antenatal history:

- *Age of mother*: Early age or late age pregnancy may be associated with complications.
- *Consanguinity marriage*: Chances of genetic disorder are very high.
- *Any drugs taken during pregnancy*: May lead to teratogenic effect and lead to CNS damage.
- *Any trauma and stress*: Head injury or other trauma to CNS may affect normal development.
- *Any addiction*: Smoking or alcoholism.
- History of rubella, toxoplasmosis infection.
- History of previous abortions, or death after birth.
- *Multiple pregnancies (duration between pregnancies)*: If may cause malnourishment and retardation of growth.
- Status and cast of the mother.
- Baby born after how many years of marriage.

Perinatal or natal history:

- Number of fetuses.
- Place of delivery
  - Home
  - Primary care center
  - Hospital
- History preterm or full term delivery
- History of asphyxia at birth
  - Type of delivery
    - Normal or vertex delivery
    - Forceps delivery
    - Breech delivery
    - Cesarean
    - Vacuum delivery
- *Delivered by*:
  - Trained dai
  - Untrained dai
  - Nurse
  - Doctor
- *Labor hours*: Prolong second stage of labor may lead to birth asphyxia

- Cord around the neck-knotted umbilical cord or cord around the neck is main cause of birth asphyxia
- Any excessive bleeding after delivery
- Condition of mother at the time of delivery
  Postnatal history:
  - Delayed birth cry
  - Weight of the child at birth
  - History of trauma to brain during the first 2 years of life
  - History of neonatal meningitis, jaundice, or hypoglycemia
  - Hydrocephalus or microcephaly
  - Nutritional habits of the child (malnutrition)
  - Feeding difficulties
  - Color of the child
- APGAR score from the case sheet
- Any medical or surgical treatment taken
- Any physiotherapy treatment previously taken
- *Chief complaints*:
  - Delayed mile stones
  - Seizures
  - Walking difficulties
- Parents observation
- *Investigations*: If any describe
  - X-rays
  - CT scan
  - MRI
  - NCV
  - EMG
  - Others—blood, CSF
- *Prognosis*:
  - Objective examinations
  - On observation
- *Behavior of the child*:
  - Whether child is alert, irritable or fearful in the session or during particular activities
  - Child becomes fatigued easily or not doing activity
- *Communication of the child*:
  - How child communicates with the parents
  - Whether child imitates or responds with sounds, hand or finger pointing, eye pointing or use words and speech

- *Attention span*:
  - For how much time child's attention is maintained on particular thing
- *Position of the child*:
  - Which position does the child prefer to be in?
  - Can child get into that position on his own or with help?
  - If involuntary movements present, then in which positions these movements are decreased or increased
- *Postural control and alignment*:
  - Supine position
  - Prone position
  - Standing position
    - How much parental support is given
    - Proper and equal weight-bearing
- *Use of limbs and hands*:
  - Limb pattern
  - Attitude of limbs during playing
  - Whether one or both hands are used, type of grasp and release
  - Any involuntary movements, tremors or spasms which interfere with action
- *Sensory aspects*: (Distal senses) observe child's all things in relevant tasks
  - Use of vision
  - Hearing
  - Of touch
  - Smell
  - Temperature
- *Form of locomotion*:
  - How child is carried
  - Any use of wheelchair or walking aids
- *Deformities*:
  - Observe any recurring position of the whole child
- Type of grasp
- Skin changes
- Gait
- Play with toys

ON EXAMINATION

- *Sensory assessment*:
  - Core senses
  - Tactile, vestibular
  - Proprioceptive senses
- *Motor assessment*:
  - Growth parameters
  - Height of the child

Height	*Centimeters or inches*
At birth	50 or 20
At 1 year	75 or 30
2–12 years	(age in years x 6) + 77 or (age in years x 2) +30

  - Weight of the child

Weight	*Kilograms*
At birth	3.25
3–12 months	(age in months + 9)/2
1–6 years	(age in years x 2) + 8
7–12 years	{(age in years x 7) + 5}/2

  - Developmental milestone assessment

Age	*Developmental milestones*	*Present*	*Absent*
4–6 weeks	Social smile		
3 months	Head holding		
6 months	Sits with support		
7 months	Sits without support		
5–6 months	Reaches out for a bright object and gets it		
6–7 months	Transfers object from one hand to other		
6–7 months	Starts imitating cough		
8–10 months	Crawls		
10–11 months	Creeps		
9 months	Standing holding furniture		

12 months	Walks holding furniture		
10–11 months	Stands without support		
13 months	Walks without much of a support		
12 months	Says one word with meaning		
13 months	Says three words with meaning		
15–18 months	Joints 2 or 3 words into sentence		
13 months	Feeds self with spoon		
15–18 months	Climbs stair		
15–18 months	Takes shoes and socks off		
24 months	Puts shoes and socks on		
24 months	Takes some clothes off		
3–4 years	Dresses self fully		
2 years	Plays with other children		
3 years	Group play		
3 years	Knows full name and sex		
3 years	Rides tricycle		

- Head circumference of the child

Head circumference	*Centimeters*	
At birth	35	
3 months	40	
1 year	45	
2 years	48	
12 years	52	

- Joint range of motion

Joint	*ROM*				*Deformity Present/ absent*	*Contracture Present/ absent*
	Active		*Passive*			
	Right	*Left*	*Right*	*Left*		
Shoulder						
Elbow						
Wrist						
MP Joint						

IP Joint						
Trunk						
Hip						
Knee						
Ankle						
Foot						

- Limb length discrepancy

Limb length discrepancy	*Right (cm)*	*Left (cm)*
Apparent (umbilicus to lateral malleolus)		
True (ASIS to medial malleolus)		

- Active movement
  - Mirror movements
  - Associated abnormal postures
  - Co-ordination
- Motor functions

Body parts	*Tone*	*Volume control spasticity*	*Shortening Present/ absent*	*Wasting Present/ absent*
Arm				
Forearm				
Hand				
Fingers				
Thigh				
Leg				
Foot				
Toes				

- Reflexes
- Superficial reflexes—normal, abnormal
  - Corneal
  - Abdominal
  - Plantar (Babinski)—check after 1 year
- Deep tendon reflexes

Jerks	*Grades*	
	Right	*Left*
Biceps (C5, C6)		
Brachioradialis (C5, C6)		
Triceps (C8, T1)		
Knee (L3, L4)		
Ankle (S1, S2)		

- Primitive reflexes

Reflexes	*Positive sign*	*Negative sign*
Moro reflex (0–3 months)		
Palmer grasp reflex (3 months)		
Plantar grasp reflex (10 months)		
Sucking reflex (3 months)		
Rooting reflex (3 months)		
Spinal level reflexes		
Flexor withdrawal reflex (0–2 months)		
Crossed extension (0–2 months)		
Extensor thrust (0–4 months)		
Brainstem level reflexes		
ATNR (0–3 months)		
STNR (0–3 months)		
TLR (0–3 months)		
Midbrain level reflexes		
Neck righting (0–6 months)		
Body righting (6 months–4 years)		
Labyrinthine righting (3 months–1 year)		
Optical righting (3 months–1 year)		
Cortical level		
Cortical (all position)		

- *Clonus*
  - Ankle clonus
  - patellar clonus
  - wrist clonus

- *Associated symptoms*: Yes or no
  - Hearing
  - Vision
  - Speech
  - Drooling of saliva
  - Mental retardation
  - Skeletal system
- *Seizures*:
  - Partial
  - Generalized
  - Absence
- Early hand preference
- *Higher functions*: Good, fair, poor
  - Interaction with examiner
  - Interest in surroundings
  - Over all activities
  - Exact IQ
- *Speech*:
  - Appropriate for age
  - Delayed
- *Hearing*:
  - Normal
  - Abnormal
- *Vision*:
  - Fixation
  - Squint
  - Abnormalities in fundi
  - Involuntary eye movements
- *Cranial nerve abnormalities:* If present, describe.
- *Involuntary movements*:
  - Chorea
  - Athetosis
  - Dystonia
  - Choreoathetosis
  - Mixed
- *Gait*: Possible or not possible
  - Tendom walk
  - Toe walk
  - Heel walk

- *Rise from squatting*
  - Independent
  - With assistance
  - Absent
- *Gait pattern*
  - Non-ambulant
  - *Spastic*: Scissoring gait
  - Gait typifying spastic cerebral palsy (i.e. hip flexed and internally rotated; knee flexed; ankle plantarflexed); the patient takes small steps, walking stiffly on tiptoe with bent knees and no heel contact
  - Ataxic
  - Dystonic
  - Mixed
  - Normal
- *Modified gait abnormal rating scale (GARS)*:
  - *Variability*: Stepping with arm movement
  - *Guardedness*: Difficulty in initiating
  - *Staggering*: Imbalance, especially while turning
  - *Foot contact*: Heel strike, flat foot, on toes
  - Hip ROM-at least 15^{0} flex
  - *Shoulder extension*: 10–15° from neutral
  - Arm heel strike synchrony

  Total score = 21
- *Functional ability and limitation in motor function in child*:
  - Walk without restrictions
  - Walks without assistive devices
  - Walk with assistive devices
  - Transported carried around (use any external aid)
  - Severely limited dependent on wheel chair
- Transfer activities
- *Balance*: Good, poor
  - Sitting balance
  - Standing balance
- *Assessment of daily activities*: Good, fair, poor
  - Feeding
  - Dressing
  - Washing
  - Toileting
  - Playing
  - Hand function

- *Cerebellar system*: Yes or no or cannot be tested
- Finger nose incoordination
- Heel knee incoordination
- *Bowel*
  - Regular
  - Intermittent incontinence
  - Continuous incontinence
  - Constipation
- *Bladder*
  - Intermittent dribbling
  - Continuous dribbling

TREATMENT PLAN/MANAGEMENT

- *Medical treatment*
  - Medication
- *Surgical treatment*
  - Surgery
- *Physiotherapy treatment*
  - Problem list
  - Aims
  - Goals
    - Short-term goals
    - Long-term goals
    - Follow-up
    - *Any new problems*: Describe

ATAXIA ASSESSMENT FORMAT

Date of Examination

- Name : ____________________
- Age : ____________________
- Sex : ____________________
- Occupation : ____________________
- Address : ____________________
- General condition : ____________________
- Socio-economic condition : ____________________
- Diagnosis : ____________________
- Chief complaint : ____________________

- History : ________________
- Past history : ________________
- Personal history : ________________
- Family history : ________________
- Doctor's notes : ________________

On Observation

- *Posture*:
  - Lying : ________________
  - Sitting : ________________
  - Standing : ________________
- Postural deviation : ________________
- Postural deformity : ________________
- Gait : ________________
- External aids : ________________
- Swelling : ________________
- Wasting : ________________
- Scar : ________________
- *Trophic changes:*
  - Skin : ________________
  - Nails : ________________
- Breathing pattern : ________________
- Patient's attitude : ________________
- Nystagmus : ________________
- Tremors : ________________

On Palpation

- Temperature : ________________
- Tenderness : ________________
- Swelling : ________________
- Spasm : ________________
- Scar : ________________

On Examination

- *Pain*:
  - Site
  - Type

- Aggravating factor
- Relieving factor

- *Motor assessment*:
  - Range of motion (ROM)-check passive
  - Tone (According to clinical rating)
  - Manual muscle testing (MMT)
  - Soft tissue tightness
    - Hamstrings
    - Tendo-Achilles
    - Rectus femoris
    - Illiopsoas
    - Thoracolumbar fascia
    - Tensor facia lata
    - Sartorius
    - Latissimus dorsi
    - Biceps
    - Triceps
    - Pectoralis major
    - Scalene
- *Other motor assessment*
- *Tremors*:

– Intention tremor – Kinetic tremor – Postural tremor – Titubation	If associated with involvement of postural truncal tremor extra-pyramidal system

- *Dysmetria*:
  - Hypermetria (overshoot)
  - Hypometria (undershoot)
- *Riddoch's test (limb ataxia)*:
  - Outstretched arm tends to be hyper-pronated at rest and at slightly higher level than the unaffected side and rebounds when examiner applied resistance on arm and sudden relieve the pressure.
- *Dyssynergia and visuomotor incoordination*: Task will be broken down into its component of parts.
- *Dysdiadochokinesia*: Inability to perform rapid alternating movements.
- *Gait examination*: The ataxia of cerebellar disease tends to produce a broad-based, lurching, reeling or drunken kind of gait. The ataxia often involves the trunk with titubation. The symptoms of imbalance

are usually manifest while trying to stand with the feet together even with the eyes open.

- Walk with wide base of support
- Incoordination between trunk and limb
- Difficulty in turning
- Increases arm swing
- Unequal steps
- Speed-slow
- High-risk of fall

- *Sensory assessment*
  - Superficial
    - Pain
    - Touch
    - Temperature
    - Pressure
  - Deep
    - Joint position
    - Joint movement
    - Vibration
  - Combined cortical
    - Tactile localization
    - Two point discrimination
    - Stereognosis
    - Barognosis
    - Graphesthesia
    - Recognition of texture

One of the most common causes of ataxia is loss of proprioception in the feet.

- *Reflex assessment*:
  - *Superficial reflexes*:
    - Corneal
    - Babinski sign
    - Abdominal
  - *Deep tendon reflexes*:
    - Biceps
    - Triceps
    - Brachioradialis
    - Patellar
    - Ankle

  - *Pathological reflexes*:
    - TLR
    - ATNR
    - STNR
- *Co-ordination tests*: It may be affected
  - Both equilibrium and nonequilibrium tests should be checked.
- ADL or transfer activity
- *Balance*:
  - *Romberg's sign*: Examining the patient's posture when standing with the feet together is important. If they are steady with the eyes open but not with the eyes closed (Romberg sign), loss of proprioception in the feet should be suspected.
- *Grips*:
  - Power
    - Spherical
    - Cylindrical
    - Lumbrical
    - Hook
  - Precision
    - Pulp
    - Pinch
    - Lateral prehension.
- *Physiotherapy treatment*:
  - Problem list
  - Aims
  - Goals
  - Short-term
  - Long-term
  - Follow-up
  - Any new problem list

PARKINSON'S DISEASE ASSESSMENT FORMAT

Date of examination

- Name : ______________________
- Age : ______________________
- Sex : ______________________
- Occupation : ______________________
- Address : ______________________

- Primary language : ____________________
- Hand dominance : ____________________
- General condition : ____________________
- Socio-economic condition : ____________________
- VDR number : ____________________
- IPD number : ____________________
- Diagnosis : ____________________
- Chief complaint : ____________________
- History : ____________________
- Past history : ____________________
- Personal history : ____________________
- Family history : ____________________
- Doctor's notes : ____________________

On Observation

- Posture
- *Lying*: Phantom pillow appearance may present
  - *Sitting*: Pocking chin appearance
  - *Standing*: Pictorial gradation
- *Postural deviation*
- *Postural deformity*: Kyphosis or scoliosis may present
- *Gait*: Festinating gait
- *External aids*: May use walker
- Swelling
- Wasting
- Scar
- *Trophic changes*:
  - Skin
  - Nails
- *Breathing pattern*: Mostly abdominal breathing due to stoop posture and kyphosis
- *Facial grimace*: Mask like face
  - Sometimes drooling of saliva may present
- *Tremors*: May be resting or postural
- *Site*: Present in upper limb and lower limb
- Pill rolling movements of fingers may be present
- Patient's attitude

On Palpation

- Temperature
- Tenderness
- Swelling
- Spasm
- Scar

On Examination

- *Higher mental function examination*:
  - Level of consciousness:
    - Awake and alert
    - Agitated
    - Lethargic—arousal with voice
    - Gentle stimulation
    - Painful/vigorous stimulation comatose
  - Language:
    - Fluency
    - Naming
    - Repetition
    - Reading
    - *Writing*: Micrographia will be present characterized by abnormal small handwritings.
    - *Comprehension*: Aphasia/dysarthria
    - Scanning speech may be present
  - Orientation:
    - Person
    - Place
    - Time

    } Not affected
  - Other cognitive functions
    - Calculation
    - Abstraction
    - Similarities/differences
    - Judgment
    - *Personality/behavior*: Depression is common
    - *Attention*: Divided and selective attention may be affected.

- Memory:
  - Immediate
  - Short-term
  - Long-term

  } If associated with Alzheimer's it may be affected
- *Pain*:
  - Location
  - Intensity
- *Sensory assessment*:
  - Superficial
    - Pain
    - Touch
    - Temperature
    - Pressure
  - Deep
    - Joint position
    - Joint movement
    - Vibration
  - Combined cortical
    - Tactile localization
    - Two point discrimination
    - Stereognosis
    - Barognosis
    - Graphesthesia
    - Recognition of texture
- *Musculoskeletal assessment*: ROM, MMT, TONE, voluntry movements
- *Reflex assessment*:
  - Superficial reflexes
    - Corneal
    - Babinski sign
    - Abdominal
  - Deep tendon reflexes
    - Biceps
    - Triceps
    - Brachioradialis
    - Patellar
    - Ankle

    } Brisk or exaggerated
  - Pathological reflexes
    - TLR
    - ATNR
    - STNR

- Tightness/flexibility (Commonly present)
  - Hamstrings
  - Tendo-Achilles
  - Rectus femoris
  - Illiopsoas
  - Thoracolumbar fascia
  - Tensor facia lata
  - Sartorius
  - Latissimus dorsi
  - Biceps
  - Triceps
  - Pectoralis major
  - Scalene
- *Motor function assessments*:
  - *Rigidity*: Lead pipe (sustained)/cog wheel (intermittent)
  - *Bradykinesia*:
    - *Movement time*: A stop watch is used to quantify detectable slowing of movement.
    - *Reaction time*: Elapsed time between the patients desire to move and the actual movement response.
    - *Finger dexterity*: Assessed by allowing a maximum of 3 minutes to button up three shirt buttons. The number of buttons and time taken should be noted.
  - *Tremor*:
    - Location
    - Persistence
    - *Severity (amplitude)*: 4–6 Hz.
    - *Pattern*: Pin rolling tremor of hand, or forearm supination-pronation.
    - *Rest tremor/activity tremor*: Typically at rest
    - *Aggravating factor*: Emotional stress or fatigue
    - *Relieving factor*: Relaxed, unoccupied, voluntary effort and sleep.
  - *Postural instability (balance)*:
    - *Retropulsion test*: Sudden sternal push or shoulder pull, observe patient's stability
    - Functional reach test
    - Timed up and go test
    - Berg balance scale

- *Gait*:
  - Assistive aid
  - *Speed of walking*: Number of steps and time taken to cover the distance.
  - Stride length
  - Cadence
  - *Heel strike*: 1. Heel-toe, 2. Flat-footed, 3. Toe-heel.
  - *Dual task walking*: (walkie-talkie test, walking while carrying objects on a tray)
  - *Freezing episodes*:
    - Frequency
    - Duration
    - Triggering stimuli (auditory or visual cues that release the patient and allow initiation of movement).
- *Fall frequency*: Fall risk diary.

Heel to Toe Characteristics

In Parkinsonian gait, motion is characterized by flat foot strike patients with Parkinson's disease (PD) have reduced impact at heel strike and this mechanism has been found to be related to the disease severity with impact decreasing as the disease progresses.

In addition, PD patients have reduced foot lifting during the swing phase of gait, which produces smaller clearance between the toes and the ground.

Also, Parkinson patients show a trend towards higher relative loads in the forefoot regions combined with a load shift towards medial foot areas.

This load shift is believed to help in compensating for postural imbalance. The intra-individual variability in foot strike pattern is found to be surprisingly lower in PD patients compared with normal people.

Vertical Ground Reaction Force

The shape of the vertical GRF signal is abnormal in PD. In the earlier stages of the disease, reduced forces (or peak heights) are found for heel contact and the push-off phase resembling that of elderly subjects. In the more advanced stages of the disorder where gait is characterized by small shuffling steps, PD patients show only one narrow peak in the vertical GRF signal.

Falls and Freezing of Gait

Falls and freezing of gait are two episodic phenomena that are common in Parkinsonian gait. Falls and freezing of gait in PD are generally thought to be closely intertwined for several reasons, most importantly: both symptoms are common in the advanced stages of the disease and are less common in the earlier stages, with freezing of gait leading to falls in many instances. Both symptoms often respond poorly and sometimes *paradoxically* to treatment with dopaminergic medication, perhaps pointing to a common underlying *pathophysiology*.

Freezing of gait: Freezing of gait (FOG) is typically a transient episode-lasting less than a minute, in which gait is halted and the patient complains that his/her feet are glued to the ground. When the patient overcomes the block, walking can be performed relatively smoothly. The most common form of FOG is 'start hesitation' (which happens when the patient wants to start walking) followed in frequency by 'turning hesitation FOG can also be experienced in narrow or tight quarters such as a doorway, whilst adjusting one's steps when reaching a destination, and in stressful situations such as when the telephone or the doorbell rings or when the elevator door opens. As the disease progresses, FOG can appear spontaneously even in an open runway space.

Falls: Falls, like FOG are rare in the earlier stages of the disorder and becomes more frequent as the disease progresses. Falls result mainly due to sudden changes in posture, in particular turning movements of the trunk, or attempts to perform more than one activity simultaneously with walking or balancing. Falls are also common during transfers, such as rising from a chair or bed. PD patients fall mostly forward (45% of all falls) and about 20% fall laterally.

Postural Sway

Postural instability in upright stance is common in end-stage PD and compromises the ability to maintain balance during everyday tasks such as walking, turning and standing up from sitting. An inability to adequately balance the body's center of mass over the base of support combined with inflexibility in body movements (due to increased rigidity) causes patients with advanced PD to fall. Whereas postural sway in normal stance usually increases in patients with balance disorders arising from stroke, head injury and cerebellar ataxia it is often reduced in patients with PD. The reason for this because in PD the problem appears to be a lack of flexibility in shifting postural responses. This inflexibility increases the tendency to fall in these patients.

- *Autonomic function*:
  - *Salivation*: Excessive drooling
  - *Sweating*: Excess sweating during "on" state is linked to presence of dyskinesia.
  - *Dizziness*
  - *Orthostatic hypotension*: In advances PD, blood pressure is significantly lower in "on" state than "off" state leading to frequent dizziness and orthostatic hypotension.
- *Cardiopulmonary function*:
  - *Chest expansion*: Affected
  - *Respiratory rate*: May be increase
  - Heart rate
- *Integumentary integrity*:
  - *Pressure areas*: Bruising and skin breakdown
- *Functional status*:
  - Functional independence measure (FIM)
- *Physiotherapy treatment:*
  - Problem list
  - Aims
  - Goals
  - Short-term
  - Long-term
  - Follow-up

SPINAL CORD INJURY ASSESSMENT FORMAT

Date of examination:

- Name : ______________________
- Age : ______________________
- Sex : ______________________
- Occupation : ______________________
- Address : ______________________
- General condition : ______________________
- Socio-economic condition : ______________________
- Diagnosis : ______________________
- Chief complain : ______________________
- History : ______________________

- Past history : ______________________
- Personal history : ______________________
- Family history : ______________________
- Doctor's notes : ______________________

On Observation

- *Posture*
  - *Lying*: Boot foot platoflex, hip externally rotated
  - Sitting
  - Standing
- Postural deviation
- Postural deformity
- *Gait*: In paraplegics with orthoses
- *External aids*: Catheter, orthoses
- Swelling
- Wasting
- *Scar*: Present if spinal stabilization has been done.
- *Trophic changes*:
  - *Skin*: Glossy skin, thickening of skin of sole
  - *Nails*: Become brittle
- Breathing pattern
- Patient's attitude

On Palpation

- *Temperature*: Normal or increase
  - Compare the temperature above and below the level of lesion
- Tenderness
- Swelling
- Spasm
- *Scar*: Mobile/adherent
  - Heal/unhealed.

On Examination

Sensory assessment (dermatome chart):

- *Superficial*
  - Pain
  - Touch

- Temperature
- Pressure
- *Deep*
  - Joint position
  - Joint movement
  - Vibration.

Assessment of sensory function helps to identify the different pathways for light touch, proprioception, vibration, and pain. Use a pinprick to evaluate pain sensation.

Sensory level is the most caudal dermatome with a normal score of 2/2 for pinprick and light touch.

Sensory index scoring is the total score from adding each dermatomal score with a possible total score of 112 each for pinprick and light touch.

Sensory testing is performed at the following levels:

- C2: Occipital protuberance
- C3: Supraclavicular fossa
- C4: Top of the acromioclavicular joint
- C5: Lateral side of antecubital fossa
- C6: Thumb
- C7: Middle finger
- C8: Little finger
- T1: Medial side of antecubital fossa
- T2: Apex of axilla
- T3: Third intercostal space
- T4: Fourth intercostal space at nipple line
- T5: Fifth intercostal space (midway between T4 and T6)
- T6: Sixth intercostal space at the level of the xiphisternum
- T7: Seventh intercostal space (midway between T6 and T8)
- T8: Eighth intercostal space (midway between T6 and T10)
- T9: Ninth intercostal space (midway between T8 and T10)
- T10: 10th intercostal space or umbilicus
- T11: 11th intercostal space (midway between T10 and T12)
- T12: Midpoint of inguinal ligament
- L1: Half the distance between T12 and L2
- L2: Midanterior thigh
- L3: Medial femoral condyle
- L4: Medial malleolus
- L5: Dorsum of the foot at third metatarsophalangeal joint
- S1: Lateral heel

- S2: Popliteal fossa in the midline
- S3: Ischial tuberosity
- S4-5: Perianal area (taken as 1 level)
- Sensory scoring is for light touch and pinprick, as follows:
- 0: Absent; a score of zero is given if the patient cannot differentiate between the point of a sharp pin and the dull edge
- 1: Impaired or hyperesthesia
- 2: Intact.

Pain:
- Site
- Type
- Aggravating factor
- Relieving factor

Motor assessment:
- ROM
- MMT (Individual muscle MMT chart)
- TONE

Motor level is determined by the most caudal key muscles that have muscle strength of 3 or above while the segment above is normal (= 5).

Motor index scoring uses the 0–5 scoring of each key muscle, with total points being 25 per extremity and with the total possible score being 100.

Lower extremities motor score (LEMS) uses the ASIA key muscles in both lower extremities, with a total possible score of 50 (i.e., maximum score of 5 for each key muscle [L2, L3, L4, L5, and S1] per extremity). A LEMS of 20 or less indicates that the patient is likely to be a limited ambulator. A LEMS of 30 or more suggests that the individual is likely to be a community ambulator.

ASIA recommends use of the following scale of findings for the assessment of motor strength in spinal cord injury:
- 0: No contraction or movement
- 1: Minimal movement
- 2: Active movement, but not against gravity
- 3: Active movement against gravity
- 4: Active movement against resistance
- 5: Active movement against full resistance.

Reflex assessment:
- *Superficial reflexes*
  - Corneal
  - Babinski sign
  - Abdominal
- *Deep tendon reflexes*
  - Biceps
  - Triceps
  - Brachioradialis
  - Patellar
  - Ankle

Tightness
- Hamstrings
- Tendo-Achilles
- Rectus femoris
- Illiopsoas
- Thoracolumbar fascia
- Tensor facia lata
- Sartorius
- Latissimus dorsi
- Biceps
- Triceps
- Pectoralis major
- Scalene.

Respiratory examination:
- Function of respiratory muscles
- Chest expansion
- Cough
- Vital capacity

Carefully evaluate respiratory rate, chest wall expansion, abdominal wall movement, cough, and chest wall and/or pulmonary injuries. Arterial blood gas (ABG) analysis and pulse oximetry are especially useful, because the bedside diagnosis of hypoxia or carbon dioxide retention may be difficult.

The degree of respiratory dysfunction is ultimately dependent on pre-existing pulmonary comorbidity, the level of the spinal cord injury, and any associated chest wall or lung injury. Any or all of the following determinants of pulmonary function may be impaired in the setting of spinal cord injury:

- Loss of ventilatory muscle function from denervation and/or associated chest wall injury
- Lung injury, such as pneumothorax, hemothorax, or pulmonary contusion
- Decreased central ventilatory drive that is associated with head injury or exogenous effects of alcohol and drugs.

A direct relationship exists between the level of cord injury and the degree of respiratory dysfunction, as follows:

- With high lesions (i.e., C1 or C2), vital capacity is only 5–10% of normal, and cough is absent
- With lesions at C3 through C6, vital capacity is 20% of normal, and cough is weak and ineffective
- With high thoracic cord injuries (i.e., T2 through T4), vital capacity is 30–50% of normal, and cough is weak
- With lower cord injuries, respiratory function improves
- With injuries at T11, respiratory dysfunction is minimal; vital capacity is essentially normal, and cough is strong.

Other findings of respiratory dysfunction include the following:

- Agitation, anxiety, or restlessness
- Poor chest wall expansion
- Decreased air entry
- Rales, rhonchi
- Pallor, cyanosis
- Increased heart rate
- Paradoxical movement of the chest wall
- Increased accessory muscle use
- Moist cough.

Site of pressure sores

Bowel-bladder: Dysfunction as falling into 1 of 2 categories:
(1) failure to store and (2) failure to empty. These 2 categories are further subdivided based on whether the failure is due to a problem with the detrusor or due to the bladder outlet. Examples of failure to store would be detrusor hyperreflexia (or uninhibited bladder contractions) or an areflexic bladder outlet. In contrast, failure to empty may be due to an areflexic bladder or a sphincter that is unable to relax. Detrusor-sphincter dyssynergia—impaired coordination between bladder contraction and sphincter relaxation—is also a common finding in patients with SCIs. Any of these problems may occur at different stages

of the acute and chronic period of SCI. Therefore, during the course of a patient's life, bladder management may have to change depending on the bladder dysfunction.

Neurologic Level and Extent of Injury

Neurologic level of injury is the most caudal level at which motor and sensory levels are intact, with motor level as defined above and sensory level defined by a sensory score of 2.

Zone of partial preservation is all segments below the neurologic level of injury with preservation of motor or sensory findings. This index is used only when the injury is complete.

The key muscles that need to be tested to establish neurologic level are as follows:
- C5: Elbow flexors (biceps, brachialis)
- C6: Wrist extensors (extensor carpi radialis longus and brevis)
- C7: Elbow extensors (triceps)
- C8: Long finger flexors (flexor digitorum profundus)
- T1: Small finger abductors (abductor digiti minimi)
- L2: Hip flexors (iliopsoas)
- L3: Knee extensors (quadriceps)
- L4: Ankle dorsiflexors (tibialis anterior)
- L5: Long toe extensors (extensor hallucis longus)
- S1: Ankle plantar flexors (gastrocnemius, soleus).

Perform a rectal examination to check motor function or sensation at the anal mucocutaneous junction. The presence of either is considered sacral-sparing.

The sacral roots may be evaluated by documenting the following:
- Perineal sensation to light touch and pinprick
- Bulbocavernosus reflex, S3 or S4
- Anal wink, S5
- Rectal tone
- Urine retention or incontinence
- Priapism.

Functional status:
Barthel index.
Physiotherapy treatment:
- Problem list
- Aims

- Goals
- Short-term
- Long-term
- Follow-up

STROKE ASSESSMENT FORMAT

Date of examination:

- Name : ______________________
- Age : ______________________
- Sex : ______________________
- Occupation : ______________________
- Address : ______________________
- General condition : ______________________
- Socio-economic condition : ______________________
- Diagnosis : ______________________
- Chief complaint : ______________________
- History : ______________________
- Past history : ______________________
- Personal history : ______________________
- Family history : ______________________
- Doctor's notes : ______________________

On Observation

- *Posture*:
  - Lying
  - Sitting
  - Standing
- Postural deviation
- Postural deformity
- Gait
- External aids
- Swelling
- Wasting
- Scar
- *Trophic changes*:
  - Skin
  - Nails
- Breathing pattern
- Facial grimace

- Abnormal movements
- Patient's attitude

On Palpation

- Temperature
- Tenderness
- Swelling
- Spasm
- Scar

On Examination

Higher mental function examination:

- *Level of consciousness*:
  - Awake and alert
  - Agitated
  - Lethargic-arousable with voice
    - Gentle stimulation
    - Painful/vigorous stimulation comatose
- *Language*:
  - Fluency
  - Naming
  - Repetition
  - Reading
  - Writing
  - *Comprehension*: Aphasia/dysarthria
- *Orientation*:
  - Person
  - Place
  - Time
- *Other cognitive functions*:
  - Calculation
  - Abstraction
  - Similarities/differences
  - Judgment
  - Personality/behavior
- *Memory*:
  - Immediate
  - Short-term
  - Long-term

Cranial nerve assessment:
- I—olfactory
- II—optic:
  - Visual acuity
  - Visual fields
  - Fundoscopic exam
- *III/IV/VI—oculomotor, trochlear, abducens*:
  - Pupillary response
  - Eye movements
    - 9 cardinal positions
  - Observe lids for ptosis
- *V—trigeminal*:
  - Motor—jaw strength
  - Sensation all 3 divisions
- *VII—facial*:
  - Observe for facial asymmetry
  - Forehead wrinkling, eyelid closure, whistle/pucker
- *VIII—vestibular*:
  - Acuity
  - Rinne, weber
- *IX/X—glossopharyngeal, vagus*:
  - Gag
- *XI—spinal accessory*:
  - Sternocleidomastoid muscle
  - Trapezius muscle
- *XII—hypoglossal*:
  - Tongue strength
  - Right XII thrusts tongue to left

Perception assessment:
- *Body scheme and body image impairments*:
  - Unilateral neglect
  - Right left discrimination
  - Anosognosia
  - Somotognosia
  - Finger agnosia
- *Spatial relation disorders*:
  - Form discrimination
  - Figure ground discrimination

  - Depth and distance
  - Spatial relations
  - Position in space
  - Topographic disorientation
  - Vertical disorientation
- *Agnosia*:
  - Visual agnosia
  - Auditory agnosia
  - Tactile agnosia
- *Apraxia*:
  - Ideomotor apraxia
  - Ideational apraxia
  - Buccofacial apraxia

Sensory assessment
- *Superficial*
  - Pain
  - Touch
  - Temperature
  - Pressure
- *Deep*
  - Joint position
  - Joint movement
  - Vibration
- *Combined cortical*
  - Tactile localization
  - Two point discrimination
  - Stereognosis
  - Barognosis
  - Graphesthesia
  - Recognition of texture

Pain:
- Site
- Type
- Aggravating factor
- Relieving factor
- Pain over shoulder joint is most common.

Abnormal pattern:

	Flexion synergy	*Extensor synergy*
Upper extremity	• Scapular retraction and elevation • Shoulder abduction, external rotation • Elbow flexion • Forearm supination • Wrist/finger flexion	• Scapular protraction • Shoulder adduction • Internal rotation • Elbow extension • Forearm pronation • Wrist/finger flexion
Lower extremity	• Hip flexion, abduction, • External rotation • Knee flexion • Ankle dorsiflexion, inversion • Toe dorsiflexion	• Hip extension, adduction • Internal rotation • Knee extension • Ankle plantar flexion, inversion • Toe planter flexion

Motor assessment:

Reflex assessment:

- *Superficial reflexes*
  - Corneal
  - Babinski sign
  - Abdominal

  } Decrease or absent
- *Deep tendon reflexes*
  - Biceps
  - Triceps
  - Brachioradialis
  - Patellar
  - Ankle

  } Exaggerated
- *Pathological reflexes*:
  - TLR
  - ATNR
  - STNR

  } Any of these may dominant

Associated reaction:

- Souque's phenomenon
- Raimiste's phenomenon

} May be present

Tightness:

- Hamstrings
- Tendo-Achilles
- Rectus femoris
- Illiopsoas

- Thoracolumbar fascia
- Tensor facia lata
- Sartorius
- Latissimus dorsi
- Biceps
- Triceps
- Pectoralis major
- Scalene

Gait:
- Unilateral weakness on affected side
- Decrease step length, stance phase
- Arm held in pattern
- Spastic gluteal and quadriceps muscle
- Decrease hip and knee flexion
- Plantar flexion of foot
- Normal arm swing is absent

Co-ordination tests—equilibrium and non-equilibrium test

Balance:
- Static
- Dynamic

Bladder:
- Initial retention, bladder neck is closed
- Detrusor hyperreflexia and incontinence
- Continence reappears by 6 months in 80%
- Irritative lower urinary tract symptoms (LUTS)
- *Dysuria and obstructive LUTS*: DHIC, BPO, poor relaxation of external sphincter (frontoparietal and internal capsule lesion)
- *Subcortical lesion*: Areflexia, retention.

Activities of daily living (ADLs) or transfer activity

Grips:
- *Power*
  - Spherical
  - Cylindrical
  - Lumbrical
  - Hook

- Precision
  - Pulp
  - Pinch
  - Lateral prehension.
- *Physiotherapy treatment:*
  - Problem list
  - Aims
  - Goals
  - Short-term
  - Long-term
  - Follow-up

BELL'S PALSY

Date of examination:

- Name : ____________________
- Age : ____________________
- Sex : ____________________
- Occupation : ____________________
- Address : ____________________
- General condition : ____________________
- Socio-economic condition : ____________________
- Diagnosis : ____________________
- Chief complaint : ____________________
- *History*: Exposure to cold
  - Inflammation/edema
  - Herpes zoster virus
  - Facial trauma
  - Ramsay Hunt syndrome
- Past history : ____________________
- Personal history : ____________________
- Family history : ____________________
- Doctor's notes : ____________________

On Observation

- *Asymmetry of face*: Present
- *Drooping of angle of mouth*: Towards affected side
- *Deviation of angle of mouth*: Towards sound side
- *Bell's phenomenon*: Positive

- *Obliteration of nasolabial fold*: Present
- *Crocodyle'stear*: May be present.

On Palpation

- *Temperature*: Maybe increase over face region
- *Tenderness*: May be present where the facial trunk immerges
- *Spasm*: May be present over face
- *Swelling*: May or may not be present.

On Examination

- Pain
- Site
- Type
- Aggravating factor
- Relieving factor
- Facial muscle testing
- Jaw jerk
- Bell's phenomena
- Tinnitus
- Crocodile's tear
- Hyperacusis

Differential diagnosis of facial nerve lesion

Nuclear: No localize associated findings, dysfunction frequently bilateral

Intrapontine fibers:
- *Physiotherapy treatment:*
  - Problem list
  - Aims
  - Goals
  - Short-term
  - Long-term
  - Follow-up

POLIOMYELITIS

Assessment

- Name : ____________________
- Age : ____________________

- *Sex*: : Victim is a male child
- Occupation : ____________________
- Address : ____________________
- General condition : ____________________
- Socio-economic condition : ____________________
- Diagnosis : ____________________

Chief complaint: Mother tells that child developed mild pyrexia associated with diarrhea followed by inability to move a part or the whole limb.

History

Accute flaccid paralysis (AFP) refers to acute onset (<4 weeks) flaccid or floppy or limp paralysis of the affected limb.

A case of AFP is defined as any child aged <15 years who has acute onset of flaccid paralysis for which no obvious cause (such as severe trauma or electrolyte imbalance) is found. Or paralytic illness in a person at any age in which polio is suspected.

The lower limbs are affected most commonly. Paralysis is of varying severity and asymmetrical in distribution. In extreme cases the respiratory muscles may also be paralyzed.

Progression of paralysis: 24–28 hours onset to full paralysis.

Fever onset: High grade, always present at onset of flaccid paralysis, gone the following day.

On Examinaton

- Glasgow coma scale (GCS) to check the level of consciousness. Usually the patient is conscious, cooperative and follows verbal command.
- *Muscle tone*: Diminished
- *Flaccidity*: Acute, asymmetrical and proximal
- *Deep tendon reflexes*: Decreased or absent
- *Muscle power/MMT*: Lower limbs affected commonly
- Strength of hip/knee and ankle-bilaterally
- Quadriceps—mostly partially paralyzed
- Tibialis anterior—complete paralysis.

In Late Stage

- Paralysis may result in wasting, weakness and deformities of limb
- Deformity—because of imbalance between opposite group of muscle, action of gravity on paralyzed limb and prolonged flexed positions.
- With the time deformity becomes permanent due to contracture of soft tissues and abnormal joint position.

Common Deformities

1. *Hip*: Flexion, abduction and external rotation
2. *Knee*: Flexion/hyperextension, rotation of tibia
3. *Patella*: Small and mobility affected
4. *Foot*: Equinovarus is common, equinovalgus, calcaneovarus or valgus
5. *Triple deformity*: Flexion, posterior subluxation and external rotation
6. *Spine*: Scoliosis, pelvic tilt
7. *UL*: Shoulder and elbow may get affected
8. *LLD*: True or apparent shortening of affected side may seen

Girth Examination

For muscle wasting

Tightness/Contracture

May develop

Sensation

Severe myalgia and backache no sensory changes

Cranial Nerves

Only when balbar and bulbospinal

Respiratory Insufficiency

Only when balbar and bulbospinal

Bladder Dysfunction

Absent.

INVESTIGATIONS

- *CSF*: High WBCs
- *Protein*: Normal or slightly increased
- Nerve conduction velocity.

Third week: Abnormal anterior horn cell disease (normal during first two weeks)

- *EMG*
- *3 weeks*: Abnormal
- *Sequelae at 3 months and up to a year*: Severe, asymmetrical atrophy, skeletal deformities developing later.
- *Physiotherapy treatment:*
  - Problem list
  - Aims
  - Goals
  - Short-term
  - Long-term
  - Follow-up

DUCHENNE MUSCULAR DYSTROPHY

Assessment

- Name : ______________________
- Age : ______________________
- *Sex*: : Victim is a male child
- Occupation : ______________________
- Address : ______________________
- General condition : ______________________
- Socio-economic condition : ______________________
- Diagnosis : ______________________
- *Chief complaint*: Mother tells that child is walking on toes or difficulty in getting up from sitting or history of frequent fall associated with fatigue symptoms.

History

Duchenne muscular dystrophy (DMD) refers to gradual onset of muscle weakness starts with bilateral lower limbs.

Muscle weakness is progressive in nature and involves proximal muscle more than distal.

Parents presented with the complains that child is walking on toes, mainly difficulty in getting up from sitting, history of frequent fall while walking.

History of fatigue that is progressive in nature.

The lower limbs are affected first then gradually involve upper limbs, neck and trunk. Paralysis is of varying severity and symmetrical in distribution. In later stages the respiratory muscles are involved.

On Examinaton

- Glasgow coma scale (GCS) usually patient is conscious, cooperative and follows verbal command
- *Posture*: Shoulder girdle retracted, sway back, protruded abdomen—increased lumbar lardosis, weak abdominals and hip extensors, tight hip flexors and back extensors
- Pseudohypertrophy of calf and tongue
- *Muscle tone*: Not affected
- *Deep tendon reflexes*: Intact or may be diminished in later stages
- *Muscle power/MMT*: Lower limbs affected first then upper limb (UL), neck and trunk
- Strength of hip, knee and ankle—bilaterally (proximal > distal)
- Abdominals and trunk muscle—affected
- Strength of shoulder, elbow and wrist
  - Muscle wasting begins in the legs and pelvis
    - Progresses to the muscles of the shoulders and neck
    - Then arm muscles and respiratory muscles.
  - Awkward manner of walking, stepping, or running. Toe walking
  - A positive *Gowers' sign* reflects the more severe impairment of the lower extremities muscles.

Deformity: Because of imbalance between opposite group of muscle, action of gravity on paralyzed limb and prolonged flexed positions.

With the time deformity becomes permanent due to contracture of soft tissues and abnormal joint position.

Common Deformities

- *Hip*: Flexion
- *Knee*: Flexion/hyperextension
- *Spine*: Hyperlordosis/scoliosis
- *Girth examination*: For muscle wasting

- *Tightness/contracture*: May develop
- *Respiratory insufficiency*: Respiratory muscle paralyzed in later stages.

INVESTIGATIONS

- Creatinine phosphokinase
- Electromyography
- Muscle biopsy.
- *Physiotherapy treatment:*
  - Problem list
  - Aims
  - Goals
  - Short-term
  - Long-term
  - Follow-up

Peripheral Nerve Injury

Date of examination:

- Name : ____________________
- Age : ____________________
- Sex : ____________________
- Occupation : ____________________
- Address : ____________________
- General condition : ____________________
- Socio-economic condition : ____________________
- Diagnosis : ____________________
- Chief complaint : ____________________

For median nerve: Patient is unable to pick-up objects like key, spoon. Patient cannot feel sensation like hot, cold, pain over the palmar aspect of hand.

Possible History

- Compression due to muscle hypertrophy.
- Anomalous fibrous band connecting pronator teres to the tendinous arch of FDS
- Thickening at the bicipital aponeurosis.
- Noncompression due to trauma.

On Observation

- Position of limb
- Deformity
- Trick movement
- Trophic changes
  - Skin
  - Nail
- Color of skin

On Palpation

- Temperature
- Tenderness
- Swelling
- Wasting
- Scar

On Examination

- *Muscle tone*: Hypotonicity noted
- *MMT*: Weakness of muscle supplied by that nerve
- ROM

ROM (Elbow, Wrist and Fingers)

- Active range is limited. Take both active and passive range.
- *Reflexes*: It reveals normal
- DTR
- Sensation
- Special test
- Tinel's sign
- Test for pseudo motor activity:
- *Investigation*: Electromyogram (EMG), Nelve conduction velocity (NCV), strength duration (SD) curve.
- *Physiotherapy treatment:*
  - Problem list
  - Aims
  - Goals
  - Short-term
  - Long-term
  - Follow-up

19 Disease-specific Scales

ASSESSMENT SCALES FOR SPINAL CORD INJURY

- *Classification of spinal cord injuries*:
  - American Spinal Injury Association (ASIA) impairment scale
- *Functional ability*:
  - Functional independence measure (FIM) for spinal cord injury with five additional mobility and locomotor items.
  - Quadriplegic index of function, self-care assessment tool.
- *Manual wheelchair user's skill*
  - Wheelchair skills test
- *Walking ability after spinal cord injury (SCI)*:
  - Walking index for spinal cord injury (WISCI)
  - Spinal cord injury-functional ambulation inventory (SCI-FAI)
  - ASIA standard neurological classification for spinal cord injury
  - The American Spinal Injury Association (ASIA) Standard Neurological Classification of spinal cord injury is a standard method of assessing the neurological status of a person who has sustained a spinal cord injury.
  - Scale assessments are usually carried out by specialist medical staff at the hospital the person is admitted to, using this ASIA Impairment Scale worksheet.
  - It is important to include the score on the ASIA Impairment Scale in the referral for a spinal injured client. This score can usually be found in the medical notes of a client who has been admitted into either of the spinal units.
  - The five categories of the ASIA impairment scale are shown in **Table 19.1**.

Table 19.1: Five categories of the ASIA Impairment Scale	
Category	*Description*
A = Complete	No motor or sensory function (for definitions, see note below) is preserved in the sacral segments S4-S5
B = Incomplete	Sensory but not motor function is preserved below the neurological level and includes the sacral segments S4-S5
C = Incomplete	Motor function is preserved below the neurological level, and more than half of key muscles below the neurological level have a muscle grade of less than 3
D = Incomplete	Motor function is preserved below the neurological level, and at least half of the key muscles below the neurological level have a muscle grade of 3 or more
E = Normal	Motor and sensory functions are normal

Note: 'Loss of motor function' means a person has no voluntary control of his muscles. 'Loss of sensory function' means a person has no sense of touch and cannot feel hot or cold, pain, or pressure. They also have no sense of where, in space their limbs are.

ASSESSMENT SCALES FOR PARKINSON'S DISEASE

- *Cognitive function*:
  - Mini-mental status exam (MMSE)
- *Psychosocial function*:
  - Geriatric depression scale
  - Beck depression inventory
- *Pain*:
  - McGill pain questionnaire
  - Visual analogue scale (VAS)
- *Postural instability*:
  - Functional reach test (FR)
  - Multidirectional reach test (MDRT)
  - Clinical test for sensory integration in balance (CTSIB)
  - Modified test for sensory integration in balance (m-CTSIB)
  - Timed up and go test
  - Tinetti's performance-oriented mobility assessment (POMA).

- *Gait*:
  - 10-meter walk test
  - Walkie-talkie test
- *Cardiopulmonary function*:
  - 12-minute walk test
  - 6-minute walk test
- *Perceived exertion*:
  - Borg's rating of perceived exertion scale (RPE scale)
- *Functional status*:
  - Functional independence measure (FIM)
- *Global health and disease-specific measures*:
  - Rand 36-item health survey
  - Sickness impact profile
  - Unified Parkinson's disease rating scale (UPDRS)
  - Parkinson's disease questionnaire (PDQ-39).

Hoehn and Yahr Staging of Parkinson's Disease

- *Stage one*:
  - Signs and symptoms on one side only
  - Symptoms mild
  - Symptoms inconvenient but not disabling
  - Usually presents with tremor of one limb
  - Friends have noticed changes in posture, locomotion and facial expression
- *Stage two*:
  - Symptoms are bilateral
  - Minimal disability
  - Posture and gait affected
- *Stage three*:
  - Significant slowing of body movements
  - Early impairment of equilibrium on walking or standing
  - Generalized dysfunction that is moderately severe
- *Stage four*:
  - Severe symptoms
  - Can still walk to a limited extent
  - Rigidity and bradykinesia
  - No longer able to live alone
  - Tremor may be less than earlier stages

- *Stage five*:
  - Cachectic stage
  - Invalidism complete
  - Cannot stand or walk
  - Requires constant nursing care

Unified Parkinson's Disease Rating Scale

Mentation, Behavior and Mood

1. *Intellectual Impairment*
   0 = None.
   1 = Mild. Consistent forgetfulness with partial recollection of events and no other difficulties.
   2 = Moderate memory loss, with disorientation and moderate difficulty handling complex problems. Mild but definite impairment of function at home with need of occasional prompting.
   3 = Severe memory loss with disorientation for time and often to place. Severe impairment in handling problems.
   4 = Severe memory loss with orientation preserved to person only. Unable to make judgements or solve problems. Requires much help with personal care. Cannot be left alone at all.
2. *Thought Disorder* (Due to dementia or drug intoxication)
   0 = None.
   1 = Vivid dreaming.
   2 = "Benign" hallucinations with insight retained.
   3 = Occasional to frequent hallucinations or delusions; without insight; could interfere with daily activities.
   4 = Persistent hallucinations, delusions, or florid psychosis. Not able to care for self.
3. *Depression*
   1 = Periods of sadness or guilt greater than normal, never sustained for days or weeks.
   2 = Sustained depression (1 week or more).
   3 = Sustained depression with vegetative symptoms (insomnia, anorexia, weight loss, loss of interest).
   4 = Sustained depression with vegetative symptoms and suicidal thoughts or intent.

4. *Motivation/Initiative*
   0 = Normal.
   1 = Less assertive than usual; more passive.
   2 = Loss of initiative or disinterest in elective (nonroutine) activities.
   3 = Loss of initiative or disinterest in day-to-day (routine) activities.
   4 = Withdrawn, complete loss of motivation.

Activities of Daily Living (for both "on" and "off")

5. *Speech*
   0 = Normal.
   1 = Mildly affected. No difficulty being understood.
   2 = Moderately affected. Sometimes asked to repeat statements.
   3 = Severely affected. Frequently asked to repeat statements.
   4 = Unintelligible most of the time.
6. *Salivation*
   0 = Normal.
   1 = Slight but definite excess of saliva in mouth; may have night time drooling.
   2 = Moderately excessive saliva; may have minimal drooling.
   3 = Marked excess of saliva with some drooling.
   4 = Marked drooling requires constant tissue or handkerchief.
7. *Swallowing*
   0 = Normal.
   1 = Rare choking.
   2 = Occasional choking.
   3 = Requires soft food.
   4 = Requires NG tube or gastrostomy feeding.
8. *Handwriting*
   0 = Normal.
   1 = Slightly slow or small.
   2 = Moderately slow or small; all words are legible.
   3 = Severely affected; not all words are legible.
   4 = The majority of words are not legible.
9. *Cutting Food and Handling Utensils*
   0 = Normal.
   1 = Somewhat slow and clumsy, but no help needed.
   2 = Can cut most foods, although clumsy and slow; some help needed.

3 = Food must be cut by someone, but can still feed slowly.
4 = Needs to be fed.

10. *Dressing*
0 = Normal.
1 = Somewhat slow, but no help needed.
2 = Occasional assistance with buttoning, getting arms in sleeves.
3 = Considerable help required, but can do some things alone.
4 = Helpless.

11. *Hygiene*
0 = Normal.
1 = Somewhat slow, but no help needed.
2 = Needs help to shower or bathe; or very slow in hygienic care.
3 = Requires assistance for washing, brushing teeth, combing hair, going to bathroom.
4 = Foley catheter or other mechanical aids.

12. *Turning in Bed and Adjusting Bed Clothes*
0 = Normal.
1 = Somewhat slow and clumsy, but no help needed.
2 = Can turn alone or adjust sheets, but with great difficulty.
3 = Can initiate, but not turn or adjust sheets alone.
4 = Helpless.

13. *Falling (Unrelated to Freezing)*
0 = None.
1 = Rare falling.
2 = Occasionally falls, less than once per day.
3 = Falls an average of once daily.
4 = Falls more than once daily.

14. *Freezing when Walking*
0 = None.
1 = Rare freezing when walking; may have start hesitation.
2 = Occasional freezing when walking.
3 = Frequent freezing. Occasionally falls from freezing.
4 = Frequent falls from freezing.

15. *Walking*
0 = Normal.
1 = Mild difficulty. May not swing arms or may tend to drag leg.
2 = Moderate difficulty, but requires little or no assistance.
3 = Severe disturbance of walking, requiring assistance.
4 = Cannot walk at all, even with assistance.

16. *Tremor (Symptomatic complaint of tremor in any part of the body.)*
    - 0 = Absent.
    - 1 = Slight and infrequently present.
    - 2 = Moderate; bothersome to patient.
    - 3 = Severe; interferes with many activities.
    - 4 = Marked; interferes with most activities.
17. *Sensory Complaints Related to Parkinsonism*
    - 0 = None.
    - 1 = Occasionally has numbness, tingling, or mild aching.
    - 2 = Frequently has numbness, tingling, or aching; not distressing.
    - 3 = Frequent painful sensations.
    - 4 = Excruciating pain.

Motor Examination

18. *Speech*
    - 0 = Normal.
    - 1 = Slight loss of expression, diction and/or volume.
    - 2 = Monotone, slurred but understandable; moderately impaired.
    - 3 = Marked impairment, difficult to understand.
    - 4 = Unintelligible.
19. *Facial Expression*
    - 0 = Normal.
    - 1 = Minimal hypomimia, could be normal "Poker Face."
    - 2 = Slight but definitely abnormal diminution of facial expression
    - 3 = Moderate hypomimia; lips parted some of the time.
    - 4 = Masked or fixed facies with severe or complete loss of facial expression; lips parted 1/4 inch or more.
20. *Tremor at Rest (head, upper and lower extremities)*
    - 0 = Absent.
    - 1 = Slight and infrequently present.
    - 2 = Mild in amplitude and persistent. Or moderate in amplitude, but only intermittently present.
    - 3 = Moderate in amplitude and present most of the time.
    - 4 = Marked in amplitude and present most of the time.
21. *Action or Postural Tremor of Hands*
    - 0 = Absent.
    - 1 = Slight; present with action.
    - 2 = Moderate in amplitude, present with action.

3 = Moderate in amplitude with posture holding as well as action.
4 = Marked in amplitude; interferes with feeding.

22. *Rigidity (Judged on passive movement of major joints with patient relaxed in sitting position. Cogwheeling to be ignored).*
    0 = Absent.
    1 = Slight or detectable only when activated by mirror or other movements.
    2 = Mild to moderate.
    3 = Marked, but full range of motion easily achieved.
    4 = Severe, range of motion achieved with difficulty.
23. *Finger Taps (Patient taps thumb with index finger in rapid succession).*
    0 = Normal.
    1 = Mild slowing and/or reduction in amplitude.
    2 = Moderately impaired. Definite and early fatiguing. May have occasional arrests in movement.
    3 = Severely impaired. Frequent hesitation in initiating movements or arrests in ongoing movement.
    4 = Can barely perform the task.
24. *Hand Movements (Patient opens and closes hands in rapid succession).*
    0 = Normal.
    1 = Mild slowing and/or reduction in amplitude.
    2 = Moderately impaired. Definite and early fatiguing. May have occasional arrests in movement.
    3 = Severely impaired. Frequent hesitation in initiating movements or arrests in ongoing movement.
    4 = Can barely perform the task.
25. *Rapid Alternating Movements of Hands (Pronation–supination movements of hands, vertically and horizontally, with as large an amplitude as possible, both hands simultaneously)*
    0 = Normal.
    1 = Mild slowing and/or reduction in amplitude.
    2 = Moderately impaired. Definite and early fatiguing. May have occasional arrests in movement.
    3 = Severely impaired. Frequent hesitation in initiating movements or arrests in ongoing movement.
    4 = Can barely perform the task.
26. *Leg Agility (Patient taps heel on the ground in rapid succession picking up entire leg. Amplitude should be at least 3 inches)*

0 = Normal.
1 = Mild slowing and/or reduction in amplitude.
2 = Moderately impaired. Definite and early fatiguing. May have occasional arrests in movement.
3 = Severely impaired. Frequent hesitation in initiating movements or arrests in ongoing movement.
4 = Can barely perform the task.

27. *Arising from Chair (Patient attempts to rise from a straightbacked chair, with arms folded across chest).*
0 = Normal.
1 = Slow; or may need more than one attempt.
2 = Pushes self up from arms of seat.
3 = Tends to fall back and may have to try more than one time, but can get up without help.
4 = Unable to arise without help.

28. *Posture*
0 = Normal erect.
1 = Not quite erect, slightly stooped posture; could be normal for older person.
2 = Moderately stooped posture, definitely abnormal; can be slightly leaning to one side.
3 = Severely stooped posture with kyphosis; can be moderately leaning to one side.
4 = Marked flexion with extreme abnormality of posture.

29. *Gait*
0 = Normal.
1 = Walks slowly, may shuffle with short steps, but no festination (hastening steps) or propulsion.
2 = Walks with difficulty, but requires little or no assistance; may have some festination, short steps, or propulsion.
3 = Severe disturbance of gait, requiring assistance.
4 = Cannot walk at all, even with assistance.

30. *Postural Stability (Response to sudden, strong posterior displacement produced by pull on shoulders while patient erect with eyes open and feet slightly apart. Patient is prepared)*
0 = Normal.
1 = Retropulsion, but recovers unaided.
2 = Absence of postural response; would fall if not caught by examiner.

3 = Very unstable, tends to lose balance spontaneously.
4 = Unable to stand without assistance.

31. *Body Bradykinesia and Hypokinesia (Combining slowness, hesitancy, decreased arm swing, small amplitude, and poverty of movement in general)*
    0 = None.
    1 = Minimal slowness, giving movement a deliberate character; could be normal for some persons. Possibly reduced amplitude.
    2 = Mild degree of slowness and poverty of movement which is definitely abnormal. Alternatively, some reduced amplitude.
    3 = Moderate slowness, poverty or small amplitude of movement.
    4 = Marked slowness, poverty or small amplitude of movement.

Complications of Therapy (In the Past Week)

A. Dyskinesias

32. *Duration: What proportion of the waking day are dyskinesias present? (Historical information)*
    0 = None
    1 = 1–25% of the day.
    2 = 26–50% of the day.
    3 = 51–75% of the day.
    4 = 76–100% of the day.
33. *Disability: How disabling are the dyskinesias? (Historical information; may be modified by office examination).*
    0 = Not disabling.
    1 = Mildly disabling.
    2 = Moderately disabling.
    3 = Severely disabling.
    4 = Completely disabled.
34. *Painful Dyskinesias: How painful are the dyskinesias?*
    0 = No painful dyskinesias.
    1 = Slight.
    2 = Moderate.
    3 = Severe.
    4 = Marked.
35. *Presence of Early Morning Dystonia (Historical information).*
    0 = No
    1 = Yes

B. Clinical Fluctuations

36. *Are "off" periods predictable?*
    - 0 = No
    - 1 = Yes
37. *Are "off" Periods Unpredictable?*
    - 0 = No
    - 1 = Yes
38. *Do "off" Periods Come on Suddenly within a Few Seconds?*
    - 0 = No
    - 1 = Yes
39. *What Proportion of the Waking Day is the Patient "off" on an Average?*
    - 0 = None
    - 1 = 1–25% of the day.
    - 2 = 26–50% of the day.
    - 3 = 51–75% of the day.
    - 4 = 76–100% of the day.

C. Other Complications

40. *Does the patient have Anorexia, Nausea, or Vomiting?*
    - 0 = No
    - 1 = Yes
41. *Any Sleep Disturbances, such as Insomnia or Hypersomnolence?*
    - 0 = No
    - 1 = Yes
42. *Does the Patient have Symptomatic Orthostasis? (Record the patient's blood pressure, height and weight on the scoring form)*
    - 0 = No
    - 1 = Yes

Modified Hoehn and Yahr Staging

Stage 0 = No signs of disease.
Stage 1 = Unilateral disease.
Stage 1.5 = Unilateral plus axial involvement.
Stage 2 = Bilateral disease, without impairment of balance.
Stage 2.5 = Mild bilateral disease, with recovery on pull test.
Stage 3 = Mild to moderate bilateral disease; some postural instability; physically independent.
Stage 4 = Severe disability; still able to walk or stand unassisted.
Stage 5 = Wheelchair bound or bedridden unless aided.

Schwab and England Activities of Daily Living Scale

100% = Completely independent. Able to do all chores without slowness, difficulty or impairment. Essentially normal. Unaware of any difficulty.

90% = Completely independent. Able to do all chores with some degree of slowness, difficulty and impairment. Might take twice as long. Beginning to be aware of difficulty.

80% = Completely independent in most chores. Takes twice as long. Conscious of difficulty and slowness.

70% = Not completely independent. More difficulty with some chores. Three to four times as long in some. Must spend a large part of the day with chores.

60% = Some dependency. Can do most chores, but exceedingly slowly and with much effort. Errors; some impossible.

50% = More dependent. Help with half, slower, etc. Difficulty with everything.

40% = Very dependent. Can assist with all chores, but few alone.

30% = With effort, now and then does a few chores alone or begins alone. Much help needed.

20% = Nothing alone. Can be a slight help with some chores. Severe invalid.

10% = Totally dependent, helpless. Complete invalid.

0% = Vegetative functions such as swallowing, bladder and bowel functions are not functioning. Bedridden.

Name ______________________ Unit Number ____________

Date																
DOPA mg/day hrs DOPA lasts																
	ON	OFF	ON	OFF	ON	OFF	ON	OFF	ON	OFF	ON	OFF	ON	OFF	ON	OFF
1. Mentation																
2. Thought disorder																
3. Depression																
4. Motivation/ initiative																

Contd...

Contd...

	ON	OFF	ON	OFF	ON	OFF	ON	OFF	ON	OFF	ON	OFF	ON	OFF	ON	OFF
Subtotal 1 – 4 (maximum = 16)																
5. Speech																
6. Salivation																
7. Swallowing																
8. Handwriting																
9. Cutting food																
10. Dressing																
11. Hygiene																
12. Turning in bed																
13. Falling																
14. Freezing																
15. Walking																
16. Tremor																
17. Sensory symptoms																
Subtotal 5 – 17 (maximum = 52)																
18. Speech																
19. Facial expression																
20. Tremor at rest: face, lips, chin																
Hands: right																
left																
Feet: right																
left																
21. Action tremor: right																
left																

Contd...

Contd...

	ON	OFF	ON	OFF	ON	OFF	ON	OFF	ON	OFF	ON	OFF	ON	OFF	ON	OFF
22. Rigidity: neck																
Upper extremity: right																
left																
Lower extremity: right																
left																
23. Finger taps: right																
left																
24. Hand grips: right																
left																
25. Hand pronate/ supinate: right																
left																
26. Leg agility: right																
left																
27. Arise from chair																
28. Posture																
29. Gait																
30. Postural stability																
31. Body bradykinesia																
Sub-total: 18–31 (maximum = 108) Total points: 1–31 (max = 176)																
32. Dyskinesia (duration)																

Contd...

Contd...

	ON	OFF	ON	OFF	ON	OFF	ON	OFF	ON	OFF	ON	OFF	ON	OFF	ON	OFF
33. Dyskinesia (disability)																
34. Dyskinesia (pain)																
35. Early morning dystonia																
36. "Offs" (predictable)																
37. "Offs" (unpredictable)																
38. "Offs" (sudden)																
39. "Offs" (duration)																
40. Anorexia, nausea, vomiting																
41. Sleep disturbance																
42. Sympto-matic orthostasis																
Blood pressure: *seated*																
supine																
standing																
Weight																
Pulse: *seated*																
standing																
Name of Examiner																
	Best	Worst	Best	Worst	Best	Worst	Best	Worst	Best	Worst	Best	Worst	Best	Worst	Best	Worst
Hoehn and Yahr Stage																
% ADL Score (PD)																
% ADL (with dyskinesia)																

Source: Fahn S, Elton R. Members of the UPDRS Development Committee. In: Fahn S, Marsden CD, Calne DB, Goldstein M, eds. Recent Developments in Parkinson's Disease, Vol 2. Florham Park, NJ. Macmillan Health Care Information 1987. pp. 153-63, 293-304.

STROKE SCALES

- *Prehospital stroke assessment tools*
  - Cincinnati stroke scale
  - Los Angeles prehospital stroke screen (LAPSS)
  - ABCD score
- *Disease specific-health related*
  - Stroke-specific quality of life scale (SSQOL)
  - Stroke impact scale (SIS)
  - National Institutes of Health Stroke Scale (NIHSS)
  - Fugl-Meyer assessment of motor recovery after stroke (FMA)
- *Upper extremity (UE) function*
  - Wolf motor function test
  - Chedoke arm and hand activity inventory (CAHAI)
  - Action research arm test (ARAT)
  - Arm motor ability test
  - Box and block test
  - Fugl-Meyer test
- *Activity outcome measures*
  - Barthel index (BI)
  - Functional independence measure (FIM)
- *Balance assessment*
  - Berg balance scale (BBS)
  - Timed "up and go" test (TUG)
  - POMA (performance-oriented mobility assessment, Tinetti)
  - Functional reach test
- *Lower extremity*
  - Lower extremity motor coordination test
  - Modified motor assessment scale
- *Depression*
  - Beck depression inventory (BDI)
  - Hamilton depression rating scale (HDRS)
- *Fatigue*
  - Fatigue severity scale
- *Gait index*
  - Dynamic gait index
- *Functional exercise capacity*
  - Six-minute walk test (6 MWT)
- *Intelligence*
  - Mini-mental state examination (MMSE)
- *Motor function*
  - Stroke rehabilitation assessment of movement (STREAM).

Stroke Rehabilitation Assessment of Movement (STREAM)

Patient last name: ____________________ Date of birth: ______________
Patient first name: ____________________ Date: ____________________

General Comments:	*Score date 1*	*Score date 2*	*Score date 3*	*Score date 4*
SUPINE				
1. Protracts scapula un supine "Lift your shoulder blade so that your hand moves towards the ceiling" Note: therapist stabilizes arm with shoulder 90° flexed and elbow extended.	/2			
2. Extends elbow in supine (starting with elbow fully flexed) "Lift your hand towards the ceiling, straightening your elbow as much as you can" Note: therapist stabilizes arm with shoulder 90° flexed; strong associated shoulder extension and/or abduction= marked deviation (score la or le).	/2			
3. Flexes hip and knee in supine (attains half crook lying) "Bend your hip and knee so that your foot rests flat on the bed"	/2			
4. Rolls onto side (starting from supine) "Roll onto your side" Note: may roll onto either side; pulling with arms to turn over = aid (score 2).	/3			
5. Raises hips off bed in crook lying (bridging) "Lift your hips as high as you can" Note: therapist may stabilize foot, but if knee pushes strongly into extension with bridging = marked deviation (score 1a or 1c); if requires aid (external or from therapist) to maintain knees in midline = aid (score 2).	/3			
6. Moves from lying supine to sitting (with feet on the floor) "Sit up and place your feet on the floor" Note: may sit up to either side using any functional and safe method; longer than 20 seconds = marked deviation (score 1a or 1c); pulling up using bedrail or edge of plinth= aid (score 2).	/3			
SITTING (feet supported ; hands resting on pillow on lap for items 7–14)				
7. Shrugs shoulders (scapular elevation) "Shrug your shoulders as high as you can" Note: both shoulders are shrugged simultaneously.	/2			

Contd...

Contd...

General Comments:	*Score date 1*	*Score date 2*	*Score date 3*	*Score date 4*
8. Raises hand to touch top of the head "Raise your hand to touch the top of your head"	/2			
9. Places hand on sacrum "Reach behind your back and as far across toward the other side as you can"	/2			
10. Raises arm overhead to fullest elevation "Reach your hand as high as you can towards the ceiling"	/2			
11. Supinates and pronates forearm (elbow flexed at 90°) "Keeping your elbow bent and close to your side, turn your forearm over so that your palm faces up, then turn your forearm over so that your palm faces down" Note: movement in one direction only = partial movement (score 1a or 1b).	/2			
12. Closes hand from fully opened position "Make a fist, keeping your thumb on the outside" Note: must extend wrist slightly (i.e., wrist cocked) to obtain full marks; full fist with lack of wrist extension = partial movement (score 1a or 1b).	/2			
13. Opens hand from fully closed position "Now open your hand all the way".	/2			
14. Opposes thumb to index finger (tip to tip) "Make a circle with your thumb and index finger".	/2			
15. Flexes hip in sitting "Lift your knee as high as you can"	/2			
16. Extends knee in sitting "Straighten your knee by lifting your foot up".	/2			
17. Flexes knee in sitting "Slide your foot back under you as far as you can" Note: start with affected foot forward (heel in line with toes of other foot).	/2			
18. Dorsiflexes ankle in sitting "Keep your heel on the ground and lift your toes off the floor as far as you can" Note: affected foot is placed slightly forward (heel in line with toes of other foot).	/2			
19. Plantar flexes ankle in sitting "Keep your toes on the groud and lift your heel off the floor as far as you can".	/2			

Contd...

Contd...

General Comments:	*Score date 1*	*Score date 2*	*Score date 3*	*Score date 4*
20. Extends knee and dorsiflexes ankle in sitting "Straighten your knee and bring your toes towards you" Note: extension of knee without dorsiflexion of ankle = partial movement (score 1a or 1b).	/2			
21. Rises to standing from sitting "Stand up; try to take equal weight on both legs" Note: pushing up with hand(s) to stand = aid (score 2); asymmetry such as trunk lean, Trendelenburg position, hip retraction, or excessive flexion or extension of the affected knee = marked deviation (score 1a or 1c).	/3			
STANDING				
22. Maintains standing for 20 counts "Stand on the spot while I count to twenty"	/3			
STANDING (holding onto a stable support to assist balance for items 23–25)				
23. Abducts affected hip with knee extended "Keep your knee straight and your hips level, and raise your leg to the side"	/2			
24. Flexes affected knee with hip extended "Keep your hip straight, bend your knee back and bring your heel towards your bottom"	/2			
25. Dorsiflexes affected ankle with knee extended "Keep your heel on the ground and lift your toes off the floor as far as you can" Note: affected foot is placed slightly forward in position of a small step (heel in line with toes of other foot).	/2			
STANDING AND WALKING ACTIVITIES				
26. Places affected foot onto first step (or stool 18 cm high) "Lift your foot and place it onto the first step (or stool) in front of you" Note: returning the foot to the ground is not scored; use of handrail = aid (score 2).	/3			
27. Takes 3 steps backwards (one and a half gait cycles) "Take three average sized steps backwards, placing one foot behind the other"	/3			
28. Takes 3 steps sideways to affected side "Take three average sized steps sideways towards your weak side"	/3			

Contd...

Contd...

General Comments:	*Score date 1*	*Score date 2*	*Score date 3*	*Score date 4*
29. Walks 10 meters indoors (on smooth, obstacle = free surface) "Walk in a straight line over to ... (a specified point 10 meters away)" Note: orthotic= aid (score 2); longer than 20 seconds = marked deviation (score 1c).	/3			
30. Walks down 3 stairs alternating feet "Walk down three stairs; place only one foot at a time on each step if you can" Note: handrail = aid (score 2); non-alternating feet = marked deviation (score 1a or 1c).	/3			
Scores				

	I. Voluntary Movement of the Limbs
0	Unable to perform the test movement through any appreciable range (includes flicker or slight movement)
1	a. Able to perform only part of the movement, and with marked deviation from normal pattern
	b. Able to perform only part of the movement, but in a manner that is comparable to the unaffected side
	c. Able to complete the movement, but only with marked deviation from normal pattern
2	Able to complete the movement in a manner that is comparable to the unaffected side
X	Activity nontested (specify why; ROM, pain, other (reason))
	II. Basic Mobility
0	Unable to perform the test activity through any appreciable range (i.e., minimal active participation)
1	a. Able to perform only part of the activity independently (requires partial assistance or stabilization to complete), with or without an aid, and with marked deviation from normal pattern
	b. Able to perform only part of the activity independently (requires partial assistance or stabilization to complete), with or without an aid, but with a grossly normal movement pattern
	c. Able to complete the activity independently, with or without an aid, but only with marked deviation from normal pattern
2	Able to complete the activity independently with a grossly normal movement pattern, but requires an aid
3	Able to complete the activity independently with a grossly normal movement pattern, without an aid
X	Activity non-tested (specify why; ROM, pain, other (reason))

Amplitude of Active Movement			
Movement Quality	None	Partial	Complete
Marked Deviation	0	1 a	1 c
Grossly Normal	0	1 b	2 (3)

COMA SCALES

- Coma/near coma scale
- Coma recovery scale
- Glasgow epilepsy outcome scale
- Western neurosensory stimulation profile.

Glasgow Coma Scale for Head Injury

The Glasgow coma scale or GCS is a neurological scale that aims to give a reliable, objective way of recording the conscious state of a person for initial as well as subsequent assessment. A patient is assessed against the criteria of the scale, and the resulting points give a patient score between 3 (indicating deep unconsciousness) and either 14 (original scale) or 15 (the more widely used modified or revised scale).

Glasgow coma scale was initially used to assess level of consciousness after head injury, and the scale is now used by first aid, EMS, nurses and doctors as being applicable to all acute medical and trauma patients. In hospitals it is also used in monitoring chronic patients in intensive care.

Glasgow coma scale is used as part of several ICU scoring systems, including APACHE II, SAPS II, and SOFA, to assess the status of the central nervous system, as it was designed for. The initial indication for use of the GCS was serial assessments of patients with traumatic brain injury and coma for at least 6 hours in the neurosurgical ICU setting, though it is commonly used throughout hospital departments. A similar scale, the Rancho Los Amigos Scale is used to assess the recovery of traumatic brain injury patients.

Eye Response (E)

There are four grades starting with the most severe:

1. No eye opening
2. Eye opening in response to pain stimulus (A peripheral pain stimulus, such as squeezing the lunula area of the patient's fingernail is more

effective than a central stimulus such as a trapezius squeeze, due to a grimacing effect).

3. Eye opening to speech (Not to be confused with the awakening of a sleeping person; such patients receive a score of 4, not 3).
4. Eyes opening spontaneously.

Verbal Response (V)

There are five grades starting with the most severe:

1. No verbal response.
2. Incomprehensible sounds (Moaning but no words).
3. Inappropriate words. (Random or exclamatory articulated speech, but no conversational exchange. Speaks words but no sentences).
4. Confused (The patient responds to questions coherently but there is some disorientation and confusion).
5. Oriented (Patient responds coherently and appropriately to questions such as the patient's name and age, where they are and why, the year, month, etc.).

Motor Response (M)

There are six grades:

1. No motor response
2. *Decerebrate posturing accentuated by pain (extensor response*: Adduction of arm, internal rotation of shoulder, pronation of forearm and extension at elbow, flexion of wrist and fingers, leg extension, plantarflexion of foot).
3. Decorticate posturing accentuated by pain (flexor response: internal rotation of shoulder, flexion of forearm and wrist with clenched fist, leg extension, plantarflexion of foot).
4. Withdrawal from pain (Absence of abnormal posturing; unable to lift hand past chin with supraorbital pain but does pull away when nailbed is pinched).
5. Localizes to pain (Purposeful movements towards painful stimuli; e.g., brings hand up beyond chin when supraorbital pressure applied).
6. Obeys commands (the patient does simple things as asked).

Interpretation: Individual elements as well as sum of the scores are important. Hence, the score is expressed in the form "GCS 9 = E2 V4 M3 at 07:35".

Generally, brain injury is classified as:

- Severe, with GCS < 8–9
- Moderate, GCS 8 or 9–12 (controversial)
- Minor, GCS ≥ 13.

Generally when a patient is in a decline of his GCS score, the nurse or medical staff should assess the cranial nerves and determine which of the twelve have been affected.

Tracheal intubation and severe facial/eye swelling or damage make it impossible to test the verbal and eye responses. In these circumstances, the score is given as 1 with a modifier attached, e.g. 'E1c' where 'c' = closed, or 'V1t' where t = tube. A composite might be 'GCS 5tc'. This would mean, for example, eyes closed because of swelling = 1, intubated = 1, leaving a motor score of 3 for 'abnormal flexion'. Often the 1 is left out, so the scale reads Ec or Vt.

Ranchos Los Amigos Scale

Level of Cognitive Functioning Scale (LCFS)

- *Level I: No Response.*
  Patient does not respond to external stimuli and appears asleep.
- *Level II: Generalized Response.*
  Patient reacts to external stimuli in nonspecific, inconsistent, and nonpurposeful manner with stereotypic and limited responses.
- *Level III: Localized Response.*
  Patient responds specifically and inconsistently with delays to stimuli, but may follow simple commands for motor action.
- *Level IV: Confused, Agitated Response.*
  Patient exhibits bizarre, nonpurposeful, incoherent or inappropriate behaviors, has no short-term recall, attention is short and nonselective.
- *Level V: Confused, Inappropriate, Nonagitated Response.*
  Patient gives random, fragmented, and nonpurposeful responses to complex or unstructured stimuli—Simple commands are followed consistently, memory and selective attention are impaired, and new information is not retained.
- *Level VI: Confused, Appropriate Response.*
  Patient gives context appropriate, goal-directed responses, dependent upon external input for direction. There is carry-over for relearned, but not for new tasks, and recent memory problems persist.

- *Level VII: Automatic, Appropriate Response.*
  Patient behaves appropriately in familiar settings, performs daily routines automatically, and shows carry-over for new learning at lower than normal rates. Patient initiates social interactions, but judgment remains impaired.
- *Level VIII: Purposeful, Appropriate Response.*
  Patient oriented and responds to the environment but abstract reasoning abilities are decreased relative to premorbid levels.

MULTIPLE SCLEROSIS

- *Pain*:
  - Dallas pain questionnaire
- *Cognitive function*:
  - Minimal assessment of cognitive function in MS
- *Spasticity*:
  - Modified Ashworth scale
- *Hand dexterity*:
  - Box and block test
- *Balance*:
  - Berg balance test
- *Functional assessment*:
  - Barthel index
  - Kurtzke functional system scores
  - Multiple sclerosis functional composite
  - Tinetti assessment tool
- *Quality of life*:
  - Multiple sclerosis quality of life
  - Multiple sclerosis quality.

Kurtzke Expanded Disability Status Scale (EDSS)

0 Normal neurological exam (all grade 0 in Functional Systems (FS); cerebral grade 1 acceptable).

1 No disability, minimal signs in one FS (i.e., one grade 1 excluding cerebral grade 1).

1.5 No disability, minimal signs in more than one FS (more than one grade 1 excluding cerebral grade 1).

2.0 Minimal disability in one FS (one FS grade 2, others 0 or 1).

2.5 Minimal disability in two FS (two FS grade 2, others 0 or 1).

3.0 Moderate disability in one FS (one FS grade 3, others 0 or 1), or mild disability in three or four FS (three-four FS grade 2, others 0 or 1).

3.5 Fully ambulatory but with moderate disability in one FS (one grade 3 and one or two FS grade 2) or two FS grade 3, others 0 or 1, or five FS grade 2, others 0 or 1.

4.0 Fully ambulatory without aid, self-sufficient, up and about some 12 hours a day despite relatively severe disability consisting of one FS grade 4 (others 0 or 1), or combinations of lesser grades exceeding limits of previous steps. Able to walk without aid or rest some 500 meters (0.3 miles).

4.5 Fully ambulatory without aid, up and about much of the day, able to work a full day, may otherwise have some limitation of full activity or require minimal assistance; characterized by relatively severe disability. [Usually consisting of one FS grade 4 (others 0 or 1) or combinations of lesser grades exceeding limits of previous steps. Able to walk without aid or rest for some 300 meters (975 ft.)].

5.0 Ambulatory without aid or rest for about 200 meters (650 ft.); disability severe enough to impair full daily activities (e.g., to work full day without special provisions). (Usual FS equivalents are one grade 5 alone (others 0 or 1); or combinations of lesser grades usually exceeding specifications for step 4.0).

5.5 Ambulatory without aid or rest for about 100 meters (325 ft); disability severe enough to impair full daily activities. (Usual FS equivalents are one grade 5 alone (others 0 or 1); or combinations of lesser grades usually exceeding specifications for step 4.0).

6.0 Intermittent or constant unilateral assistance (cane, crutch, or brace) required to walk about 100 meters (325 ft.) with or without resting (Usual FS equivalents are combinations with more than two FS grade 3+).

6.5 Constant bilateral assistance (canes, crutches, or braces) required to walk about 20 meters (65 ft.). (Usual FS equivalents are combinations with more than two FS grade 3+).

7.0 Unable to walk beyond about 5 meters (16 ft.) event with aid, essentially restricted to wheelchair, wheels self in standard wheelchair a full day and transfers alone; up and about in wheelchair some 12 hours a day. (Usual FS equivalents are combinations with more than one FS grade 4+; very rarely pyramidal grade 5 alone).

7.5 Unable to take more than a few steps; restricted to wheelchair; may need aid in transfers, wheels self but cannot carry on in standard wheelchair a full day; may require motorized wheelchair. (Usual FS equivalents are combinations with more than one FS grade 4+).

8.0 Essentially restricted to bed or chair or perambulated in wheelchair; but may be out of bed much of the day; retains many self-care functions; generally has effective use of arms. (Usual FS equivalents are combinations, generally grade 4+ in several systems).

8.5 Essentially restricted to bed for much of the day; has some effective use of arm (s); retains some self-care functions. (Usual FS equivalents are combinations, generally grade 4+ in several systems).

9.0 Helpless bed patient; can communicate and eat. (Usual FS equivalents are combinations, mostly grade 4).

9.5 Totally helpless bed patient; unable to communicate or effectively eat/swallow. (Usual FS equivalents are combinations, almost all grade 4+).

10 Death due to MS.

HOUSE BRACKMANN SCALE FOR FACIAL PALSY

Facial nerve dysfunction (facial paralysis) manifests in various symptom patterns. To objectively describe facial function, clinicians use a number of standardized scales—the most common being the House-Brackmann facial nerve grading system.

Symptoms of facial nerve injury may vary due to age, facial anatomy and the extent of nerve damage. Frequent patient concerns relate to brow position, movement abnormalities, eyelid closure issues, inability to smile, mid-facial asymmetries, poor oral function and lower lip asymmetry.

A light degree of facial nerve weakness may only be visible as subtle asymmetries following repeated and exhausting muscle function, whereas severe dysfunction can be easily recognized even at rest.

Many of these symptoms will change over time, for example following a spontaneous recovery of nerve function or as a result of different therapeutic modalities (i.e after surgical treatment).

House-Brackmann (HB) is one of several analysis tools developed to quantify facial function and provide reproducible information. It is a widely accepted system, simple, sensitive, accurate and reliable—grading facial function in six steps froms normal (HB I) to total paralysis (HB VI).

At the Sorensen clinic, we routinely use the House-Brackmann scale to evaluate new and existing patients. In addition, we include a description of segmental weakness (zone-specific information), changes in the facial soft tissues and synkinesis.

- House-Brackmann facial nerve grading system

Grade I—Normal facial function in all areas

Grade II—Slight dysfunction

- *Gross*: Slight weakness noticeable on close inspection; may have very slight synkinesis
- *At rest*: Normal symmetry and tone
- *Motion*: Forehead—moderate-to-good function; eye—complete closure with minimum effort; mouth—slight asymmetry.

Grade III—Moderate dysfunction

- *Gross*: Obvious but not disfiguring difference between two sides; noticeable but not severe synkinesis, contracture, and/or hemifacial spasm.
- *At rest*: Normal symmetry and tone
- *Motion*: Forehead—slight-to-moderate movement; eye—complete closure with effort; mouth—slightly weak with maximum effort.

Grade IV—Moderate severe dysfunction

- *Gross*: Obvious weakness and/or disfiguring asymmetry
- *At rest*: Normal symmetry and tone
- *Motion*: Forehead—none; eye—incomplete closure; mouth—asymmetric with maximum effort.

Grade V—Severe dysfunction

- *Gross*: Only barely perceptible motion
- *At rest*: Asymmetry
- *Motion*: Forehead—none; eye—incomplete closure; mouth—slight movement

Grade VI—Total paralysis

- No movement.

NORTH STAR AMBULATORY ASSESSMENT

We have attempted to give clear explanations of the methods employed to achieve motor goals, but it is not possible to be exhaustive in the descriptions, particularly of modifications to activity. Whilst DMD children may generally present with recognizable adaptations to activity due to the underlying progressive muscular weakness, they may modify their activity to achieve functional goals in slightly differing ways. Generally, activities are graded in the following manner:

2: 'Normal'—no obvious modification of activity

1: Modified method but achieves goal independent of physical assistance from another

0: Unable to achieve independently.

Gowers' Maneuver (Figs 19.1A to H)

Definition of Gowers' Maneuver

The child turns towards the floor (generally into a four-point kneeling position) to place hands on the floor to assist rising, walks hands back in towards him then uses arms to 'climb up' legs to achieve upright standing. A wide base of support is often assumed through the phases of rising from the floor.

Stair Climb

As it is not possible to ensure standardization or availability of flights of stairs, we are asking that a box step (approximately 15 cm high) is used to assess single-step climb and descend. A plinth or other immovable object may need to be available to provide support.

The following gives test details and instructions for the patient and a scoring sheet with details for grading. They should be used in conjunction. Please familiarize yourself with the test detail before starting to evaluate the patients **(Table 19.2)**.

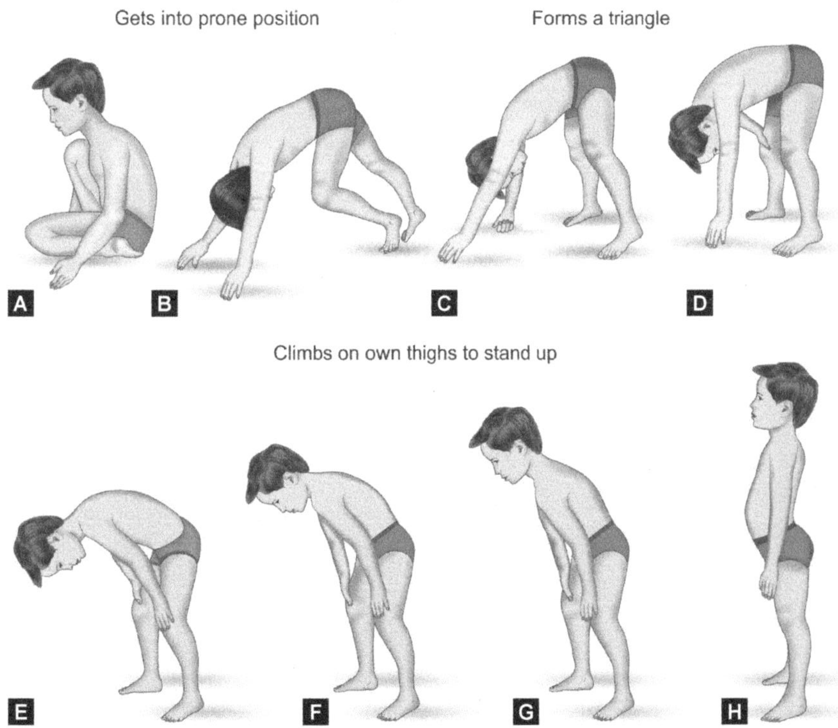

Figs 19.1A to H Gowers' maneuver (*Source:* WR Gowers' pseudohypertrophic muscular paralysis, 1879)

Table 19.2: Test detail and instructions to patient

Activity	*Instructions to patient*	*Start position/test detail*	*Comments*
Stand	Can you stand up tall for me for as long as you can and as still as you can	Feet should be close together and heels on the ground if possible. Arms by sides. No shoes should be worn	Best done on the floor rather than on a mat. Whichever is chosen, maintain consistency through repeated testing sessions. Minimum count of 3 seconds to score 2.
Walk	Can you walk from A to B (state to and where from) for me	Walk without shoes/socks on. Should be enough of a distance to observe 'normal gait' for that subject	A value judgement needs to be made in scoring—if the patient generally toe walks but occasionally gets heels flat, or can, on request, but does not usually, they should score 1
Stand up from chair	Stand up from the chair keeping your arms folded if you can	Starting position 90° hips and knees, feet on floor/supported on a box step	A size-appropriate chair or height adjustable plinth should be used. Arms should be kept crossed throughout the activity to score 2.
Stand on one leg–Right	Can you stand on your right leg for as long as you can?	Minimum count of 3 seconds to score 2. No shoes should be worn.	Best done on the floor rather than on a mat. Whichever is chosen, maintain consistency through repeated testing sessions.
Stand on one leg–Left	Can you stand on your left leg for as long as you can?	Minimum count of 3 seconds to score 2. No shoes should be worn.	Best done on the floor rather than on a mat. Whichever is chosen, maintain consistency through repeated testing sessions.
Climb box step–Right	Can you step onto the top of the box using your right leg first?	Stands facing the box step. Step should be approximately 15 cm high	Support may be provided by the use of a height adjustable plinth, or, if not available, a 'neutral' hand from the therapist.

Contd...

Contd...

Activity	*Instructions to patient*	*Start position/test detail*	*Comments*
Climb box step–Left	Can you step onto the top of the box using your left leg first?	Stands facing the box step. Step should be approximately 15 cm high.	Support may be provided by the use of a height adjustable plinth, or, if not available a 'neutral' hand from the therapist.
Descend box step–Right	Can you step down from the box using your right leg first?	Stands on top of the box step facing forwards. Step should be approximately 15 cm high.	Support may be provided by the use of a height adjustable plinth, or if not available, a 'neutral' hand from the therapist.
Descend box step–Left	Can you step down from the box using your left leg first?	Stands on top of the box step facing forwards. Step should be approximately 15 cm high.	Support may be provided by the use of a height adjustable plinth, or if not available, a 'neutral' hand from the therapist.
Gets to sitting	Can you get from lying to sitting?	Starting position supine on a mat. No pillow should be used under head.	If patient turns into prone or towards the floor to work their way into sitting 1 should be scored.
Rise from floor	Get up from the floor using as little support as possible and as fast as you can (from supine)	Starting position supine with arms by sides, legs straight. No pillow to be used.	Activity should be attempted without use of furniture in the first instance. Do not note time if a chair has to be used.
Lifts head	Lift your head to look at your toes keeping your arms folded	Supine on a mat. No pillow should be used.	Ask patient to keep arms crossed over chest during the activity to avoid self-assist. Also ask to look at toes to ensure neck is flexed—should be a chin to chest maneuver.

Contd...

Contd...

Activity	*Instructions to patient*	*Start position/test detail*	*Comments*
Stands on heels	Can you stand on your heels?	Standing on the floor. No shoes to be worn.	Watch for inversion. If substantial inversion but forefeet are still lifted – score 1. If only inversion with lateral border of foot still on the ground score.
Jump	How high can you jump?	Standing on the floor, feet fairly close together.	Want height, not forward movement. Small amount of forward movement acceptable.
Hop right leg	Can you hop on your right leg?	Starting position standing on floor on right leg. No shoes should be worn.	Needs obvious floor clearance to score 2.
Hop left leg	Can you hop on your left leg?	Starting position standing on floor on right leg. No shoes should be worn.	Needs obvious floor clearance to score 2.
Run (10 m)	Run as fast as you can to……(give point)	A straight 10 m walkway should be clearly marked in a quiet department or corridor. A stopwatch should be used to time the walk. Be consistent as to whether shoes are worn or not. Ensure safety of patient. They should self select speed after being asked to go 'as fast as they can'.	'Duchenne jog'—not a true run (there probably IS a double support phase), but more than a walk. Typically characterized by excessive use of arms, trunk rotation, substantial 'waddle'. No real 'push-off'.

SCALE FOR THE ASSESSMENT AND RATING OF ATAXIA (SARA)

Rater:__________________ date: _________ patient:________________

Gait

Patient is asked (1) to walk at a safe distance parallel to a wall, including a half-turn (turn around to face the opposite direction of gait) and (2) to walk in tandem (heels to toes) without support.

0 Normal, no difficulties in walking, turning and walking tandem (up to one mis-step allowed)
1 Slight difficulties, only visible when walking 10 consecutive steps in tandem
2 Clearly abnormal, tandem walking >10 steps not possible
3 Considerable staggering, difficulties in half-turn, but without support
4 Marked staggering, intermittent support of the wall required
5 Severe staggering, permanent support of one stick or light support by one arm required
6 Walking >10 m only with strong support (two special sticks or stroller or accompanying person)
7 Walking <10 m only with strong support (two special sticks or stroller or accompanying person)
8 Unable to walk, even supported.

Score	

Stance

Patient is asked to stand (1) in natural position, (2) with feet together in parallel (big toes touching each other) and (3) in tandem (both feet on one line, no space between heel and toe). Patient does not wear shoes, eyes are open. For each condition, three trials are allowed. Best trial is rated.

0 Normal, able to stand in tandem for >10 s
1 Able to stand with feet together without sway, but not in tandem for >10s
2 Able to stand with feet together for >10 s, but only with sway

3 Able to stand for >10 s without support in natural position, but not with feet together
4 Able to stand for >10 s in natural position only with intermittent support
5 Able to stand >10 s in natural position only with constant support of one arm
6 Unable to stand for >10 s even with constant support of one arm

Score	

Sitting

Patient is asked to sit on an examination bed without support of feet, eyes open and arms outstretched to the front.
0 Normal, no difficulties sitting >10 sec
1 Slight difficulties, intermittent sway
2 Constant sway, but able to sit >10 s without support
3 Able to sit for >10 s only with intermittent support
4 Unable to sit for >10 s without continuous support

Score	

Speech Disturbance

Speech is assessed during normal conversation.
0 Normal
1 Suggestion of speech disturbance
2 Impaired speech, but easy to understand
3 Occasional words difficult to understand
4 Many words difficult to understand
5 Only single word understandable
6 Speech unintelligible/anarthria

Score	

Finger Chase

Rated Separately for Each Side

Patient sits comfortably. If necessary, support of feet and trunk is allowed. Examiner sits in front of patient and performs 5 consecutive sudden and fast pointing movements in unpredictable directions in a frontal plane, at about 50% of patient's reach. Movements have an amplitude of 30 cm and a frequency of 1 movement every 2s. Patient is asked to follow the movements with his index finger, as fast and precisely as possible. Average performance of last 3 movements is rated.

0 No dysmetria
1 Dysmetria, under/overshooting target <5 cm
2 Dysmetria, under/overshooting target <15 cm
3 Dysmetria, under/overshooting target >15 cm
4 Unable to perform 5 pointing movements

Score	Right	Left
Mean of both sides (R+L)/2		

Nose-Finger Test

Rated Separately for Each Side

Patient sits comfortably. If necessary, support of feet and trunk is allowed. Patient is asked to point repeatedly with his index finger from his nose to examiner's finger which is in front of the patient at about 90% of patient's reach. Movements are performed at moderate speed. Average performance of movements is rated according to the amplitude of the kinetic tremor.

0 No tremor
1 Tremor with an amplitude <2 cm
2 Tremor with an amplitude <5 cm
3 Tremor with an amplitude >5 cm
4 Unable to perform 5 pointing movements

Score	Right	Left
Mean of both sides (R+L)/2		

Fast Alternating Hand Movements

Rated Separately for Each Side

Patient sits comfortably. If necessary, support of feet and trunk is allowed. Patient is asked to perform 10 cycles of repetitive alternation of pro- and supinations of the hand on his/her thigh as fast and as precise as possible. Movement is demonstrated by examiner at a speed of approx. 10 cycles within 7 s. Exact times for movement execution have to be taken.

0 Normal, no irregularities (performs <10s)
1 Slightly irregular (performs <10s)
2 Clearly irregular, single movements difficult to distinguish or relevant interruptions, but performs <10s
3 Very irregular, single movements difficult to distinguish or relevant interruptions, performs >10s
4 Unable to complete 10 cycles

Score	Right	Left
Mean of both sides (R+L)/2		

Heel-shin Slide

Rated Separately for Each Side

Patient lies on examination bed, without sight of his legs. Patient is asked to lift one leg, point with the heel to the opposite knee, slide down along the shin to the ankle, and lay the leg back on the examination bed. The task is performed 3 times. Slide-down movements should be performed within 1s. If patient slides down without contact to shin in all three trials, rate 4.

0 Normal
1 Slightly abnormal, contact to shin maintained
2 Clearly abnormal, goes off shin up to 3 times during 3 cycles
3 Severely abnormal, goes off shin 4 or more times during 3 cycles
4 Unable to perform the task

Score	Right	Left
Mean of both sides (R+L)/2		

20 Scales Used for Neurological Assessment

MINI-MENTAL STATE EXAMINATION (MMSE)

- Patient's Name : ______________________
- Date : ______________________

Instructions: Ask the questions in the order listed. Score one point for each correct response within each question or activity.

Maximum Score	*Patient's Score*	*Questions*
5		"What is the year? Season? Date? Day of the week? Month?"
5		"Where are we now: State? Country? Town/city? Hospital? Floor?"
3		The examiner names three unrelated objects clearly and slowly, then asks the patient to name all three of them. The patient's response is used for scoring. The examiner repeats them until the patient learns all of them, if possible. Number of trials: ________
5		"I would like you to count backward from 100 by sevens." (93, 86, 79, 72, 65, ...). Stop after five answers.
3		"Earlier I told you the names of three things. Can you tell me what were those?"
2		Show the patient two simple objects, such as a wristwatch and a pencil, and ask the patient to name them.
1		Repeat the phrase: "No ifs, ands, or buts."
3		"Take the paper in your right hand, fold it in half, and put it on the floor." (The examiner gives the patient a piece of blank paper)
1		"Please read this and do what it says." (Written instruction is "Close your eyes")
1		"Make up and write a sentence about anything." (This sentence must contain a noun and a verb)

Contd...

Contd...

Maximum Score	*Patient's Score*	*Questions*
1		"Please copy this picture." (The examiner gives the patient a blank piece of paper and asks him/her to draw the symbol below. All 10 angles must be present and two must intersect) 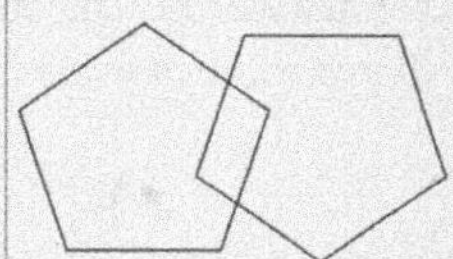
30		TOTAL

(Adapted from Rovner and Folstein, 1987)

Instructions for Administration and Scoring of the MMSE

Orientation (10 Points)

- Ask for the date. Then specifically ask for parts omitted (e.g., "Can you also tell me what season is it?"). One point for each correct answer.
- Ask in turn, "Can you tell me the name of this hospital (town, county, etc.)?" One point for each correct answer.

Registration (3 Points)

- Say the names of three unrelated objects clearly and slowly, allowing approximately one second for each. After you have said all three, ask the patient to repeat them. The number of objects the patient names correctly upon the first repetition determines the score (0–3). If the patient does not repeat all three objects the first time, continue saying the names until the patient is able to repeat all three items, up to six trials. Record the number of trials it takes for the patient to learn the words. If the patient does not eventually learn all the three, recall cannot be meaningfully tested.
- After completing this task, tell the patient, "Try to remember the words, as I will ask for them in a little while."

Attention and Calculation (5 Points)

- Ask the patient to begin with 100 and count backward by sevens. Stop after five subtractions (93, 86, 79, 72, 65). Score the total number of correct answers.
- If the patient cannot or will not perform the subtraction task, ask the patient to spell the word "world" backwards. The score is the number of letters in correct order (e.g., dlrow=5, dlorw=3).

Recall (3 Points)

Ask the patient if he or she can recall the three words you previously asked him or her to remember. Score the total number of correct answers (0–3).

Language and Praxis (9 Points)

- *Naming*: Show the patient a wrist watch and ask the patient what it is. Repeat with a pencil. Score one point for each correct naming (0–2).
- *Repetition*: Ask the patient to repeat the sentence after you ("No ifs, ands, or buts"). Allow only one trial. Score 0 or 1.
- *Three-stage Command*: Give the patient a piece of blank paper and say, "Take this paper in your right hand, fold it in half, and put it on the floor." Score one point for each part of the command correctly executed.
- *Reading*: On a blank piece of paper print the sentence, "Close your eyes," in letters large enough for the patient to see clearly. Ask the patient to read the sentence and do what it says. Score one point only if the patient actually closes his or her eyes. This is not a test of memory, so you may prompt the patient to "do what it says" after the patient reads the sentence.
- *Writing*: Give the patient a blank piece of paper and ask him or her to write a sentence for you. Do not dictate a sentence; it should be written spontaneously. The sentence must contain a subject and a verb and make sense. Correct grammar and punctuation are not necessary.
- *Copying*: Show the patient the picture of two intersecting pentagons and ask the patient to copy the figure exactly as it is. All ten angles must be present and two must intersect to score one point. Ignore tremor and rotation.

  (Folstein, Folstein and McHugh, 1975).

Interpretation of the MMSE

Method	*Score*	*Interpretation*
Single cutoff	<24	Abnormal
Range	<21 >25	Increased odds of dementia Decreased odds of dementia
Education	21 <23 <24	Abnormal for 8th grade education Abnormal for high school education Abnormal for college education
Severity	24–30 18–23 0–17	No cognitive impairment Mild cognitive impairment Severe cognitive impairment

McGILL PAIN QUESTIONNAIRE

(*Courtesy:* Ronald Melzack)

Patient's Name: ______________ Date: __________ Time: ______ am/pm

PRI: S ________ A ________ E ________ M ________ PRI(T) ________ PPI ________

(1–10) (11–15) (16) (17–20) (1–20)

1. Flickering	_	11. Tiring	_
Quivering	_	Exhausting	_
Pulsing	_	12. Sickening	_
Throbbing	_	Suffocating	_
Beating	_	13. Fearful	_
Pounding	_	Frightful	_
2. Jumping	_	Terrifying	_
Flashing	_	14. Punishing	_
Shooting	_	Gruelling	_
3. Pricking	_	Cruel	_
Boring	_	Vicious	_
Drilling	_	Killing	_
Stabbing	_	15. Wretched	_
Lancinating	_	Blinding	_
4. Sharp	_	16. Annoying	_
Cutting	_	Troublesome	_
Lacerating	_	Miserable	_
5. Pinching	_	Intense	_
Pressing	_	Unbearable	_
Gnawing	_	17. Spreading	_
Champing	_	Radiating	_
Crushing	_	Penetrating	_
6. Tugging	_	Piercing	_
Pulling	_	18. Tight	_
Wrenching	_	Numb	_
7. Hot	_	Drawing	_
Burning	_	Squeezing	_
Scalding	_	Tearing	_
Searing	_	19. Cool	_
8. Tingling	_	Cold	_
Itchy	_	Freezing	_
Smarting	_	20. Nagging	_
Stinging	_	Nauseating	_
9. Dull	_	Agonizing	_
Sore	_	Dreadful	_
Hurting	_	Torturing	_
Aching	_	*PPI*	
Heavy	_	0. No pain	_
10. Tender	_	1. Mild	_
Taut	_	2. Discomforting	_
Rasping	_	3. Distressing	_
Splitting	_	4. Horrible	_
		5. Excruciating	_

Brief	_	Rhythmic	_	Continuous	_
Momentary	_	Periodic	_	Steady	_
Transient	_	Intermittent	_	Constant	_

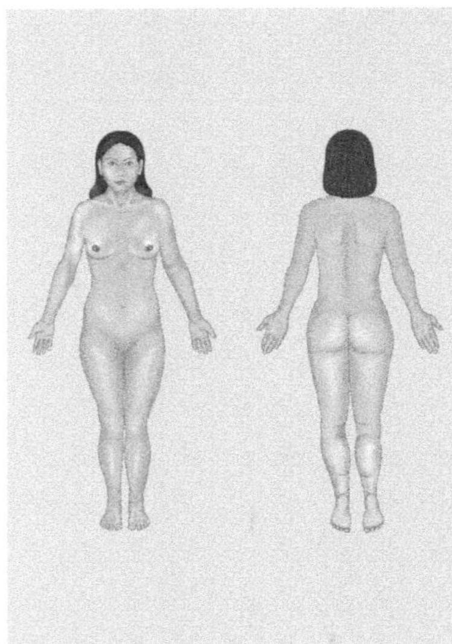

E = External
I = Internal

Comments:

BERG BALANCE SCALE

The Berg Balance Scale (BBS) was developed to measure balance among older people with impairment in balance function by assessing the performance of functional tasks. It is a valid instrument used for evaluation of the effectiveness of interventions and for quantitative descriptions of function in clinical practice and research. The BBS has been evaluated in several reliability studies. A recent study of the BBS, which was completed in Finland, indicates that a change of eight (8) BBS points is required to reveal a genuine change in function between two assessments among older people who are dependent in ADL and living in residential care facilities.

Description

14-item scale designed to measure balance of the older adult in a clinical setting.

Equipment needed: Ruler, two standard chairs (one with arm rests, one without), footstool or step, stopwatch or wrist watch, 15 ft walkway.

Completion

- *Time*: 15–20 minutes
- *Scoring*: A five-point scale, ranging from 0–4. "0" indicates the lowest level of function and "4" the highest level of function. Total score = 56
- *Interpretation*: 41–56 = low fall risk
  21–40 = medium fall risk
  0–20 = high fall risk

A change of 8 points is required to reveal a genuine change in function between 2 assessments.

Name : ____________________ Date : ________________________
Location : ____________________ Rater : ________________________

Item Description — Score (0–4)

- Sitting to standing ________________________
- Standing unsupported ________________________
- Sitting unsupported ________________________
- Standing to sitting ________________________

- Transfers ______
- Standing with eyes closed ______
- Standing with feet together ______
- Reaching forward with outstretched arm ______
- Retrieving object from floor ______
- Turning to look behind ______
- Turning 360° ______
- Placing alternate foot on stool ______
- Standing with one foot in front ______
- Standing on one foot ______

Total ______

General Instructions

Please document each task and/or give instructions as written. When scoring, please record the lowest response category that applies for each item.

In most items, the subject is asked to maintain a given position for a specific time. Progressively more points are deducted, if:

- The time or distance requirements are not met
- The subject's performance warrants supervision
- The subject touches an external support or receives assistance from the examiner.

Subject should understand that they must maintain their balance while attempting the tasks. The choices of which leg to stand on or how far to reach are left to the subject. Poor judgment will adversely influence the performance and the scoring.

Equipment required for testing is a stopwatch or watch with a second hand, and a ruler or other indicator of 2, 5, and 10 inches. Chairs used during testing should be a reasonable height. Either a step or a stool of average step height may be used for item # 12.

Sitting to Standing

Instructions: Please stand up. Try not to use your hand for support.

( ) 4 able to stand without using hands and stabilize independently
( ) 3 able to stand independently using hands
( ) 2 able to stand using hands after several tries
( ) 1 needs minimal aid to stand or stabilize
( ) 0 needs moderate or maximal assist to stand

Standing Unsupported

Instructions: Please stand for two minutes without holding on.

( ) 4 able to stand safely for 2 minutes
( ) 3 able to stand for 2 minutes with supervision
( ) 2 able to stand for 30 seconds unsupported
( ) 1 needs several tries to stand for 30 seconds unsupported
( ) 0 unable to stand for 30 seconds unsupported

If a subject is able to stand for 2 minutes unsupported, score full points for sitting unsupported. Proceed to item #4.

Sitting with Back Unsupported but Feet Supported on the Floor or on a Stool

Instructions: Please sit with arms folded for 2 minutes

( ) 4 able to sit safely and securely for 2 minutes
( ) 3 able to sit for 2 minutes under supervision
( ) 2 able to sit for 30 seconds
( ) 1 able to sit for 10 seconds
( ) 0 unable to sit without support for 10 seconds

Standing to Sitting

Instructions: Please sit down.

( ) 4 sits safely with minimal use of hands
( ) 3 controls descent by using hands
( ) 2 uses back of legs against chair to control descent
( ) 1 sits independently but has uncontrolled descent
( ) 0 needs assist to sit

Transfers

Instructions: Arrange chair (s) for pivot transfer. Ask the subject to transfer one way toward a seat with armrests and one way toward a seat without armrests. You may use two chairs (one with and one without armrests) or a bed and a chair.

( ) 4 able to transfer safely with minor use of hands
( ) 3 able to transfer safely with definite need of hands
( ) 2 able to transfer with verbal cuing and/or supervision
( ) 1 needs one person to assist
( ) 0 needs two people to assist or supervise to be safe

Standing Unsupported with Eyes Closed

Instructions: Please close your eyes and stand still for 10 seconds.

( ) 4 able to stand for 10 seconds safely
( ) 3 able to stand for 10 seconds with supervision
( ) 2 able to stand for 3 seconds
( ) 1 unable to keep eyes closed for 3 seconds but stays safely
( ) 0 needs help to keep from falling

Standing Unsupported with Feet Together

Instructions: Place your feet together and stand without holding on.

( ) 4 able to place feet together independently and stand for 1 minute safely
( ) 3 able to place feet together independently and stand for 1 minute with supervision
( ) 2 able to place feet together independently but unable to hold for 30 seconds
( ) 1 needs help to attain position but able to stand for 15 seconds with feet together
( ) 0 needs help to attain the position and unable to hold for 15 seconds

Reaching Forward with Outstretched Arm while Standing

Instructions: Lift arm to 90°. Stretch out your fingers and reach forward as far as you can. (Examiner places a ruler at the end of fingertips when arm is at 90°. Fingers should not touch the ruler while reaching forward. The recorded measure is the distance forward that the fingers reach while the subject is in the most forward lean position. When possible, ask the subject to use both arms when reaching to avoid rotation of the trunk).

( ) 4 can reach forward confidently 25 cm (10 inches)
( ) 3 can reach forward 12 cm (5 inches)
( ) 2 can reach forward 5 cm (2 inches)
( ) 1 reaches forward but needs supervision
( ) 0 loses balance while trying/requires external support

Pick up Object from the Floor from a Standing Position

Instructions: Pick up the shoe/slipper, which is in front of your feet.

( ) 4 able to pick up slipper safely and easily
( ) 3 able to pick up slipper but needs supervision
( ) 2 unable to pick up but reaches 2–5 cm (1–2 inches) from slipper and keeps balance independently
( ) 1 unable to pick up and needs supervision while trying
( ) 0 unable to try/needs assist to keep from losing balance or falling

Turning to Look Behind over Left and Right Shoulders while Standing

Instructions: Turn to look directly behind you over toward the left shoulder. Repeat to the right. (Examiner may pick an object to look at directly behind the subject to encourage a better twist turn).

( ) 4 looks behind from both sides and weight shifts well
( ) 3 looks behind one side only other side shows less weight shift
( ) 2 turns sideways only but maintains balance
( ) 1 needs supervision when turning
( ) 0 needs assist to keep from losing balance or falling

Turn 360 Degrees

Instructions: Turn completely around in a full circle. Pause. Then turn a full circle in the other direction.

( ) 4 able to turn 360° safely in 4 seconds or less
( ) 3 able to turn 360° safely one side only for 4 seconds or less
( ) 2 able to turn 360° safely but slowly
( ) 1 needs close supervision or verbal cuing
( ) 0 needs assistance while turning

Place Alternate Foot on a Step or Stool while Standing Unsupported

Instructions: Place each foot alternately on the step/stool. Continue until each foot has touched the step/stool four times.

( ) 4 able to stand independently and safely and complete 8 steps in 20 seconds

( ) 3 able to stand independently and complete 8 steps in > 20 seconds
( ) 2 able to complete 4 steps without aid with supervision
( ) 1 able to complete > 2 steps needs minimal assist
( ) 0 needs assistance to keep from falling/unable to try

Standing Unsupported One Foot in Front

Instructions: (Demonstrate to subject) Place one foot directly in front of the other. If you feel that you cannot place your foot directly in front, try to step far enough ahead that the heel of your forward foot is ahead of the toes of the other foot. (To score 3 points, the length of the step should exceed the length of the other foot and the width of the stance should approximate the subject's normal stride width).

( ) 4 able to place foot in tandem independently and hold for 30 seconds
( ) 3 able to place foot ahead independently and hold for 30 seconds
( ) 2 able to take small step independently and hold for 30 seconds
( ) 1 needs help to step but can hold for 15 seconds
( ) 0 loses balance while stepping or standing

Standing on One Leg

Instructions: Stand on one leg as long as you can without holding on.

( ) 4 able to lift leg independently and hold for > 10 seconds
( ) 3 able to lift leg independently and hold for 5–10 seconds
( ) 2 able to lift leg independently and hold for ≥ 3 seconds
( ) 1 tries to lift leg unable to hold for 3 seconds but remains standing independently
( ) 0 unable to try of needs assist to prevent fall
( ) Total score (Maximum = 56)

TINETTI BALANCE ASSESSMENT TOOL

(Tinetti ME, Williams TF, Mayewski R. Fall Risk Index for elderly patients based on number of chronic disabilities. Am J Med. 1986;80:429-34.)

Patient's Name : ____________________________

DoB : ____________________________

Ward : ____________________________

Balance Section

Patient is seated in hard, armless chair:

	Date		
Sitting balance	Leans or slides in chair = 0 Steady, safe = 1		
Rises from chair	Unable, without help = 0 Able, uses arms to help = 1 Able, without use of arms = 2		
Attempts to rise	Unable to, without help = 0 Able, requires > 1 attempt = 1 Able to rise, 1 attempt = 2		
Immediate standing balance (first 5 seconds)	Unsteady (staggers, moves feet, trunk sway) = 0 Steady but uses walker or other support = 1 Steady without walker or other support = 2		
Standing balance	Unsteady = 0 Steady but wide stance and uses support = 1 Narrow stance without support = 2		
Nudged	Begins to fall = 0 Staggers, grabs, catches self = 1 Steady = 2		
Eyes closed	Unsteady = 0 Steady = 1		
Turning 360°	Discontinuous steps = 0 Continuous = 1		
	Unsteady (grabs, staggers) = 0 Steady = 1		
Sitting down	Unsafe (misjudged distance, falls into chair) = 0 Uses arms or not a smooth motion = 1 Safe, smooth motion = 2		
	Balance score	/16	/16

Gait Section

The patient stands with therapist, walks across room (+/- aids), first at usual pace, then at rapid pace.

	Date		
Indication of gait (Immediately after told to 'go')	Any hesitancy or multiple attempts = 0 No hesitancy = 1		
Step length and height	Step to = 0 Step through R = 1 Step through L = 1		
Foot clearance	Foot drop = 0 L foot clears floor = 1 R foot clears floor = 1		
Step symmetry	Right and left step length not equal = 0 Right and left step length appear equal = 1		
Step continuity	Stopping or discontinuity between steps = 0 Steps appear continuous = 1		
Path	Marked deviation = 0 Mild/moderate deviation or uses w. aid = 1 Straight without w. aid = 2		
Trunk	Marked sway or uses w. aid = 0 No sway but flex. knees or back or uses arms for stability = 1 No sway, flex., use of arms or w. aid = 2		
Walking time	Heels apart = 0 Heels almost touching while walking = 1		
	Gait score	/12	/12
	Balance score carried forward	/16	/16
	Total score = Balance + Gait score	/28	/28

Risk Indicators:

Tinetti Tool Score	Risk of Falls
≤18	High
19–23	Moderate
≥24	Low

THE BARTHEL INDEX

Patient name : ______________________________
Rater name : ______________________________
Date : ______________________________

Activity *Score*

FEEDING
- 0 = unable
- 5 = needs help in cutting, spreading butter, etc., or requires modified diet
- 10 = independent ________

BATHING
- 0 = dependent
- 5 = independent (or in shower) ________

GROOMING
- 0 = needs help with personal care
- 5 = independent face/hair/teeth/shaving (implements provided) ________

DRESSING
- 0 = dependent
- 5 = needs help but can do about half unaided
- 10 = independent (including buttons, zips, laces, etc.) ________

BOWELS
- 0 = incontinent (or needs to be given enemas)
- 5 = occasional accident
- 10 = continent ________

BLADDER
- 0 = incontinent, or catheterized and unable to manage alone
- 5 = occasional accident
- 10 = continent ________

TOILET USE
- 0 = dependent
- 5 = needs some help, but can do something alone
- 10 = independent (on and off, dressing, wiping) ________

TRANSFERS (BED TO CHAIR AND BACK)
- 0 = unable, no sitting balance
- 5 = major help (one or two people, physical), can sit
- 10 = minor help (verbal or physical)
- 15 = independent ________

MOBILITY (ON LEVEL SURFACES)

0 = immobile or < 50 yards
5 = wheelchair independent, including corners, > 50 yards
10 = walks with help of one person (verbal or physical) > 50 yards
15 = independent (but may use any aid; for example, stick) > 50 yards ________

STAIRS

0 = unable
5 = needs help (verbal, physical, carrying aid)
10 = independent ________

TOTAL (0–100): ____________

The Barthel Activities of Daily Living (ADL) Index: Guidelines

- The index should be used as a record of what a patient does, not as a record of what a patient could do.
- The main aim is to establish degree of independence from any help, physical or verbal, however minor and for whatever reason.
- The need for supervision renders the patient not independent.
- A patient's performance should be established using the best available evidence. Asking the patient, friends/relatives and nurses is the usual source, but direct observation and common sense are also important. However, direct testing is not needed.
- Usually the patient's performance over the preceding 24–48 hours is important, but occasionally longer periods will be relevant.
- Middle categories imply that the patient supplies over 50% of the effort.
- Use of aids to be independent is allowed.

FUNCTIONAL INDEPENDENCE MEASURE™ AND FUNCTIONAL ASSESSMENT MEASURE

Brain Injury

Scale

7 Complete independence (timely, safely)
6 Modified independence (extra time, devices)
5 Supervision (cuing, coaxing, prompting)
4 Minimal assist (performs 75% or more of task)
3 Moderate assist (performs 50–74% of task)
2 Maximal assist (performs 25–49% of task)
1 Total assist (performs less than 25% of task)

SELF-CARE ITEMS	Adm	Goal	D/C	F/U
1. Feeding				
2. Grooming				
3. Bathing				
4. Dressing upper body				
5. Dressing lower body				
6. Toileting				
7. Swallowing*				
SPHINCTER CONTROL				
8. Bladder management				
9. Bowel management				
MOBILITY ITEMS (Type of Transfer)				
10. Bed, chair, wheelchair ____________				
11. Toilet ____________				
12. Tub or shower ____________				
13. Car transfer* ____________				
LOCOMOTION				
14. Walking/Wheelchair (circle)				
15. Stairs				
16. Community access*				

COMMUNICATION ITEMS

17. Comprehension–Audio/Visual (circle)
18. Expression–Verbal, Non-verbal (circle)
19. Reading*
20. Writing*
21. Speech intelligibility*

PSYCHOSOCIAL ADJUSTMENT

22. Social interaction
23. Emotional status*
24. Adjustment to limitations*
25. Employability*

COGNITIVE FUNCTION

26. Problem solving
27. Memory
28. Orientation*
29. Attention*
30. Safety judgement*

**FAM items*

	Admt	Date	D/C	Date		Admt	Date	D/C	Date
RN	____	____	____	____	ST	____	____	____	____
PT	____	____	____	____	PSY	____	____	____	____
OT	____	____	____	____	REC	____	____	____	____

FUGL-MEYER ASSESSMENT OF PHYSICAL PERFORMANCE

General Procedure and Rules	
Procedure	*General Rules*
Description: This assessment is a measure of upper extremity (UE) and lower extremity (LE) motor and sensory impairment. *Equipment:* A chair, bedside table, reflex hammer, cotton ball, pencil, small piece of cardboard or paper, small can, tennis ball, stop watch, and blindfold. *Administration:* The complete assessment usually requires 45 minutes.	Perform the assessment in a quiet area when the patient is maximally alert. *Volitional movement assessment:* This includes flexor synergy, extensor synergy, movement combining synergies, movement out of synergy, wrist, hand, and coordination/speed. For all tests of volitional motion, these guidelines are to be followed: 1. Give clear and concise instructions. Mime as well as verbal instructions permissible. 2. Have patient perform the movement with non-affected extremity first. On affected side, check for available passive range of motion (PROM) prior to asking patient to perform the movement. 3. Repeat each movement 3x on the affected side and score best performance. If full score is attained on trials 1 or 2, do not have to repeat 3 times. Only test Coordination/speed, one time. 4. Do not assist patient, however verbal encouragement is permitted. 5. Test the wrist and hand function independently of the arm. During the wrist tests, support under the elbow may be provided to decrease demand at the shoulder; however, the patient should be activating the elbow flexors during the elbow at 90° tests and activating the elbow extensors during the elbow at 0 ° tests. In contrast, assistance can be provided to the arm at the elbow and just proximal to the wrist in order to position the arm during the hand tests.

Fugl-Meyer Motor Assessment		
Lower extremity		
Item	*Procedure*	*Scoring*
I. Reflex activity	• Patient is supine or sitting. • Attempt to elicit the Achilles and patellar reflexes. • Assess the unaffected side first. • Test affected side.	• *Scoring* (Maximum possible score = 4): – (0)—No reflex activity can be elicited; – (2)—Reflex activity can be elicited. Items to be scored are Achilles and patellar reflexes.
IIA. Flexor synergy	• Patient is supine. • Have patient perform movement with unaffected side first. • On the affected side, check patient's available PROM at each joint to be tested. • Start with leg fully extended at hip, knee, and ankle. Instruct the patient to "bring your knee to your chest and pull up your toes" (therapist is observing for evidence of hip, knee, ankle flexion in order to assess the presence of all components of the flexor synergy). Therapist can cue the patient to move any missing component. • Test 3x on the affected side and score best movement at each joint.	• *Scoring* (Maximum possible score = 6): – (0)—Cannot be performed at all – (1)—Partial motion – (2)—Full motion • Items to be scored are: Hip flexion, knee flexion, ankle dorsiflexion.
IIB. Extensor synergy	• Patient is sidelying. • Have patient perform movement with unaffected side first. • On the affected side, check patient's available PROM at each joint to be tested. • Start in 90° hip flexion, 90° knee flexion and ankle dorsiflexion.	• *Scoring* (Maximum possible score = 8): – (0)—No motion – (1)—Partial motion – (2)—Full motion • Items to be scored are: Hip extension, hip adduction, knee extension, ankle plantar flexion.

Contd...

Contd...

Item	*Procedure*	*Scoring*
	• Instruct the patient to "push your foot down and kick down and back" (Ankle plantar flexion, knee extension, hip adduction and hip extension) • Slight resistance should be applied in adduction which is gravity-assisted in this position to ensure patient is actively adducting. • Test 3x on the affected side and score best movement at each joint.	
III. Movement combining synergies (in sitting)	*3a. Knee flexion beyond 90°:* • Patient is sitting, feet on floor, with knees free of chair. Knee to be tested is slightly extended beyond 90° knee flexion. Calf muscles should not be on stretch. To decrease friction, patient's shoes can be removed, but socks should remain on. • Have patient perform movement with unaffected side first. • Check patient's available PROM on the affected side for this motion. • Patient is instructed to "pull your heel back and under the chair." • Test 3x on the affected side and score best movement.	• *Scoring (Maximum possible score = 2)*: – (0)—No active motion – (1)—From slightly extended position, knee can be flexed but not beyond 90° or hip flexes while attempting to flex knee – (2)—Knee flexion beyond 90°
	3b. Ankle dorsiflexion: • Patient is sitting, feet on floor, with knees free of chair. Calf muscles should not be on stretch. • Have patient perform movement with unaffected side first. • On the affected side, check patient's available PROM at the ankle joint. • Patient is instructed to "keeping your heel on the floor, lift your foot." • Test 3x on the affected side and score best movement.	• *Scoring (Maximum possible score = 2)*: – (0)—No active motion – (1)—Incomplete active flexion (heel must remain on floor with medial and lateral borders of the forefoot clearing the floor during dorsiflexion) – (2)—Normal dorsiflexion (full within available ROM, heel remains on the floor)

Contd...

Contd...

Item	*Procedure*	*Scoring*
IV. Movement out of synergy (Standing, hip at 0°)	*4a. Knee Flexion:* • Patient is standing, hip at 0° (or full available ROM up to 0°). On leg that is being tested, hip is at 0° (or full available ROM up to 0°), but the knee is flexed, and the patient's toes are touching the floor slightly behind. Evaluator can provide assistance to maintain balance and patient can rest hands on a table. • Have patient perform movement with unaffected side first. • Check patient's available PROM on the affected side for this motion. • Patient is instructed to "keeping your hip back, kick your bottom with your heel." • Test 3x on the affected side and score best movement.	• *Scoring (Maximum possible score = 2)*: – (0)—Knee cannot flex without hip flexion – (1)—Knee flexion begins without hip flexion but does not reach to 90° or hip begins to flex in later phase of motion – (2)—Knee flexion beyond 90° (Knee flexion beyond 90° with hip maintained in extension)
	4b. Ankle dorsiflexion: • Patient is standing, hip at 0°. If patient's calf muscle length is limiting active dorsiflexion in this starting position, then leg that is being tested can be positioned forward, so the hip is at approximately 5° of flexion, and calf muscles are in lengthened position. Knee must stay fully extended. Evaluator can provide assistance to maintain balance and patient can rest hands on a table. • Have patient perform movement with unaffected side first. • On the affected side, check patient's available dorsiflexion PROM. • Patient is instructed to "keeping your knee extended and your heel on the floor, lift your foot." • Test 3x on the affected side and score best movement	• *Scoring (Maximum possible score = 2)*: – (0)—No active motion – (1)—Partial motion (less than full available range with knee extended; heel must remain on floor with medial and lateral borders of the forefoot clearing the floor during dorsiflexion, or hip and/or knee flexes during motion while attempting dorsiflexion) – (2)—Full motion (within available dorsiflexion range with knee extended and heel on the floor)

Contd...

Contd...

Item	*Procedure*	*Scoring*
V. *Normal reflexes (sitting)*:	• This item is only included if the patient achieves a maximum score on all previous lower extremity items, otherwise score 0. • The examiner shall elicit patellar and Achilles phasic reflexes with a reflex hammer and knee flexors with quick stretch of the affected leg and note if the reflexes are hyperactive or not.	• *Scoring (Maximum possible score = 2)*: – (0)—At least 2 of the 3 phasic reflexes are markedly hyperactive – (1)—One reflex is markedly hyperactive or at least 2 reflexes are lively – (2)—No more than one reflex is lively and none are hyperactive
VI. *Coordination/ speed—Sitting*: Heel to opposite knee repetitions in rapid succession	• Patient positioned in sitting with eyes open. • Starting position is with heel to be tested resting on opposite ankle. • Have patient perform movement with unaffected side first. • Check available PROM on the affected side. • Patient is instructed to "Bring your heel from your opposite ankle to your opposite knee, keeping your heel on your shin bone, move as fast as possible." • Use a stopwatch to time how long it takes the patient to do 5 full (ankle to knee to ankle) repetitions.	• *Scoring Tremor (Maximum possible score = 2)*: – (0)—Marked tremor – (1)—Slight tremor – (2)—No tremor • *Scoring Dysmetria* (Maximum possible score = 2): – (0)—Pronounced or unsystematic dysmetria – (1)—Slight or systematic dysmetria – (2)—No dysmetria

Contd...

Contd...

Item	*Procedure*	*Scoring*
	• Use the full achieved active ROM on the unaffected limb as the comparison for the affected limb. If active ROM of affected limb is significantly less than that of unaffected limb, patient should be scored "0" for speed. • Repeat the same movement with the affected leg. Record the time for both the unaffected and affected sides. Observe for evidence of tremor or dysmetria during the movement • *Note:* This item attempts to discriminate between basal ganglia, thalamic, or cerebellar strokes in which tremor or dysmetria may result as a direct result of lesion to these areas. The majority of stroke cases are in the middle cerebral artery or basilar artery distributions where we expect to observe paralysis that affects movement speed but does not cause tremor or dysmetria. In cases of complete paralysis, observe for any indication of tremor or dysmetria that may be evident in face, voice, arms or legs. If there are no indicators of tremor or dysmetria, then score these items 2 and score speed 0.	• *Scoring Speed* (Maximum possible score = 2): – (0)—Activity is more than 6 seconds longer than unaffected leg – (1)—2–5.9 seconds longer than unaffected leg – (2)—less than 2 seconds difference

Upper Extremity		
Item	*Instructions*	*Scoring*
I. Reflex activity	• Patient is sitting. • Attempt to elicit the biceps and triceps reflexes. • Test reflexes on unaffected side first. • Test affected side.	• *Scoring (Maximum possible score = 4)*: – (0)—No reflex activity can be elicited – (2)—Reflex activity can be elicited
II. Flexor synergy	• Patient is sitting. • Have patient perform movement with unaffected side first. • On the affected side, check patient's available PROM at each joint to be tested. • The starting position should be that of full extensor synergy. If the patient cannot actively achieve the starting position, the limb may be passively placed extended towards opposite knee in shoulder adduction/internal rotation, elbow extension, and forearm pronation. • Instruct the patient to fully supinate his/her forearm, flex the elbow, and bring the hand to the ear of the affected side. The shoulder should be abducted at least 90°. • Test 3x on the affected side and score best movement at each joint	• *Scoring (Maximum possible score = 12)*: – (0)—Cannot be performed at all – (1)—Performed partly – (2)—Performed faultlessly • Items to be scored are: Elevation (scapular), shoulder retraction (scapular), shoulder abduction (at least 90°) and external rotation, elbow flexion, and forearm supination.

Contd...

Contd...

Item	*Instructions*	*Scoring*
III. Extensor synergy	• Patient is sitting. • Have patient perform movement with unaffected side first. • On the affected side, check patient's available PROM at each joint to be tested. • The starting position should be that the limb is passively placed at patient's side in elbow flexion and supination. The examiner must ensure that the patient does not rotate and flex the trunk forward, thereby allowing gravity to assist with the movement. The pectoralis major and triceps brachii tendons may be palpated to assess active movement. • Instruct the patient to adduct and internally rotate the shoulder, extend his arm towards the unaffected knee with the forearm pronated. • Test 3x on the affected side and score best movement at each joint.	• *Scoring (Maximum possible score = 6)*: – (0)—Cannot be performed at all – (1)—Performed partly – (2)—Performed faultlessly • Items to be scored are: Shoulder adduction/internal rotation, elbow extension, and forearm pronation.
IV. Movement combining synergies The patient is asked to perform three separate movements (4a, 4b, 4c).	*4a. Hand to lumbar spine:* • Patient is sitting with arm at side, shoulder at 0°, elbow at 0°. • Have patient perform movement with unaffected side first. • Check patient's available PROM on the affected side for this motion. • Patient is instructed to actively position the affected hand on the lumbar spine by asking them to "put your hand behind your back". • Test 3x on the affected side and score best movement.	• Scoring *(Maximum possible score = 2)*: – (0)—No specific action is performed (or patient moves but does not reach ASIS) – (1)—Hand must pass anterior superior iliac spine (performed partly) – (2)—Performed faultlessly (patient clears ASIS and can extend arm behind back towards sacrum; full elbow extension is not required to score a 2)

Contd...

Contd...

Item	*Instructions*	*Scoring*
	4b. Shoulder flexion to 90°, elbow at 0°: • Patient is sitting with hand resting on lap. • Have patient perform movement with unaffected side first. • On the affected side, check patient's available PROM for shoulder flexion to 90° and full elbow extension. • Patient is instructed to flex the shoulder to 90°, keeping the elbow extended. The elbow must be fully extended throughout the shoulder flexor movement; the forearm can be in pronation or in a mid-position between pronation and supination. • Test 3x on the affected side and score best movement.	• *Scoring (Maximum possible score = 2):* – (0)—Arm is immediately abducted, or elbow flexes at start of motion – (1)—Abduction or elbow flexion occurs in later phase of motion – (2)—Performed faultlessly (patient can flex shoulder keeping elbow extended)
	4c. Pronation/supination of forearm, elbow at 90°, shoulder at 0°: • Patient is sitting with arm at side, elbow flexed, and forearm in supination. • Have patient perform movement with unaffected side first. • On the affected side, check patient's available PROM for end range of pronation and supination. • Patient is instructed to actively flex the elbow to 90° and pronate/supinate the forearm through the full available ROM. • Test 3x on the affected side and score best movement.	• *Scoring (Maximum possible score = 2):* – (0)—Correct position of shoulder held in adduction at side of body and elbow flexion, and/or pronation or supination cannot be performed. – (1)—Active pronation or supination can be performed even within a limited range of motion, with elbow flexed at 90° and arm at side. – (2)—Complete pronation and supination with elbow flexed at 90° and arm at side.

Contd...

Contd...

Item	*Instructions*	*Scoring*
V. *Movement out of synergy*: The patient is asked to perform three separate movements (5a, 5b, 5c).	*5a. Shoulder abduction to 90°, elbow at 0°, and forearm pronated:* • Patient is sitting with arm and hand resting at side. • Have patient perform movement with unaffected side first. • Check patient's available PROM on the affected side for this motion. • Patient is instructed to abduct the shoulder to 90°, in a pure abduction motion, with the elbow fully extended and the forearm pronated. • Test 3x on the affected side and score best movement.	• *Scoring (Maximum possible score = 2)*: – (0)—Initial elbow flexion occurs, or any deviation from pronated forearm occurs – (1)—Motion can be performed partly, or, if during motion, elbow is flexed, or forearm cannot be kept in pronation; – (2)—Performed faultlessly (patient can fully abduct shoulder, keeping forearm pronated with no elbow flexion)
	5b. Shoulder flexion from 90–180°, elbow at 0°, and forearm in mid-position: • Patient is sitting with elbow extended, hand resting on knee. • Have patient perform movement with unaffected side first. • Check patient's available PROM on the affected side for this motion. • Patient is instructed to flex the shoulder above 90°, with the elbow fully extended and the forearm in the mid-position between pronation and supination. • Test 3x on the affected side and score best movement.	• *Scoring (Maximum possible score = 2)*: – (0)—Initial flexion of elbow or shoulder abduction occurs (arm is immediately abducted, or elbow flexes at start of motion) – (1)—Elbow flexion or shoulder abduction occurs during shoulder flexion (in later phases of motion) – (2)—Performed faultlessly (patient can flex shoulder above, with forearm in mid-position and no elbow flexion)

Contd...

Contd...

Item	*Instructions*	*Scoring*
	5c. Pronation/supination of forearm, elbow at 0°, and shoulder at 30–90° of flexion: • Patient is sitting with elbow extended, shoulder between 30–90° of flexion. • Have patient perform movement with unaffected side first. • Check patient's available PROM on the affected side for this motion. • Patient is instructed to pronate and supinate the forearm as the shoulder remains flexed between 30–90° and the elbow is fully extended. • Test 3x on the affected side and score best movement.	• *Scoring (Maximum possible score = 2)*: – (0)—Supination and pronation cannot be performed at all, or elbow and shoulder positions cannot be attained – (1)—Elbow and shoulder properly positioned and supination performed in a limited range – (2)—Performed faultlessly (complete pronation and supination with correct positions at elbow and shoulder)
VI. *Normal Reflexes (sitting)*:	• This item is only included if the patient achieves a maximum score on all previous upper extremity items, otherwise score 0. • The examiner shall elicit biceps and triceps phasic reflexes with a reflex hammer and finger flexors with quick stretch and note if the reflexes are hyperactive or not.	• *Scoring (Maximum possible score = 2)*: – (0)—At least 2 of the 3 phasic reflexes are markedly hyperactive – (1)—One reflex is markedly hyperactive or at least 2 reflexes are lively – (2)—No more than one reflex is lively, and none are hyperactive

Contd...

Contd...

Item	*Instructions*	*Scoring*
VII. *Wrist*: During the wrist tests, support under the elbow to may be provided to decrease demand at the shoulder; however, the patient should be activating the elbow flexors during the elbow at 90° tests and activating the elbow extensors during the elbow at 0° tests. The patient is asked to perform five separate movements (7a, 7b, 7c, 7d, 7e).	*7a. Stability, elbow at 90°, and shoulder at 0°*: • Patient is sitting with arm and hand resting at side. • Have patient perform movement with unaffected side first. • Check patient's available PROM on the affected side for this motion. • Patient is instructed to dorsiflexion (extend) the wrist to the full range of 15° (or full available range) with the elbow at 90° flexion and the shoulder at 0°. If full range of dorsiflexion is attained, slight resistance is given. • Test 3x on the affected side and score best movement.	• *Scoring (Maximum possible score = 2)*: – (0)—Patient cannot dorsiflexion wrist to required 15° – (1)—Dorsiflexion is accomplished, but no resistance is taken – (2)—Position can be maintained with some (slight) resistance
	7b. Flexion/extension, elbow at 90°, and shoulder at 0°: • Patient is sitting with arm and hand resting at side. • Have patient perform movement with unaffected side first. • Patient is instructed to perform repeated smooth alternating movements from 15° of flexion (wrist extension) to 15° of extension. • Test 3x on the affected side and score best movement	• *Scoring (Maximum possible score = 2)*: – (0)—Volitional movement does not occur – (1)—Patient cannot actively move through the wrist joint throughout the total range of motion – (2)—Faultless, smooth movement (repetitive through full available ROM)

Contd...

Contd...

Item	*Instructions*	*Scoring*
	7c. Stability, elbow at 0°, and shoulder at 30° flexion: • Patient is sitting with elbow extended, hand resting on knee and forearm pronated. • Have patient perform movement with unaffected side first. • Check patient's available PROM on the affected side for this motion. • Patient is instructed to dorsiflexion (extend) the wrist to the full range of 15° (or full available range) with the elbow fully extended and the shoulder at 30° flexion. If full range of dorsiflexion is attained, slight resistance is given. • Test 3x on the affected side and score best movement.	• *Scoring (Maximum possible score = 2)*: – (0)—Patient cannot dorsiflexion wrist to required 15° – (1)—Dorsiflexion is accomplished, but no resistance is taken – (2)—Position can be maintained with some (slight) resistance
	7d. Flexion/extension, elbow at 0°, and shoulder at 30° flexion: • Patient is sitting with elbow extended, hand resting on knee and forearm pronated. • Have patient perform movement with unaffected side first. • Patient is instructed to perform repeated smooth alternating movements from maximum dorsiflexion to maximum volar flexion with the fingers somewhat flexed to the full range of 15° (or full available range) with the elbow fully extended and the shoulder at 30° flex. • Test 3x on the affected side and score best movement.	• *Scoring (Maximum possible score = 2)*: – (0)—Volitional movement does not occur – (1)—Patient cannot actively move throughout the total range of motion; – (2)—Faultlessly, smooth movement (repetitive through full ROM)

Contd...

Contd...

Item	*Instructions*	*Scoring*
	7e. Circumduction: • Patient is sitting with arm at side elbow flexed to 90°, and forearm pronated. • Have patient perform movement with unaffected side first. • Check patient's available PROM on the affected side for this motion. • Patient is instructed to circumduct the wrist with smooth alternating movements throughout the full range of circumduction. • Test 3x on the affected side and score best movement.	• *Scoring (Maximum possible score = 2)*: – (0)—Cannot be performed (volitional movement does not occur) – (1)—Jerky motion or incomplete circumduction – (2)—Complete motion with smoothness (performs faultlessly, smooth, repetitive movement through full ROM)
VIII. *Hand*: During the hand tests, assistance can be provided to the arm at the elbow and just proximal to the wrist in order to position the arm for the grasp tasks.	*8a. Finger mass flexion:* 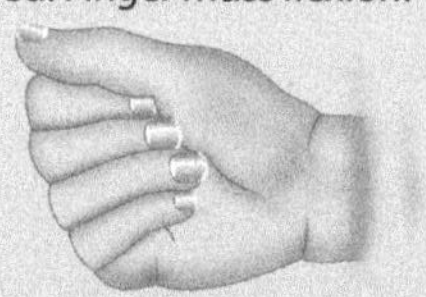 • Patient is sitting with arm on bedside table or lap. • Have patient perform movement with unaffected side first. • Check patient's available PROM on the affected side for this motion. • Starting from the position of finger extension (this may be attained passively, if necessary), instruct the patient to fully flex all fingers. • Test 3x on the affected side and score best movement	• *Scoring (Maximum possible score = 2)*: – (0)—No flexion occurs – (1)—Some flexion, but not full motion – (2)—Completed active flexion (compared to unaffected hand)

Contd...

Contd...

Item	*Instructions*	*Scoring*
The patient is asked to perform seven separate movements (8a, 8b, 8c, 8d, 8e, 8f, 8g). The object is not placed in the hand but presented to the patient so that it requires sufficient opening to grasp test object, closure on object, ability to hold against a slight tug.	*8b. Finger mass extension:* 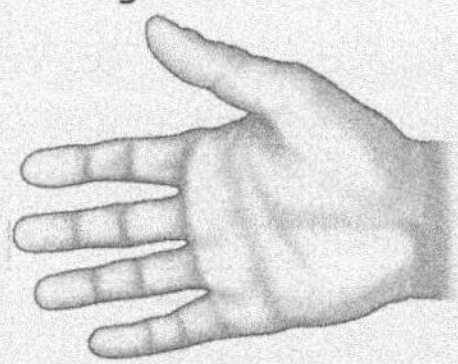 • Patient is sitting with arm on bedside table or lap. • Have patient perform movement with unaffected side first. • Check patient's available PROM on the affected side for this motion. • Starting from the position of finger flexion (this may be attained passively, if necessary), instruct the patient to fully extend all fingers. • Test 3x on the affected side and score best movement.	• *Scoring (Maximum possible score = 2):* – (0)—No extension occurs – (1)—Patient can release an active mass flexion grasp – (2)—Full active extension (compared to unaffected side)
	8c. Grasp I: • Patient is sitting with arm on bedside table. • Have patient perform movement with unaffected side first. • Check patient's available PROM on the affected side for this motion.	• *Scoring (Maximum possible score = 2):* – (0)—Required position cannot be attained – (1)—Grasp is weak – (2)—Grasp can be maintained against relatively great resistance

Contd...

Contd...

Item	*Instructions*	*Scoring*
	• Instruct the patient to extend the metacarpophalangeal joints of digits II-V and flex the proximal and distal interphalangeal joints. Test this grip against resistance. You can tell the patient "pretend you are holding the handle of a briefcase." • Test 3x on the affected side and score best movement.	
	8d. Grasp II: 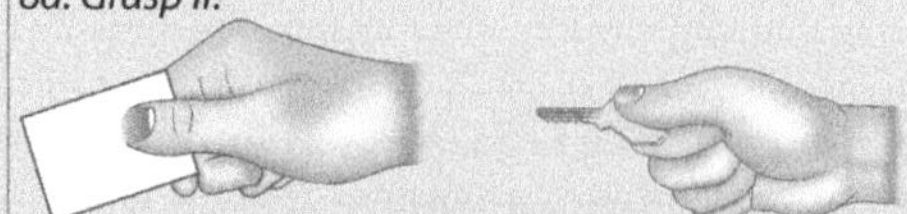 • Patient is sitting with arm on bedside table. • Have patient perform movement with unaffected side first. • Instruct the patient to abduct the thumb to grasp a piece of paper. Then ask the patient to perform pure thumb adduction with the scrap of paper interposed between the thumb and first digit (as in figure). Test this grip against resistance by asking the patient to hold as you attempt to pull the paper out with a slight tug. • Test 3x on the affected side and score best movement.	• *Scoring (Maximum possible score = 2)*: – (0)—Function cannot be performed – (1)—Scrap of paper interposed between the thumb and index finger can be kept in place, but not against a slight tug – (2)—Paper is held firmly against a tug

Contd...

Contd...

Item	*Instructions*	*Scoring*
	8e. Grasp III: 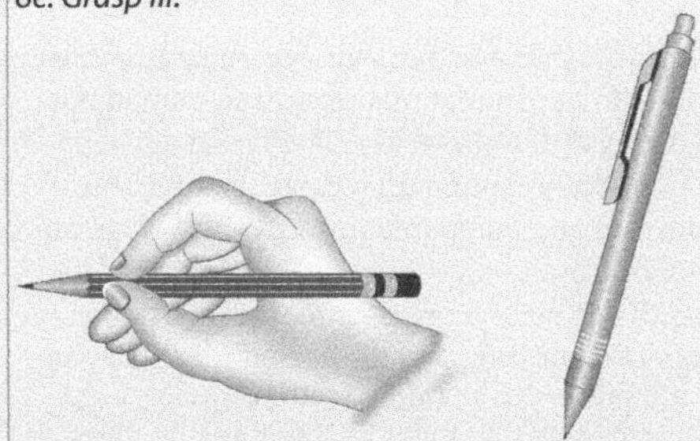 • Patient is sitting with arm on bedside table. • Have patient perform movement with unaffected side first. • Instruct the patient to grasp a pen or pencil by opposing the thumb and index finger pads around the pen. The tester may support the patient's arm but may not assist with the hand function required for the retrieval task. The pen may not be stabilized by the therapist or the patient's other hand. To minimize excessive movement, however, a pen with a 'pocket clip' that prevents rolling more than 180° may be used. • Once the pencil is retrieved, instruct the patient to oppose the thumb pad against the pad of the index finger with a pencil interposed. Test this grip against resistance by asking the patient to hold as you attempt to pull the pencil out with a slight tug upwards. • Test 3x on the affected side and score best movement.	• *Scoring (Maximum possible score = 2)*: – (0)—Function cannot be performed – (1)—A pencil interposed between the thumb pad and the pad of the index finger can be kept in place, but not against a slight tug – (2)—Pencil is held firmly against a tug

Contd...

Contd...

Item	*Instructions*	*Scoring*
	8f. Grasp IV: 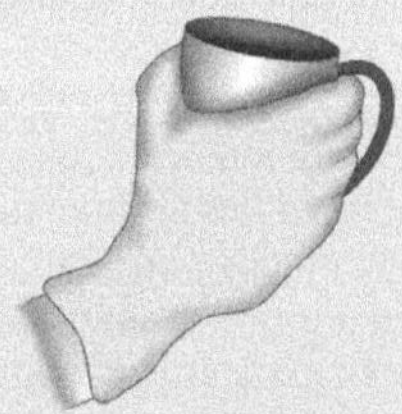 • Patient is sitting with arm on bedside table. • Have patient perform movement with unaffected side first. • Instruct the patient to grasp a small can (placed upright on a table without stabilization) by opening the fingers and opposing the volar surfaces of the thumb and digits. The arm may be supported but the tester may not assist with hand function. • Once the can is grasped, test this grip against resistance by asking the patient to hold as you attempt to pull the can out with a slight tug. Test 3x on the affected side and score best movement.	• *Scoring (Maximum possible score = 2)*: – (0)—Function cannot be performed – (1)—A can interposed between the thumb and index finger can be kept in place, but not against a slight tug – (2)—Can is held firmly against a tug – *Note:* the hand must open and close on the can; it is not acceptable to have the patient grasp can by coming down from the top of the can.

Contd...

Contd...

Item	*Instructions*	*Scoring*
	8g. Grasp V: 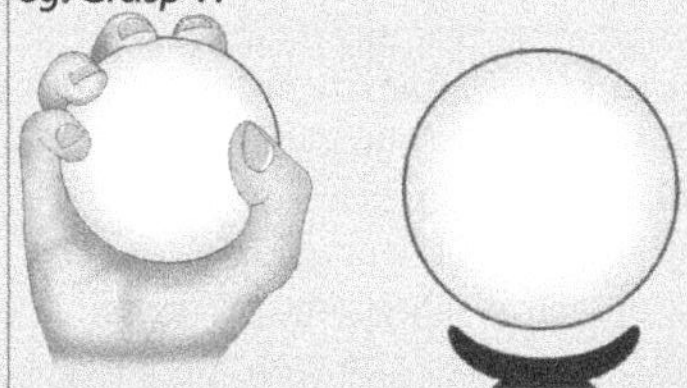 • Patient is sitting with arm on bedside table. • Have patient perform movement with unaffected side first. • Instruct the patient to perform a spherical grasp by grasping a tennis ball. The tester may support the patient's arm but may not assist with the hand function required for the retrieval task. The ball may not be stabilized by the therapist or the patient's other hand. To minimize excessive movement, the ball can be placed on an object that reduces rolling. An inverted medium-sized bottle cap placed under the ball to prevent rolling is acceptable. Once the tennis ball is grasped, test this grip against resistance by asking the patient to hold as you attempt to pull the ball out with a slight tug. • Test 3x on the affected side and score best movement.	• *Scoring (Maximum possible score = 2):* – (0)—Function cannot be performed – (1)—A tennis ball can be kept in place with a spherical grasp, but not against a slight tug – (2)—Tennis ball is held firmly against a tug

Contd...

Contd...

Item	*Instructions*	*Scoring*
IX. *Coordination and speed—Sitting*: Finger to nose (5 repetitions in rapid succession)	• Patient positioned in sitting with eyes open. • Starting position is with hand on lap. • Have patient perform movement with unaffected side first. • Check patient's available PROM on the affected side for this motion. • Patient is instructed to "bring your finger from your knee to your nose, as fast as possible." • Use a stopwatch to time how long it takes the patient to do 5 repetitions. • Repeat the same movement with the affected arm. Record the time for both the unaffected and affected sides. Observe for evidence of tremor or dysmetria during the movement. • *Note*: This item attempts to discriminate between basal ganglia, thalamic, or cerebellar strokes in which tremor or dysmetria may result as a direct result of lesion to these areas. The majority of stroke cases are in the middle cerebral artery or basilar artery where we expect to observe paralysis that affects movement speed but does not cause tremor or dysmetria. In cases of complete paralysis, observe for any indication of tremor or dysmetria that may be evident in face, voice, arms or legs. If there are no indicators of tremor or dysmetria, then score these items 2 and score speed 0. If active ROM of affected limb is significantly less than that of affected limb, patient should be scored "0" for speed.	• *Scoring Tremor (Maximum possible score = 2)*: – (0)—Marked tremor – (1)—Slight tremor – (2)—No tremor • *Scoring Dysmetria (Maximum possible score = 2)*: – (0)- Pronounced or unsystematic dysmetria – (1)—Slight or systematic dysmetria – (2)—No dysmetria • *Scoring Speed (Maximum possible score = 2)*: – (0)—Activity is more than 6 seconds longer than unaffected hand – (1)—(2–5.9) seconds longer than unaffected side – (2)—less than 2 seconds difference

Fugl-Meyer Sensory Assessment		
Light Touch	**Procedure:** • For light touch assessment, area of skin to be touched, should be free of clothing and exposed. • The procedure can be tested in the sitting or supine positions. Explain to the patient with their eyes open, "I am going to touch you with this cotton ball and I would like you to tell me if you can feel that you are being touched." Lightly touch patient with cotton ball over the unaffected muscle belly. Ask them, "Can you feel that you are being touched?" This part of the procedure confirms that the patient understands the test. • Explain to the patient, "I am going to ask you to close your eyes. Then I am going to touch you with the cotton ball on your right/left (unaffected) side followed by your right/left (affected) side. When I ask you, tell me if you can feel the touch." Ask the patient to close their eyes. Lightly touch unaffected area with cotton ball and ask, "Do you feel this?" Lightly touch affected area with cotton ball and ask "Do you feel this?" If the patient says they feel the touch on both sides, then repeat the procedure by touching first the unaffected side immediately followed by the affected side and ask the following question. "Does 'this' (unaffected area touch) feel the same as 'this' (affected area touch)?" The intent is to determine, if there are differences in the characteristics of the touch between the two sides.	• *Scoring :* – (0)—*Absent*: If the patient states that he does not feel the touch on the affected side, the score is absent. – (1)—*Impaired*: If the patient states that he feels the touch on the affected side and the touch does not feel the same between affected and unaffected sides or the response is delayed or unsure, the score is impaired. – (2)—*Intact*: If the patient states that he feels the touch on the affected side and the touch feels the same between affected and unaffected sides, the score is intact.

Contd...

Contd...

	• If the tester is not confident that the patient understands this procedure or that the response is inconsistent, the tester may confirm their impression by using the following procedure. With the eyes closed, touch the patient on the affected side and ask them to point to where they were touched with the unaffected side. If the patient does not recognize that they are being touched, the score would be absent. If they recognize the touch but are not accurate on the localization, the score will be impaired. If they recognize the touch and are accurate on the localization, the score will be intact. **Upper Extremity** • *Upper arm:* Follow above procedure by touching patient over the unaffected and affected biceps muscle belly. • *Palmar surface of the hand:* Follow above procedure by touching patient over the unaffected and affected palmar surface of the hand. **Lower Extremity** • *Thigh:* Follow above procedure by touching patient over the unaffected and affected thigh of the leg. • *Sole of foot:* Follow above procedure by touching patient over the unaffected and affected sole of the foot.	

Contd...

Contd...

Proprio-ception: The objective of this test is to determine a consistent response that is accurate and timely. If unsure, the tester can add additional repetitions to determine, if a missed response is true sensory loss or an error by the patient due to test length not sensory loss.	**Procedure:** • Proprioception can be tested in the sitting or supine positions for the upper extremity and in supine for the lower extremity. Start with the unaffected limb. Explain to the patient with their eyes open, "I am going to move your arm. This is up; this is down (demonstrate test). I want you to close your eyes and tell me if I am moving you up or down." Use the hand positions described below for each joint movement. • Move the joint through a small range of motion (approximately 10° for the limb joints and 5° for the digit joints of the hand and foot). Move the limb at least 3 times in random directions. If the patient is wrong on any direction, then add several more repetitions to determine, if the accuracy is greater than 75% (score 2) or 75% or less (score 1). • Start with the most proximal limb joint on the unaffected side. Move to the same joint on the affected side. The intent is to determine if there are differences in the perception of proprioception between the two sides. For example, if the patient identifies the movement stimulus with the same accuracy and responsiveness of the unaffected side then the score would be 2. However, if the patient is accurate but responses are delayed or unsure then the score would be 1. (At this point, you could ask the patient if the movement on this side feels the same as the other side). No perception of joint movement is scored 0.	• *Scoring*: – (0)—Absent (no sensation) – (1)—Impaired (inconsistent response or three quarters of answers are correct, but considerable difference in sensation compared with unaffected side) – (2)—Intact (all answers are correct, little or no difference).

Contd...

Contd...

	Upper Extremity • *Shoulder:* Therapist supports patient's arm by the medial and lateral epicondyles of the humerus and at the distal ulnar and radius. Have patient look at arm. Move shoulder, saying "This is up. This is down." I am now going to have you close your eyes and I am going to move your shoulder in either direction. I want you to tell me "up" or "down." Randomly move arm approximately 10°, 4 times (more if needed), keeping track of correct responses. • *Elbow:* Therapist supports patient's arm by the medial and lateral epicondyles and the distal ulnar and radius. Have patient look at elbow. Move elbow, saying "This is up. This is down." I am now going to have you close your eyes and I am going to move your elbow in either direction. I want you to tell me "up" or "down." Randomly move elbow approximately 10°, 4 times (more if needed) keeping track of correct responses. • *Wrist:* Therapist supports patient's wrist at the distal ulna and radius and the heads of the 2nd and 5th metacarpal. Have patient look at wrist. Move wrist, saying "This is up. This is down." I am now going to have you close your eyes and I am going to move your wrist in either direction. I want you to tell me "up" or "down." Randomly move wrist approximately 10°, 4 times (more if needed), keeping track of correct responses.	

Contd...

Contd...

	• *Thumb:* Therapist supports patient's thumb proximal to the interphalangeal joint and either side of the most distal aspect of the thumb. Have patient look at thumb. Move thumb at interphalangeal joint, saying "This is up. This is down." I am now going to have you close your eyes and I am going to move your thumb in either direction. I want you to tell me "up" or "down." Randomly move thumb approximately 10°, 4 times (more if needed), keeping track of correct responses. **Lower Extremity** • The hip and knee should be tested in the supine position. The ankle and toe can be tested in the supine or sitting position. • *Hip:* Therapist supports patient's leg at the femoral condyles and the medial and lateral malleolus. Have patient look at leg. Move hip, saying "This is up. This is down." I am now going to have you close your eyes and I am going to move your hip in either direction. I want you to tell me "up" or "down." Randomly move hip approximately 10°, 4 times (more if needed), keeping track of correct responses. • *Knee:* Therapist supports patient's leg at the femoral condyles and the medial and lateral malleolus. Have patient look at knee. Move knee, saying "This is up. This is down." I am now going to have you close your eyes and I am going to move your knee in either direction. I want you to tell me "up" or "down." Randomly move knee approximately 10°, 4 times (more if needed), keeping track of correct responses.	

Contd...

Contd...

	• *Ankle:* Therapist supports patient's leg at the medial and lateral malleoli and the heads of the 1st and 5th metatarsal. Have patient look at ankle. Move ankle, saying "This is up. This is down." I am now going to have you close your eyes and I am going to move your ankle in either direction. I want you to tell me "up" or "down." Randomly move ankle approximately 10°, 4 times (more if needed), keeping track of correct responses. • *Toe:* Therapist supports patient's toe at the interphalangeal joint and either side of the most distal aspect of the great toe. Have patient look at great toe. Move interphalangeal joint, saying "This is up. This is down." I am now going to have you close your eyes and I am going to move your big toe in either direction. I want you to tell me "up" or "down." Randomly move great toe approximately 10°, 4 times (more if needed), keeping track of correct responses.	

Motor Function Upper Extremity				
Test	*Item*	*Score*		*Scoring criteria*
		Pre	*Post*	
I. Reflexes	Biceps			0—No reflex activity can be elicited 2—Reflex activity can be elicited
	Triceps			
II. Flexor synergy	Elevation			0—Cannot be performed at all 1—Performed partly 2—Performed faultlessly
	Shoulder retraction			
	Abduction (at least 90°)			
	External rotation			
	Elbow flexion			
	Forearm supination			
III. Extensor Synergy	Shoulder add./int. rot.			0—Cannot be performed at all 1—Performed partly 2—Performed faultlessly
	Elbow extension			
	Forearm pronation			
IV. Movement combining synergies	Hand to lumbar spine			0—No specific action performed 1—Hand must pass anterior–superior iliac spine 2—Performed faultlessly
	Shoulder flexion to 90°, elbow at 0°			0—Arm is immediately abducted, or elbow flexes at start of motion 1—Abduction or elbow flexion occurs in later phase of motion 2—Performed faultlessly

Contd...

Contd...

Test	*Item*	*Score*		*Scoring criteria*
		Pre	*Post*	
	Pronation/supination of forearm with elbow at 90° and shoulder at 0°			0—Correct position of shoulder and elbow cannot be attained, and/or pronation or supination cannot be performed at all 1—Active pronation or supination can be performed even within a limited range of motion, and at the same time, the shoulder and elbow are correctly positioned 2—Complete pronation and supination with correct positions at elbow and shoulder
V. Movement out of synergy	Shoulder abduction to 90°, elbow at 0°, and forearm pronated			0—Initial elbow flexion occurs, or any deviation from pronated forearm occurs 1—Motion can be performed partly, or, if during motion, elbow is flexed, or forearm cannot be kept in pronation 2—Performed faultlessly
	Shoulder flexion 90–180°, elbow at 0°, and forearm in mid-position			0—Initial flexion of elbow or shoulder abduction occurs 1—Elbow flexion or shoulder abduction occurs during shoulder flexion 2—Performed faultlessly
	Pronation/supination of forearm, elbow at 0° and shoulder between 30–90° of flexion			0—Supination and pronation cannot be performed at all, or elbow and shoulder positions cannot be attained 1—Elbow and shoulder properly positioned and pronation and supination performed in a limited range 2—Performed faultlessly

Contd...

Contd...

Test	*Item*	*Score*		*Scoring criteria*
		Pre	*Post*	
VI. Normal reflex activity	Biceps and/or finger flexors and triceps (This item is only included, if the patient achieves a maximum score on all previous items, otherwise score 0)			0—At least 2 of the 3 phasic reflexes are markedly hyperactive 1—One reflex is markedly hyperactive, or at least 2 reflexes are lively 2—No more than one reflex is lively and none are hyperactive
VII. Wrist	Stability, elbow at 90°, shoulder at 0°			0—Patient cannot dorsiflexion wrist to required 15° 1—Dorsiflexion is accomplished, but no resistance is taken 2—Position can be maintained with some (slight) resistance
	Flexion/extension, elbow at 90°, shoulder at 0°			0—Volitional movement does not occur 1—Patient cannot actively move the wrist joint throughout the total ROM 2—Faultless, smooth movement
	Stability, elbow at 0°, shoulder at 30°			0—Patient cannot dorsiflexion wrist to required 15° 1—Dorsiflexion is accomplished, but no resistance is taken 2—Position can be maintained with some (slight) resistance
	Flexion/extension, elbow at 0°, shoulder at 30°			0—Volitional movement does not occur 1—Patient cannot actively move the wrist joint throughout the total ROM 2—Faultless, smooth movement
	Circumduction			0—Cannot be performed 1—Jerky motion or incomplete circumduction 2—Complete motion with smoothness

Contd...

Contd...

Test	*Item*	*Score*		*Scoring criteria*
		Pre	*Post*	
VIII. Hand	Finger mass flexion			0—No flexion occurs 1—Some flexion, but not full motion 2—Complete active flexion (compared with unaffected hand)
	Finger mass extension			0—No extension occurs 1—Patient can release an active mass flexion grasp 2—Full active extension
	Grasp I: MCP joints extended and proximal and distal IP joints are flexed; grasp is tested against resistance			0—Required position cannot be acquired 1—Grasp is weak 2—Grasp can be maintained against relatively great resistance
	Grasp II: Patient is instructed to adduct thumb, with a scrap of paper interposed			0—Function cannot be performed 1—Scrap of paper interposed between the thumb and index finger can be kept in place, but not against a slight tug 2—Paper is held firmly against a tug
	Grasp III: Patient opposes thumb pad against the pad of index finger, with a pencil interposed			0—Function cannot be performed 1—Pencil interposed between the thumb and index finger can be kept in place, but not against a slight tug 2—Pencil is held firmly against a tug
	Grasp IV: The patient should grasp a can by opposing the volar surfaces of the 1st and 2nd digits.			0—Function cannot be performed 1—A can interposed between the thumb and index finger can be kept in place, but not against a slight tug 2—Can is held firmly against a tug

Contd...

Contd...

Test	*Item*	*Score*		*Scoring criteria*
		Pre	*Post*	
	Grasp V: The patient grasps a tennis ball with a spherical grip or is instructed to place his/her fingers in a position with abduction position of the thumb and abduction flexion of the 2nd, 3rd, 4th and 5th fingers			0—Function cannot be performed 1—A tennis ball can be kept in place with a spherical grasp but not against a slight tug 2—Tennis ball is held firmly against a tug
IX. Coordination/ Speed—Finger from knee to nose (5 repetitions in rapid succession)	Tremor			0—Marked tremor 1—Slight tremor 2—No tremor
	Dysmetria			0—Pronounced or unsystematic dysmetria 1—Slight or systematic dysmetria 2—No dysmetria
	Speed			0—Activity is more than 6 seconds longer than unaffected hand 1—(2–5.9) seconds longer than unaffected hand 2—Less than 2 seconds difference
Upper extremity total		**Maximum = 66**		

Motor Function: Lower Extremity				
Test	*Item*	*Score*		*Scoring criteria*
		Pre	*Post*	
I. Reflex activity	Achilles			0—No reflex activity can be elicited 2—Reflex activity can be elicited
	Patellar			
II. A. Flexor synergy (in supine)	Hip flexion			0—Cannot be performed at all 1—Partial motion 2—Full motion
	Knee flexion			
	Ankle dorsiflexion			
II. B. Extensor synergy (in side lying)	Hip extension			0—Cannot be performed at all 1—Partial motion 2—Full motion
	Adduction Knee extension			
	Ankle plantar flexion			
III. Movement combining synergies (sitting: knees free of chair)	A. Knee flexion beyond 90°			0—No active motion 1—From slightly extended position, knee can be flexed, but not beyond 90° 2— Knee flexion beyond 90°
	B. Ankle dorsiflexion			0—No active flexion 1—Incomplete active flexion 2—Normal dorsiflexion
IV. Movement out of synergy (standing, hip at 0°)	A. Knee flexion			0—Knee cannot flex without hip flexion 1—Knee begins flexion without hip flexion, but does not reach to 90°, or hip flexes during motion 2—Full motion as described

Contd...

Contd...

Test	*Item*	*Score*		*Scoring criteria*
		Pre	*Post*	
	B. Ankle dorsiflexion			0—No active motion 1—Partial motion 2—Full motion
V. Normal reflexes (sitting)	Knee flexors Patellar Achilles (This item is only included, if the patient achieves a maximum score on all previous items, otherwise score 0)			0—At least 2 of the 3 phasic reflexes are markedly hyperactive 1—One reflex is markedly hyperactive, or at least 2 reflexes are lively 2—No more than one reflex is lively and none are hyperactive
VI. Coordination/speed—Sitting: Heel to opposite knee (5 repetitions in rapid succession)	A. Tremor			0—Marked tremor 1—Slight tremor 2—No tremor
	B. Dysmetria			0—Pronounced or unsystematic dysmetria 1—Slight or systematic dysmetria 2— No dysmetria
	C. Speed			0—Activity is more than 6 seconds longer than unaffected side 1—(2–5.9) seconds longer than unaffected side 2—Less than 2 seconds difference
Lower Extremity Total				**Maximum = 34**
Total Motor Score (UE + LE)				**Maximum = 100**

Contd...

Sensation				
Type of sensation	*Item*	*Score*		*Scoring criteria*
		Pre	*Post*	
I. Light Touch	Upper arm			0—Anesthesia 1—Hyperesthesia / dysesthesia 2—Normal
	Palm of hand			
	Thigh			
	Sole of foot			
II. Proprioception	Shoulder			0—No sensation 1—75% of answers are correct, but considerable difference in sensation relative to unaffected side 2—All answers are correct, little or no difference
	Elbow			
	Wrist			
	Thumb			
	Hip			
	Knee			
	Ankle			
	Toe			
Total Sensation Score				**Maximum = 24**
Total Motor and Sensory Score				**Maximum = 124**
Comments	Pre:			
	Post:			

FUNCTIONAL REACH TEST AND MODIFIED FUNCTIONAL REACH INSTRUCTIONS

General information: The functional reach test can be administered while the patient is standing (functional reach) or sitting (modified functional reach).

Functional Reach (Standing Instructions)

- The patient is instructed to next to, but not touching, a wall and position the arm that is closer to the wall at 90° of shoulder flexion with a closed fist.
- The assessor records the starting position at the 3rd metacarpal head on the yardstick.
- Instruct the patient to "Reach as far as you can forward without taking a step."
- The location of the 3rd metacarpal is recorded.
- Scores are determined by assessing the difference between the start and end position in the reach distance, usually measured in inches.
- Three trials are done and the average of the last two is noted.

Modified Functional Reach Test (Adapted for Individuals who are Unable to Stand)

- Performed with a leveled yardstick that has been mounted on the wall at the height of the patient's acromion level in the non-affected arm while sitting in a chair.
- Hips, knees and ankles positioned are at 90° of flexion, with feet positioned flat on the floor.
- The initial reach is measured with the patient sitting against the back of the chair with the upper-extremity flexed to 90°, measure was taken from the distal end of the third metacarpal along the yardstick.
- Consists of three conditions over three trials
  - Sitting with the unaffected side near the wall and leaning forward
  - Sitting with the back to the wall and leaning right
  - Sitting with the back to the wall leaning left.
- Instructions should include leaning as far as possible in each direction without rotation and without touching the wall.
- Record the distance in centimeters covered in each direction.

- If the patient is unable to raise the affected arm, the distance covered by the acromion during leaning is recorded.
- First trial in each direction is a practice trial and should not be included in the final result.
- A 15-second rest break should be allowed between trials.

Set-up

- A yardstick and duck tap will be needed for the assessment.
- The yardstick should be affixed to the wall at the level of the patient's acromion.

SCORE SHEET

Name: ____

Instructions

Instruct the patient to "Reach as far as you can forward without taking a step"

Score Sheet

Date	Trial one (Practice)	Trial two	Trial three	Total (average of trial 2 and 3 only

GAIT ASSESSMENT RATING SCALE (GARS)

- *General categories*:
  - Variability—a measure of inconsistency and arrhythmicity in steps and arm movements
    - 0 = Fluid and predictably paced limb movements.
    - 1 = Occasional interruptions (changes in velocity) approximately < 25% of the time.
    - 2 = Unpredictability of rhythm of movement > 25% of the time.
    - 3 = Random timing of limb movements.
  - Guardedness—hesitancy, slowness, diminished propulsion and lack of commitment stepping and arm swing.
    - 0 = Good forward momentum and lack of apprehension in propulsion.
    - 1 = Center of gravity of head, arms and trunk (HAT) projects only slightly in front of push off, but still good arm-leg coordination.
    - 2 = HAT held over anterior aspect of foot, and some moderate loss of smooth reciprocation.
    - 3 = HAT held over rear aspect of stance phase foot, and great tentativeness in stepping.
  - Weaving—an irregular line of progression.
    - 0 = Straight line of progress on frontal view.
    - 1 = Single deviation from straight line of progression.
    - 2 = Two to three deviations from straight line of progression.
    - 3 = Four or more deviations from straight line of progression.
  - Waddling—A broad based gait characterized by excessive truncal crossing of the midline and bending.
    - 0 = Narrow base of support and body held nearly vertically over feet.
    - 1 = Slight separation of medial aspects of feet and just perceptible lateral movements of head trunk.
    - 2 = 3" to 4" separation of feet and obvious bending of trunk to side so that cog of head lies well over ipsilateral stance foot.
  - Staggering—sudden and unexpected laterally directed partial losses of balance.
    - 0 = No losses of balance to side.
    - 1 = A single lurch to the side.
    - 2 = Two lurches to the side.
    - 3 = Three or more lurches to the side.

- *Lower extremity categories*:
  - Percent of time in swing—loss of percentage in the gait cycle constituted by the swing phase.
    - 0 = Approximately 3:2 ratio of stance:swing.
    - 1 = 1:1 or less ratio of stance:swing.
    - 2 = Markedly prolonged stance phase but with some obvious swing time remaining.
    - 3 = Barely perceptible portion of cycle spent in swing phase.
  - Foot contact—the degree to which the heel strikes the ground before the forefoot.
    - 0 = Very obvious angle of impact of heel on ground.
    - 1 = Barely visible contact of heel before forefoot.
    - 2 = Entire foot lands on ground.
    - 3 = Anterior aspect of foot strikes ground before heel.
  - Hip ROM—the degree of loss of hip ROM seen during a gait cycle.
    - 0 = Obvious angulation of thigh backwards during double support (~ 10 deg.)
    - 1 = Just barely visible angulation of thigh backwards from vertical.
    - 2 = Thigh in line with vertical projection from ground.
    - 3 = Thigh angled forward from vertical at maximum posterior excursion.
  - Knee ROM—the degree of loss of knee ROM seen during the gait cycle
    - 0 = Knee moves from complete extension at heel strike (and late stance) to 70 or nearly 90° during swing.
    - 1 = Slight bend in knee seen at heel strike and late stance and maximal flexion at midswing is closer to 45° than 90°.
    - 2 = Knee flexion at late stance more obvious than at heel strike, very little clearance seen for toe during swing.
    - 3 = Toe appears to touch ground during swing, knee flexion appears constant during stance, and knee angle during stance, and knee angle during swing appears 45° or less.
- *Trunk, head and upper extremity categories*:
  - Elbow extension—a measure of the decrease in elbow range of motion.
    - 0 = large peak-to-peak excursion of forearm (approximately 20°), with distinct maximal flexion at end of anterior trajectory.

  - 1 = 25° decrement of extension during maximal posterior excursion of upper extremity.
  - 2 = almost no change in elbow angle.
  - 3 = no apparent change in elbow angle (held in flexion).
- Shoulder extension—a measure of the decrease in shoulder range of motion.
  - 0 = clearly seen movement of upper arm anterior (15°) and posterior (20°) to vertical axis of trunk.
  - 1 = shoulder flexes slightly anterior to vertical axis.
  - 2 = shoulder comes only to vertical axis or slightly posterior to during flexion.
  - 3 = shoulder stays well behind vertical axis during entire excursion.
- Shoulder abduction—a measure of pathological increase in shoulder range of motion laterally.
  - 0 = shoulders held almost parallel to trunk.
  - 1 = shoulders held 5–10° to side.
  - 2 = shoulders held 10–20° to side.
  - 3 = shoulders held greater than 20° to side.
- Arm-heel strike synchrony—the extent to which the contralateral movements of an arm and leg are out of phase.
  - 0 = good temporal conjunction of arm and contralateral leg at apex of shoulder and hip excursions all of the time.
  - 1 = arm and leg slightly out of phase 25% of the time.
  - 2 = arm and leg moderately out phase 25–50% of the time.
  - 3 = little or no temporal cadence of arm and leg.
- Head held forward—a measure of the pathological forward projection of the head relative to the trunk.
  - 0 = earlobe vertically aligned with shoulder tip.
  - 1 = earlobe vertical projection falls 1" anterior to shoulder tip.
  - 2 = earlobe vertical projection falls 2" anterior to shoulder tip.
  - 3 = earlobe vertical projection falls 3" anterior to shoulder tip.
- Shoulders held elevated—the degree to which the scapular girdle is held higher than normal.
  - 0 = tip of shoulder (acromion) markedly below level of chin (1–2").
  - 1 = tip of shoulder slightly behind level of chin.
  - 2 = tip of shoulder at level of chin.
  - 3 = tip of shoulder above level of chin.

- Upper trunk flexed forward—a measure of kyphotic involvement of the trunk.
  - 0 = very gentle thoracic convexity, cervical spine flat, or almost flat.
  - 1 = emerging cervical curve, more distant thoracic convexity.
  - 2 = anterior concavity at mid-chest level apparent.
  - 3 = anterior concavity at mid-chest level very obvious.
  - > 9 = at risk for falling.

BECK'S DEPRESSION INVENTORY

This depression inventory can be self-scored. The scoring scale is at the end of the questionnaire.

1 – 0 I do not feel sad.
  – 1 I feel sad.
  – 2 I am sad all the time and I can't snap out of it.
  – 3 I am so sad and unhappy that I can't stand it.
2 – 0 I am not particularly discouraged about the future.
  – 1 I feel discouraged about the future.
  – 2 I feel I have nothing to look forward to.
  – 3 I feel the future is hopeless and that things cannot improve.
3 – 0 I do not feel like a failure.
  – 1 I feel I have failed more than the average person.
  – 2 As I look back on my life, all I can see is a lot of failures.
  – 3 I feel I am a complete failure as a person.
4 – 0 I get as much satisfaction out of things as I used to.
  – 1 I don't enjoy things the way I used to.
  – 2 I don't get real satisfaction out of anything any more.
  – 3 I am dissatisfied or bored with everything.
5 – 0 I don't feel particularly guilty.
  – 1 I feel guilty a good part of the time
  – 2 I feel quite guilty most of the time.
  – 3 I feel guilty all of the time.
6 – 0 I don't feel I am being punished.
  – 1 I feel I may be punished.
  – 2 I expect to be punished.
  – 3 I feel I am being punished.
7 – 0 I don't feel disappointed in myself.
  – 1 I am disappointed in myself.
  – 2 I am disgusted with myself.
  – 3 I hate myself.
8 – 0 I don't feel I am any worse than anybody else.
  – 1 I am critical of myself for my weaknesses or mistakes.
  – 2 I blame myself all the time for my faults.
  – 3 I blame myself for everything bad that happens.
9 – 0 I don't have any thoughts of killing myself.
  – 1 I have thoughts of killing myself, but I would not carry them out.
  – 2 I would like to kill myself.
  – 3 I would kill myself if I had the chance.

10 – 0 I don't cry any more than usual.
– 1 I cry more now than I used to.
– 2 I cry all the time now.
– 3 I used to be able to cry, but now I can't cry even though I want to.
11 – 0 I am no more irritated by things than I ever was.
– 1 I am slightly more irritated now than usual.
– 2 I am quite annoyed or irritated a good deal of the time.
– 3 I feel irritated all the time.
12 – 0 I have not lost interest in other people.
– 1 I am less interested in other people than I used to be.
– 2 I have lost most of my interest in other people.
– 3 I have lost all of my interest in other people.
13 – 0 I make decisions about as well as I ever could.
– 1 I put off making decisions more than I used to.
– 2 I have greater difficulty in making decisions more than I used to.
– 3 I can't make decisions at all any more.
14 – 0 I don't feel that I look any worse than I used to.
– 1 I am worried that I am looking old or unattractive.
– 2 I feel there are permanent changes in my appearance that make me look unattractive.
– 3 I believe that I look ugly.
15 – 0 I can work about as well as before.
– 1 It takes an extra effort to get started at doing something.
– 2 I have to push myself very hard to do anything.
– 3 I can't do any work at all.
16 – 0 I can sleep as well as usual.
– 1 I don't sleep as well as I used to.
– 2 I wake up 1–2 hours earlier than usual and find it hard to get back to sleep.
– 3 I wake up several hours earlier than I used to and cannot get back to sleep.
17 – 0 I don't get more tired than usual.
– 1 I get tired more easily than I used to.
– 2 I get tired from doing almost anything.
– 3 I am too tired to do anything.
18 – 0 My appetite is no worse than usual.
– 1 My appetite is not as good as it used to be.
– 2 My appetite is much worse now.
– 3 I have no appetite at all any more.

19 – 0 I haven't lost much weight, if any, lately.
– 1 I have lost more than five pounds.
– 2 I have lost more than ten pounds.
– 3 I have lost more than fifteen pounds.
20 – 0 I am no more worried about my health than usual.
– 1 I am worried about physical problems like aches, pains, upset stomach, or constipation.
– 2 I am very worried about physical problems and it is hard to think of much else.
– 3 I am so worried about my physical problems that I cannot think of anything else.
21 – 0 I have not noticed any recent change in my interest in sex.
– 1 I am less interested in sex than I used to be.
– 2 I have almost no interest in sex.
– 3 I have lost interest in sex completely.

Interpreting the Beck Depression Inventory

Now, that you have completed the questionnaire, add up the score for each of the twenty-one questions by counting the number to the right of each question you marked. The highest possible total for the whole test would be sixty-three. This would mean you circled number three on all twenty-one questions. Since the lowest possible score for each question is zero, the lowest possible score for the test would be zero. This would mean you circled zero on each question. You can evaluate your depression according to the table below.

Total score ____________ *Levels of depression*
- 1–10 ____________ These ups and downs are considered normal
- 11–16 ____________ Mild mood disturbance
- 17–20 ____________ Borderline clinical depression
- 21–30 ____________ Moderate depression
- 31–40 ____________ Severe depression
- Over 40 ____________ Extreme depression

FATIGUE SEVERITY SCALE (FSS)

Date: ____________________

Name: ____________________

Please circle the number between 1 and 7 which you feel best fits the following statements. This refers to your usual way of life within the last week. 1 indicates "strongly disagree" and 7 indicates "strongly agree."

Read and circle a number	*Strongly disagree → strongly agree*
1. My motivation is lower when I am fatigued	1 2 3 4 5 6 7
2. Exercise brings on my fatigue	1 2 3 4 5 6 7
3. I am easily fatigued	1 2 3 4 5 6 7
4. Fatigue interferes with my physical functioning	1 2 3 4 5 6 7
5. Fatigue causes frequent problems for me	1 2 3 4 5 6 7
6. My fatigue prevents sustained physical functioning	1 2 3 4 5 6 7
7. Fatigue interferes with carrying out certain duties and responsibilities	1 2 3 4 5 6 7
8. Fatigue is among my most disabling symptoms	1 2 3 4 5 6 7
9. Fatigue interferes with my work, family, or social life	1 2 3 4 5 6 7

Visual Analog Fatigue Scale (VAFS)

Please mark an "X" on the number line which describes your global fatigue with 0 being worst and 10 being normal.

0	1	2	3	4	5	6	7	8	9	10

SF-36 QUESTIONNAIRE

Name : ____________________
Ref. Dr : ____________________
Date : ____________________
ID# : ____________________
Age : ____________________
Gender: M/F : ____________________

Please answer the 36 questions of the Health Survey completely, honestly, and without interruptions.

General Health

1. **In general, you would say, your health is:**
   ☐ Excellent ☐ Very good ☐ Good ☐ Fair ☐ Poor
2. **Compared to one year ago, how would you rate your health in general now?**
   ☐ Much better now than one year ago
   ☐ Somewhat better now than one year ago
   ☐ About the same
   ☐ Somewhat worse now than one year ago
   ☐ Much worse than one year ago

Limitations of Activities

The following items are about activities you might do during a typical day. Does your health now limit you in these activities? If so, how much?

1. **Vigorous activities, such as running, lifting heavy objects, participating in strenuous sports:**
   ☐ Yes, limited a lot ☐ Yes, limited a little ☐ No, not limited at all
2. **Moderate activities, such as moving a table, pushing a vacuum cleaner, bowling, or playing golf:**
   ☐ Yes, limited a lot ☐ Yes, limited a little ☐ No, not limited at all
3. **Lifting or carrying groceries:**
   ☐ Yes, limited a lot ☐ Yes, limited a little ☐ No, not limited at all
4. **Climbing several flights of stairs:**
   ☐ Yes, limited a lot ☐ Yes, limited a little ☐ No, not limited at all

5. **Climbing one flight of stairs:**
☐ Yes, limited a lot ☐ Yes, limited a little ☐ No, not limited at all

6. **Bending, kneeling, or stooping:**
☐ Yes, limited a lot ☐ Yes, limited a little ☐ No, not limited at all

7. **Walking more than a mile:**
☐ Yes, limited a lot ☐ Yes, limited a little ☐ No, not limited at all

8. **Walking several blocks:**
☐ Yes, limited a lot ☐ Yes, limited a little ☐ No, not limited at all

9. **Walking one block:**
☐ Yes, limited a lot ☐ Yes, limited a little ☐ No, not limited at all

10. **Bathing or dressing yourself:**
☐ Yes, limited a lot ☐ Yes, limited a little ☐ No, not limited at all

Physical Health Problems

During the past 4 weeks, have you had any of the following problems with your work or other regular daily activities as a result of your physical health?

1. **Cut down the amount of time you spent on work or other activities:**
☐ Yes ☐ No

2. **Accomplished less than you would like:**
☐ Yes ☐ No

3. **Were limited in the kind of work or other activities:**
☐ Yes ☐ No

4. **Had difficulty performing the work or other activities (for example, it took extra effort):**
☐ Yes ☐ No

Emotional Health Problems

During the past 4 weeks, have you had any of the following problems with your work or other regular daily activities as a result of any emotional problems (such as feeling depressed or anxious)?

1. **Cut down the amount of time you spent on work or other activities:**
☐ Yes ☐ No

2. **Accomplished less than you would like:**
   ☐ Yes ☐ No
3. **Didn't do work or other activities as carefully as usual:**
   ☐ Yes ☐ No

Social Activities

1. **Emotional problems interfered with your normal social activities with family, friends, neighbors, or groups?**
   ☐ Not at all ☐ Slightly ☐ Moderately ☐ Severely ☐ Very severe

Pain

1. **How much bodily pain have you had during the past 4 weeks?**
   ☐ None ☐ Very mild ☐ Mild ☐ Moderate ☐ Severe ☐ Very severe
2. **During the past 4 weeks, how much did pain interfere with your normal work (including both work outside the home and housework)?**
   ☐ Not at all ☐ A little bit ☐ Moderately ☐ Quite a bit ☐ Extremely

Energy and Emotions

These questions are about how you feel and how things have been with you during the last 4 weeks. For each question, please give the answer that comes closest to the way you have been feeling.

1. **Did you feel full of pep?**
   ☐ All the time
   ☐ Most of the time
   ☐ A good bit of the time
   ☐ Some of the time
   ☐ A little bit of the time
   ☐ None of the time
2. **Have you been a very nervous person?**
   ☐ All the time
   ☐ Most of the time
   ☐ A good bit of the time
   ☐ Some of the time
   ☐ A little bit of the time
   ☐ None of the time

3. Have you felt so down in the dumps that nothing could cheer you up?
- ☐ All the time
- ☐ Most of the time
- ☐ A good bit of the time
- ☐ Some of the time
- ☐ A little bit of the time
- ☐ None of the time

4. Have you felt calm and peaceful?
- ☐ All the time
- ☐ Most of the time
- ☐ A good bit of the time
- ☐ Some of the time
- ☐ A little bit of the time
- ☐ None of the time

5. Did you have a lot of energy?
- ☐ All the time
- ☐ Most of the time
- ☐ A good bit of the time
- ☐ Some of the time
- ☐ A little bit of the time
- ☐ None of the time

6. Have you felt downhearted and blue?
- ☐ All the time
- ☐ Most of the time
- ☐ A good bit of the time
- ☐ Some of the time
- ☐ A little bit of the time
- ☐ None of the time

7. Did you feel worn out?
- ☐ All the time
- ☐ Most of the time
- ☐ A good bit of the time
- ☐ Some of the time
- ☐ A little bit of the time
- ☐ None of the time

8. Have you been a happy person?
- ☐ All the time
- ☐ Most of the time
- ☐ A good bit of the time

☐ Some of the time
☐ A little bit of the time
☐ None of the time

9. **Did you feel tired?**
☐ All the time
☐ Most of the time
☐ A good bit of the time
☐ Some of the time
☐ A little bit of the time
☐ None of the time

Social Activities

1. **During the past 4 weeks, how much of the time has your physical health or emotional problems interfered with your social activities (like visiting to friends, relatives, etc.)?**
☐ All the time
☐ Most of the time
☐ Some of the time
☐ A little bit of the time
☐ None of the time

General Health

How true or false is each of the following statements for you?

1. **I seem to get sick a little easier than other people:**
☐ Definitely true ☐ Mostly true ☐ Don't know
☐ Mostly false ☐ Definitely false

2. **I am as healthy as anybody I know:**
☐ Definitely true ☐ Mostly true ☐ Don't know
☐ Mostly false ☐ Definitely false

3. **I expect my health to get worse:**
☐ Definitely true ☐ Mostly true ☐ Don't know
☐ Mostly false ☐ Definitely false

4. **My health is excellent:**
☐ Definitely true ☐ Mostly true ☐ Don't know
☐ Mostly false ☐ Definitely false

DYNAMIC GAIT INDEX

Scoring Form

Gait Level Surface

Instructions: Walk at your normal pace from here to the next mark (20 feet).

Grading: Mark the lowest category that applies.

3 *Normal:* Walks 20', no assistive devices, good speed, no evidence of imbalance, normal gait pattern.

2 *Mild impairment:* Walks 20', uses assistive devices, slower speed, mild gait' deviations.

1 *Moderate impairment:* Walks 20', slow speed, abnormal gait pattern, evidence of imbalance.

0 *Severe impairment:* Walks 20' without assistance, severe gait deviations or imbalance.

Change in Gait Speed

Instructions: Begin walking at your normal pace (for 5 feet), when I tell you 'go', walk as fast as you can (for 5 feet). When I tell you 'slow', walk as slowly as you can (for 5 feet).

Grading: Mark the lowest category that applies.

3 *Normal:* Changes walking speed smoothly without loss of balance or gait deviation. Shows a significant difference in walking speeds between normal, fast, and slow.

2 *Mild impairment:* Changes speed but demonstrates mild gait deviations, or no gait deviations but unable to achieve a significant change in velocity, or uses an assistive device.

1 *Moderate impairment:* Makes only minor adjustments to walking speed, or accomplishes a change in speed with significant gait deviations, or changes speed but loses significant gait deviations, or changes speed but loses balance but is able to recover and continue walking.

0 *Severe impairment:* Unable to change speeds, or loses balance and has to reach for wall or be caught.

Gait with Horizontal Head Turns

Instructions: Begin walking at your normal pace. When I tell you 'lookright', keep walking straight and turn your head to the right. Keep looking to the right until I tell you 'lookleft', then keep walking straight and turn your head to the left. Keep your head to the left until I tell you 'lookstraight', then keep walking straight but return your head to the center.

Grading: Mark the lowest category that applies.

3 *Normal:* Turns head smoothly with no change in gait.
2 *Mild impairment:* Turns head smoothly with slight change in gait, i.e. minor disruption to smooth gait path, or uses walking aid.
1 *Moderate impairment:* Turns head smoothly with moderate change in gait, i.e. slows down, staggers but recovers, can continue to walk.
0 *Severe impairment:* Turns head smoothly with severe disruption of gait, i.e. staggers outside 15" path, loses balance, stops, reaches for wall.

Gait with Vertical Head Turns

Instructions: Begin walking at your normal pace. When I tell you 'lookup', keep walking straight and tilt your head up. Keep looking up until I tell you 'lookdown', then keep walking straight and tilt your head down. Keep looking down until I tell you 'lookstraight', then keep walking straight and return your head to the center.

Grading: Mark the lowest category that applies.

3 *Normal:* Performs head turns with no change in gail.
2 *Mild impairment:* Performs head turns with slight change in gait, i.e. minor disruption to smooth gait path or uses walking aid.
1 *Moderate impairment:* Performs head turns with moderate change in gait, i.e. slows down, staggers but recovers, can continue to walk.
0 *Severe impairment:* Performs head turns with severe disruption of gait, i.e. staggers outside a 15" path, loses balance, reaches for wall.

Gait and Pivot Turn

Instructions: Begin walking at your normal pace. When I tell you 'turnand stop',turn as quickly as you can to face the opposite direction and stop.

Grading: Mark the lowest category that applies.

3 *Normal:* Pivot turns safely within 3 seconds and stops quickly with no loss of balance.

2 *Mild impairment:* Pivot turns safely in over 3 seconds and stops with no loss in balance.

1 *Moderate impairment:* Pivot turns slowly, requires verbal cueing, requires several small steps to catch balance following turn and stop.

0 *Severe impairment:* Cannot pivot turn safely, requires assistance to turn and stop.

Step Over Obstacle

Instructions: Begin walking at your normal pace. When you come to the obstacle, step over it, not around it, and continue walking.

Grading: Mark the lowest category that applies.

3 *Normal:* Steps over box without changing gait, no evidence of imbalance.

2 *Mild impairment:* Steps over box, but must slow down and adjust steps to clear box safely.

1 *Moderate impairment:* Steps over box, but must stop before stepping over. May require verbal cueing.

0 *Severe impairment:* Cannot step over box without assistance.

Step Around Obstacles

Instructions: Begin walking at a normal speed. When you come to the first cone (about 6 feet away), walk around it on the right side. When you come to the second cone (6 feet past first one), walk around it on the left.

Grading: Mark the lowest category that applies.

3 *Normal:* Walks around cones safely without changing gait, no evidence of imbalance.

2 *Mild impairment:* Walks around both cones, but must slow down and adjust gait to clear cones.

1 *Moderate impairment:* Walks around both cones, but must significantly slow gait or requires verbal cueing.

0 *Severe impairment:* Unable to clear cones, walks into one or both, or requires physical assistance.

Steps

Instructions: Walk up these stairs as you would at home (i.e. using the rail if necessary). At the top, turn around and come down.

Grading: Mark the lowest category that applies:

3 *Normal:* Alternates feet, no rail.

2 *Mild impairment:* Alternates feet, must use rail.

1 *Moderate impairment:* Two feet to a stair, must use rail.

0 *Severe impairment:* Cannot do safely.

Bibliography

1. Ali D, Moore J. Rehab measures: Fugl-Meyer Assessment of Motor Recovery after Stroke. Retrieved from: *http://www.rehabmeasures org/Lists/RehabMeasures/DispForm.aspx?ID=908. 2010;15.*
2. Allan H Ropper, Robert H Brown. Adams and Victor's Principles of Neurology, 6th Edition. 2008.
3. Bickley L. Bates guide to Physical Examination, 11th Edition. 2011.
4. *choa.org/concussion.*
5. Collin C, Wade DT, Davies S, Horne V. The Barthel ADL Index: a reliability study. Int Disability Study.1988;10:61-3.
6. Crum RM, Anthony JC, Bassett SS, Folstein MF. Population-based norms for the mini-mental state examination by age and educational level. JAMA. 1993;269(18):2386-91.
7. Darcy Umphred. Neuro-Rehabilitation, 6th Edition. 2012.
8. Duncan PW, Weiner DK, et al. Functional reach: a new clinical measure of balance. J Gerontol. 1990;45(6):M192-7.
9. Ellen Hillegass. A Clinical Examination Pocket Guide. 2001.
10. Folstein MF, Folstein SE, McHugh PR. "Mini-mental state": a practical method for grading the cognitive state of patients for the clinician. J Psychiatr Res. 1975;12:189-98.
11. Fugl-Meyer, Jaasko AR, Leyman L, Olsson IS, Steglind S. The post-stroke hemiplegic patient: A method for evaluation of physical performance. Scandinavian Journal of Rehabilitation Medicine. 1975 7(1):13-31.
12. Geraint Fuller. Neurological Examination Made Easy, 4th Edition. 2008.
13. Gresham GE, Phillips TF, Labi ML. ADL status in stroke: relative merits of three standard indexes. Arch Phys Med Rehabil. 1980;61:355-8.
14. Jeffrey M Hausdorff, Neil B Alexander. Gait Disorders. Evaluation and Management. 2005.
15. John Spillane. Bickerstaff's Neurological Examination in Clinical Practice, 6th Edition. 1995.
16. Katz-Leurer M, Fisher I, et al. Reliability and validity of the modified functional reach test at the subacute stage post-stroke. Disabil Rehabil. 2009;31(3):243-8.
17. Loewen SC, Anderson BA. Predictors of stroke outcome using objective measurement scales. Stroke. 1990;21:78-81.
18. Mahoney FI, Barthel D. Functional evaluation: the Barthel Index. Maryland State Medical Journal. 1965;14:56-61. Used with permission.
19. Martin Kessler. Neurological Intervention for Physical Therapy. 2016.
20. Michael Donaghy. Brain's Disease of Nervous system, 12th Edition. 2009.
21. North Star Clinical Network: the North Star Ambulatory Assessment. 2016.
22. Richard J Greenwood. Neurological Rehabilitation Handbook. 2002.

23. Robert J Schwartzan. Neurological Examination. 2006.
24. Rovner BW, Folstein MF. Mini-mental state exam in clinical practice. Hosp Pract. 1987;22(1A):99,103,106,110.
25. RT Ross. How to Examine Nervous System, 4th Edition. 1998.
26. Susan B O'Sullivan. Physical Rehabilitation Assessment and Treatment, 6th Edition. 2013.
27. Susan Edward. Neurological Physiotherapy. 2002.
28. Tombaugh TN, McIntyre NJ. The mini-mental state examination: a comprehensive review. J Am Geriatr Soc. 1992;40(9):922-35.
29. Web Resources.
30. Weiner DK, Bongiorni DR, et al. Does functional reach improve with rehabilitation? Arch Phys Med Rehabil. 1993;74(8):796-800.
31. Weiner DK, Duncan PW, et al. Functional reach: a marker of physical frailty. J Am Geriatr Soc. 1992;40(3):203-7.
32. William E DeMyer. Technique of the Neurological Examination, 5th Edition. 2003.
33. William W Campbell. Dejong's Neurological Examination, 7th Edition. 2012.

Index

Page numbers followed by *f* refer to figure, and *t* refer to table

A

D

E

H

Q

R

S

T

U

V